*The Complete Editorials of*

# Dr. Lawrence H. Meskin

Editor of the Journal of the American Dental Association 1990-2001

# TABLE OF CONTENTS

**ADA** American Dental Association®

America's leading advocate for oral health

ISBN (978-1-935201-34-2)

# A man to remember

By the time I was elected to the Board of Trustees in 2004, Dr. Lawrence H. Meskin already had stepped down after 11 years as Editor of The Journal of the American Dental Association.

Larry had moved on, but his legend remained. Ably leading our prestigious journal through the tumultuous 1990s, he had written 131 editorials on a vast parade of topics. His approach in these commentaries was to begin by spotlighting a problem, but he wouldn't leave it at that. Unlike many other commentators, he would proffer a solution—sometimes more than one—and never let his readers walk away empty handed. His role, as he saw it, was to replace confusion with clarity, and he did it well.

This approach to the issues of the day earned Dr. Meskin the accolades of his peers. He would become, in time, the voice of our profession, the wise man on the hill. It was a role he reveled in, leading him to confide in his last editorial (December 2001) that writing his monthly commentaries had been "a real joy" for him, something he would miss.

In 1999, Larry Meskin was named to the American Student Dental Association's roster of 25 "dental visionaries." And when he stepped down as editor two years later, the American Association of Dental Editors honored him by establishing the Meskin Journalism Award for Excellence in Dental Student Publications. These are just two of many honors earned in a lifetime of service to dentistry.

Beyond his contributions to organized dentistry, much of Dr. Meskin's life was devoted to dental education. He received his dental degree from the University of Detroit in 1961, moving that same year to the University of Minnesota School of Dentistry where he taught for two decades.

In 1981, he was named dean of the University of

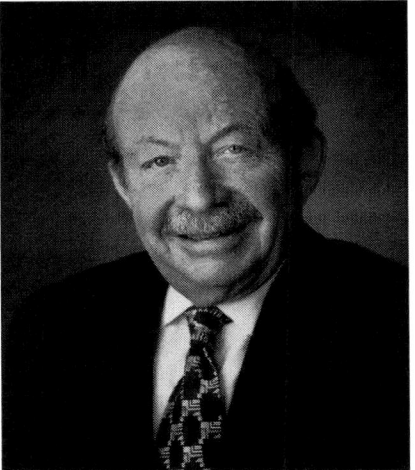

**Dr. Lawrence H. Meskin**
**1935-2007**

Colorado School of Dentistry, a post he held until 1987. He remained at Colorado thereafter, holding a number of different positions and earning, in 1988, the university's highest honor: the Thomas Jefferson Award, bestowed annually on a faculty member with broadly demonstrated interests in "literature, arts and sciences, and public affairs."

On June 26, 2007, Larry was playing tennis with Estelle, his wife of 48 years, when he suddenly collapsed. At 71, the esteemed dental educator, researcher, clinician and editor had been taken from our midst much too soon. His interment in Aurora, Colo.'s, Mount Nebo Cemetery took place just two days before Larry was officially to begin his retirement after 21 years at the University of Colorado and nearly 50 years in dental education and research.

"The outpouring of great love and support from the whole dental community, both nationally and internationally, has been incredible to us," Estelle Meskin, speaking for her family, told the ADA News. Among Dr. Meskin's survivors are his son, Scott, a physician; his daughter, Sarah, an architect; and three grandchildren, Alie, Andrew and Hailey.

This book, compiling all 131 of Dr. Meskin's JADA editorials, is presented as a celebration of his life as a dentist, as a man, as a thinking, feeling human being who loved life and who brought much wisdom and joy into the lives of all who knew and loved him.

Larry Meskin is no longer with us, but his words live on in these pages, as fresh and pertinent today as they were on the day he wrote them.

*Ron Tankersley*

**Ronald L. Tankersley, DDS**
**President**

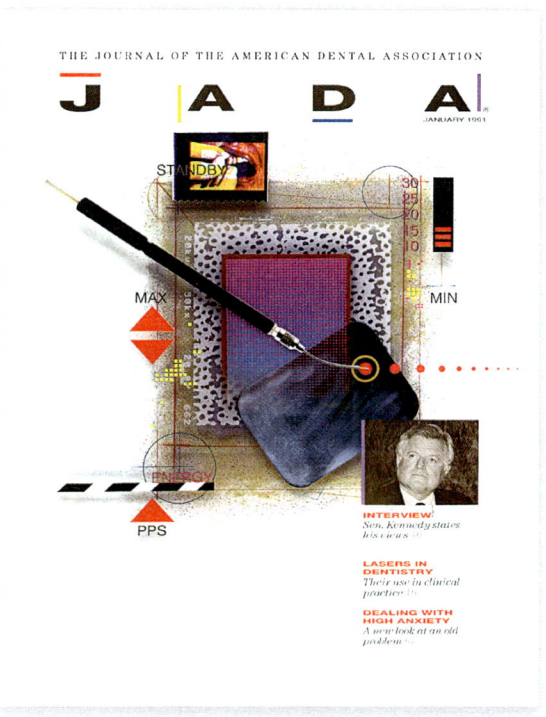

THE JOURNAL OF THE AMERICAN DENTAL ASSOCIATION

**J A D A**

JANUARY 1991

STANDBY

MAX

MIN

ENERGY

PPS

**INTERVIEW**
*Sen. Kennedy states his views*

**LASERS IN DENTISTRY**
*Their use in clinical practice*

**DEALING WITH HIGH ANXIETY**
*A new look at an old problem*

# 1991

"While I do not advocate a quota system, believing rather that individuals should be selected on merit and not on what proportion of an organization they represent, I do strongly suggest that our present ADA leadership make extraordinary efforts to recruit females for political office."

# The bottom line: relevance and readability

*Originally published in JADA 1991 122: 12-14*

Gold Hill, Colo., is a small front range mountain community that lies adjacent to the 14,000-foot peaks of Rocky Mountain National Park. Until recently this obscure town was known only to locals as a place worth a Sunday drive or perhaps a visit to one of its two restaurants. However, this summer Gold Hill has been overwhelmed by tourists, due to a syndicated Sunday newspaper article that described the history and authenticity of "magnificently scenic Gold Hill."

I am sure that visitors to Gold Hill do indeed enjoy its vistas and the cordiality of its residents. But I wonder how many visitors note the one item that makes Gold Hill unique from all other cities and towns? Road signs describing population, altitude or date of incorporation of towns are commonplace. In that regard, the Gold Hill road sign conforms to all others. What makes its sign so different is an additional entry designated as "Total" (see photo).

It often takes a second or third glance to note that the Total is just that—a simple addition of three nonrelated figures. I often use a slide of this sign in my lectures to make the point that "you shouldn't accept the bottom line until you examine its component parts."

That message is most appropriate as you peruse your NEW issues of JADA. The striking changes in format and content should be evident. The concept now used by the publisher and the executive editor is to make The Journal more readable and relevant. I'm sure that as you examine each new section you will be able to put aside your previous perceptions and develop a new "bottom line" regarding The Journal.

My role as the new Editor will be to enhance the process already in place by the solicitation of relevant material from dental leaders in all disciplines. There is new excitement that has pervaded all who have been associated with the NEW JADA. I share this enthusiasm and invite you to become a contributor to its success.

Your suggestions regarding pertinent subjects for inclusion in The Journal will assist me in ensuring that material suitable for our entire readership will be included in The Journal.

With your support, the new components of The Journal will add up to a "bottom line" that will evoke both competence and confidence as you transfer its messages to your practice and professional life. ■

*Dr. Meskin was appointed editor in October. He is dean of the Graduate School, The University of Colorado Health Sciences Center, where he is also a professor in both the School of Dentistry and in the Department of Preventative Medicine and Biometrics. Dr. Meskin is a well-known lecturer and widely published author.*

# A letter of importance

*Originally published in JADA 1991 122: 8-10*

Dear Colleague:
On Jan. 18, the Centers for Disease Control, a federal agency that monitors the morbidity and mortality of the U.S. population, released a report of the possible transmission of the AIDS virus from an HIV-positive dentist to three of his patients. This was a startling revelation since this incident would represent the first documented transmission of the AIDS virus from a health professional to a patient.

The stated association between the infected dentist and his patients was based on genetic similarities of their HIV viruses. The CDC has investigated possible routes of hypothesized transmission. Unfortunately incomplete data have impeded identification of any conclusive route of infection. Nevertheless, the potential implications of the report from the CDC cannot be ignored. The need for further study is obvious.

Unless new information becomes available, the past safety record of the health professions should provide reassurance to concerned patients. Consider, in the last decade there has not been a single documented case of a dentist, physician or other health worker who has transmitted the HIV infection to a patient. For the dental profession, that safety record has been achieved while performing uncountable numbers of invasive procedures during an estimated four billion dental visits.

This past history has guided the American Dental Association's Officers and Trustees as they deliberated on a policy that would address the unique relationship that exists between dentist and patient. Their conclusions, reproduced here as an interim policy, demonstrate a strong commitment to protect the health of the individual seeking dental care.

To ensure a continuing high level of public confidence, it is imperative that the profession respond to this new policy.

> **The potential implications of the report from the CDC cannot be ignored. The need for further study is obvious.**

## INTERIM POLICY ON HIV-INFECTED DENTISTS

The dental profession has long adhered to a moral commitment of service to the public and an ethical obligation to protect the health of the patient. An advisory opinion to the American Dental Association's Code of Professional Conduct urges dentists who become ill or impaired to limit the activities of practice to those areas that do not endanger either patients or dental staff.

Currently, there is no scientific evidence to indicate that HIV-positive health care providers pose an identifiable risk of HIV transmission to their patients. There has been only one documented case of transmission from an HIV-infected health care provider to patients during the past ten years of experience with AIDS, an indication that the risk is infinitesimal. The ADA continues to believe that the recommended infection control procedures are effective in preventing transmission of infection.

However, the recent case of possible HIV transmission from dentist to patient has raised some uncertainty about the risk of transmission from health care provider to patient. While there is evidence that this dental practice did not consistently adhere to all recommended guidelines for prevention of disease transmission, the precise mechanism of transmission in this case remains unknown. This uncertainty leads to the conclusion that the foremost concern of the dental profession must continue to be protection of the patient. Thus, until the uncertainty about transmission is resolved, the ADA believes that HIV-infected dentist should refrain from performing invasive procedures or should disclose their seropositive status.

The American Dental Association will assist and support infected dentists in sustaining meaningful professional careers. ∎

# A perception of risk

*Originally published in JADA 1991 122: 10*

The Centers for Disease Control's recent meeting on the risk of percutaneous transmission of HIV was preceded by a discussion paper that described risk models for HIV-infected provider-to-patient transmissions.

While the estimated probabilities for a patient to become infected during a random dental visit ranged between 1/263,000 to 1/1,263,000, probability that an infected surgeon would transmit HIV to at least one patient in his or her professional lifetime was estimated as 8.1 percent.

The public response to news media coverage of this document was more attendant to the "high risk" of receiving care from an HIV-infected health care worker than the low risk of infection from a visit to a randomly chosen dental provider. This perception of potential risk was accentuated by the adverse outcome resulting from an HIV infection. Since most medical and dental invasive procedures can be performed by any number of competent health providers without a major cost differential, I believe the majority of the public will want accurate information on the HIV status of physicians and dentists. This should allow them to make a se-

> **I believe the majority of the public will want accurate information on the HIV status of physicians and dentists.**

lection of health provider based on their individual perception of risk.

Would such demands have an impact on the present AMA and ADA interim policies for HIV-infected physicians and dentists? Undoubtedly! I question the public's satisfaction with voluntary disclosure of HIV status.

Their arguments for mandatory testing will include the unique fiduciary position that exists between health provider and patient and the doctrine of informed consent, which recognizes the patient's right to know all risks of treatment, including the HIV status of the health provider.

In the next months, the concept of mandatory testing of health workers who perform invasive procedures will be discussed. What will be the position of the health professions to this potential request for testing? What protection is there for HIV-infected providers in the Fourth and 14th amendments to the Constitution? What will be the position of the insurance industry in regard to malpractice coverage?

To assist in this complex issue, JADA will provide pertinent information and opportunity for dialogue by publishing your letters. ∎

1991

# "...Potential unreasonable risk..."

*Originally published in JADA 1991 122: 8-10*

The FDA recently held hearings to determine whether dental mercury, now a Class I product, and amalgam alloy, a Class II product, should be reclassified to Class III-a status that denotes a "potential unreasonable risk."[1] Such an action might well end the use of dental amalgam as the "workhorse" filling material of the dental profession. The subsequent costs to the American public would be staggering and could easily disenfranchise a significant proportion of the population.

Clearly the dental profession would never support the continued use of any product perceived as having the potential to endanger the safety of the public. Indeed, dentistry has a long history of continually reviewing and evaluating its products and techniques. The recent examination of the safety of fluoride exemplifies this ongoing activity.

It is important to note that, at present, there is virtually no scientific evidence which suggests that dental amalgam presents a health risk to normal healthy individuals. In fact, dentists themselves have served as an experimental model, handling amalgam in the course of their daily activities for several decades. And while mercury blood and urine levels in dentists are four times higher than those of the average population, there is no documentation of a higher incidence of neurologic disease.

Unfortunately, these and other pertinent facts were not reported in the highly emotional "throw your crutches away" TV presentation by the "60 Minutes" staff. Rather, by focusing on sensational and anecdotal reports, they offered false hope to thousands of chronically ill and often desperate patients. The fear generated in many viewers surely has precipitated the FDA's call for reevaluation of their standards for amalgam restorations. The consequences of this capricious action-initiated without any new, substantiated evidence of potential harm-could have a chaotic impact on the dental care delivery system.

For example, were the FDA to place amalgam into a Class III category, even for a limited time, while "additional studies are carried out," the response of many consumers would be to replace as many of their present restorations as possible. Having heard only that the FDA views amalgam as "potentially risky," they would ask no further questions; they would certainly not understand that the classification was temporary. The impact on subsequent spending for dental products would overwhelm the ability of the public to pay for the additional services.

Consider that it would take $930 to replace existing amalgam surfaces with composite in the average adult. If just 10 percent of these amalgam-filled surfaces were replaced with a necessary posterior gold restoration the cost would escalate to $1,318. With total U.S. dental expenditures at approximately $25 billion annually, if 1 percent of the adult population chose to replace their amalgams, total expenditures would increase by 10 percent; a 5 percent replacement group would increase expenditures by 50 percent. If one-tenth of our adult population acted in a similar manner, it would double the yearly spending for dental care and still leave 90 percent of our population with unsafe amalgam restorations.

It is unlikely that many Americans would be able to afford the out-of-pocket expense necessary for this replacement program. It is equally unlikely that dental insurance companies would be able to offset ANY of this additional expense without massive increases in premiums. We are left with a situation in which only the very affluent would be able to replace their restorations. Seeing that only the wealthy were able to avoid the "supposed" serious

> **Knee-jerk, emotional reactions in response to an unsubstantiated television documentary have no place in public policy decisions.**

consequences of amalgam would initiate massive public concern. The government would be called on to address their imperative need. With government spending presently limited to less than 5 percent of total dental expenditures a federal response to this public outcry would be an impossibility without a radical change in the entire dental economic delivery system.

Neither the public nor the profession should be required to address this difficult situation unless it becomes scientifically evident that those with dental amalgam restorations are, in fact, at risk. Such evidence does not exist and, in fact, research presented in the March JADA clearly refutes earlier anti-amalgam claims.

The FDA must be made aware of the chaotic potential of product reclassification. Knee-jerk, emotional reactions in response to an unsubstantiated television documentary have no place in public policy decisions. Systematic, scientific evidence must prevail in the decision-making process of our nation's health community. ∎

1. Singleton G., Executive-Secretary, Denial Products Panel, Dept HHS, FDA. Letter to panel members and consultants, Feb. 1991.

# Hold the line–an opportunity revisited

*Originally published in JADA 1991 122: 8-10*

This month the American Association of Dental Schools will report an 8 percent increase in dental school applications. This marks the second consecutive year in which an increase in applications has been noted. Until last year, the number of applicants for admission into dental schools had declined yearly, falling from over 15,000 in 1975 to 4,996 in 1989. Even worse, the applicant to enrollee ratio reached 1.3 to 1.

With concerns about continued dental school closures and reduced standards for admittance to dental school, it is understandable why this two-year reversal in applicants is considered good news by both dental education and organized dentistry.

This resurgence of interest in pursuing a professional dental career presents a major opportunity-the opportunity to reexamine the policies of a generation ago and develop strategies that will ensure they will not be repeated. Do you remember 1965? Faced with evidence of a major potential deficit in the dental workforce, the federal government subsidized building 14 new dental schools and assisted in the enlargement and renovation of existing schools. With this stimulus, first-year enrollments rose from 3,616 to a high of 6,301 in 1978. Simultaneously, the auxiliary workforce was also expanded.

Unfortunately, the predicted demand for dental care did not fully materialize. Many dentists found themselves with excess capacity to treat patients. The appointment delay factor dropped precipitously. As market forces responded to this situation, conflict often arose between educational institutions and organized dentistry.

In 1978, recognizing the need to critically discuss the issue of dental supply and demand, I wrote a paper entitled "Too many dentists? If so, what then?"[1] Published in the Journal of Dental

> **There is no evidence that the dental care delivery system requires an increased number of dental practitioners above the level now determined by the normal/tow of those entering and leaving the profession.**

Education, it contained a number of suggestions that would provide for balance in future dental workforce systems. One proposal is exceedingly important to this editorial. It recommended that future professional responses to variations in dental demand be met by using auxiliaries as the flexible portion of the delivery system-not by enlarging the pool of dental practitioners. Acceptance of this position acknowledges the importance of having dentists deliver services commensurate with their abilities and training.

Since that publication, first-year dental enrollee positions decreased from a 1978 high of 6,301 to 4,001. As mentioned earlier, numbers of applications also decreased. Presently, with dental schools under heavy financial pressures, there is some question if this trend to decrease will continue. It is conceivable that if the number of dental school applications continues to increase, there may be pressure to enlarge class size.

Recently, dental school budgets have been reduced by decreases in state appropriations and the necessity to hold tuition at reasonable levels. Additional funds must be found if dental education is to offer the quality programs necessary to maintain the high standards required by national accreditation boards. Traditionally, increasing class size often represents an opportunity to enhance the education budget since the addition of students can significantly increase resources with minimal additional expenditure.

Yet, whenever possible, dental administrators should resist increasing student numbers to increase revenues. The long-term consequences of such an action must be considered. There is no evidence that the dental care delivery system requires an increased number of dental practitioners above the level now determined by the normal flow of those entering and leaving the profession.

Indeed, today dentists are working at only 63 percent of capacity. If that capacity increases, auxiliaries can assist in meeting the additional demand. Other means of increasing dental school funding must be discovered. The mistakes of the past must not be repeated!

What can you, as a practitioner of dentistry, do to ensure that the future will not replicate the past? Two suggestions: First, participate in preserving your dental school's financial viability by contributing to its annual fund-raising efforts. Second: Continue your efforts to recruit the brightest, the most energetic and the dedicated to become future dental professionals. Both activities will build a solid base for the future of our profession. ∎

1. Meskin LH. Too many dentists? If so, what then? J Dent Educ 1977;41;601.

# Nothing new under the sun

*Originally published in JADA 1991 122: 8-10*

**N**early 6,000 dental scientists, educators and practitioners gathered recently in Acapulco, Mexico, to discuss the results of more than 2,600 research projects. A novice at an annual session of the International Association for Dental Research, someone without prior experience in conducting and disseminating research results, might easily become confused, if not overwhelmed, by the volume, specificity and apparent lack of focus of these research reports.

Such a novice might raise the question: Where in this myriad of information can I find new evidence to substantiate clinical prevention and treatment of periodontal diseases? Of dental caries? Of oral cancer? Why do these reports appear to address questions supposedly answered decades ago? Is there anything truly new, truly "breakthrough," being reported here? If there's nothing "new under the sun," why have such a research extravaganza?

Unfortunately, our novice's view reflects a basic lack of understanding of the research process. Scientific "breakthroughs," when they do occur, are rarely the result of dazzling flashes of genius. Rather, they are the culmination of painstaking, often tedious small steps taken by dozens of scientists. Each small step adds another stone to the wall of evidence and theory being developed, each a significant dimension to the final work.

Thus, taken individually, any given research presentation might seem independent of any major research goal. In point of fact, however, each presentation is a component in that larger effort directed at the eventual control of oral disease.

Understanding this research scenario should assist our novice observer in seeing the potential clinical significance of the multitude of research reports presented at the IADR meeting. Some examples:

> **Scientific "breakthroughs," when they do occur, are rarely the result of dazzling flashes of genius.**

■ A research update on sealants placed 15 years ago demonstrated high retention and continued protection against dental caries. These results may help convince the insurance companies that there is a positive cost benefit to including sealants under their preventive coverage.

■ Results from a comparison of 1986 with 1989 National Health Interview Survey data indicated an increase of better than 5 percent in the number of patients visiting a dentist at least once a year. This study also demonstrated that the elderly increased their visits to the dentist by almost 10 percent, continuing a trend first observed in 1986.

■ An investigation in The Netherlands explored the time required to produce a restoration with composite vs. amalgam. Looking at Class II restorations, the study found that nearly twice the time was required if composites were used. This study draws attention to the potential cost impact on health care financing if composites become the preferred posterior material.

■ An eight-year study of retained "hopeless" teeth and their effect on proximal periodontium gave credence to earlier observations that there is not a significant effect on the periodontium following therapy. This information should aid those practitioners who are actively engaged in periodontal therapy,

While these four short synopses represent less than one tenth of 1 percent of the total material presented at the Acapulco meeting, they serve as excellent examples of research that has immediate and direct implications for clinical practice.

The research community has become sensitized to the importance of developing mechanisms that will ensure active dialogue with dental practitioners. Your Journal will continually strive to be a vital link in that chain of communication. ■

# Risk-free in '93

*Originally published in JADA 1991 122: 10*

The 1992 presidential campaign is in its infancy. Thus far, only a few candidates have chosen to venture forth to test the public's acceptance of their political aspirations. At least another six months will pass before the strongest candidates will begin their parade toward the presidency with their platforms, promises and slogans. At this time, we have no idea what the substantive issues of the campaign will be. Some will surface in response to domestic and international circumstances; others will be created to play on the emotions of various constituencies.

After witnessing the public's reaction to several of dentistry's major issues—HIV, amalgam and fluoride—let me suggest that our presidential aspirants consider adopting the rhythmic slogan: "Risk-free in '93." Doing so should elevate its sponsor to the highest office in a landslide.

## WHY?

The ratings for the "60 Minutes" segment on the dangers of amalgam attracted more than 20 million viewers—more than any other program that week. The isolated case of an unexplained transmission of the AIDS virus to five dental patients became the focus for those who want to institute universal testing for HIV.

Recently, a nationwide Gallop poll indicated that 87 percent of those responding thought physicians and dentists should be tested for HIV.

Fluoride, too, became an issue again when, in a government study, osteogenic sarcoma appeared in four male rats fed excessive fluoride diets. The nationwide publicity that resulted gave rise to new fears regarding the safety of this proved preventive agent. Fortunately, a blue-ribbon committee upheld the value and safety of fluoride, but not until a year's worth of negative publicity stirred public concern over the potential risks of fluoride additives.

The emotional fervor of these issues focused public attention on the potential risks of a dental visit. For a profession that has worked hard to gain a long-standing reputation for quality, safety and personal integrity, these detractions have caused many in our profession to react defensively. Maintaining such a posture can only lead to erosion of public confidence in our profession.

Rather than lash out reactively, we must work to educate all members of the profession so they can assume a proactive and positive role in the public debate over these and other health issues. The American Dental Association and this Journal seek to fulfill that educational function.

Through the year, JADA has published timely and informative material on each of the major issues. At the same time, the public's desire for a risk-free health care environment continues, carrying with it a concomitant demand for better informed dental practitioners.

To provide dentists with the most recent and pertinent information, we have committed this August issue to a comprehensive review of HIV and infection control, the safety and effectiveness of fluoride and the current status of amalgam as the preferred restorative material. Pertinent ethical and legal issues are also addressed.

Some of the most knowledgeable people in the dental health field have prepared material for this important professional update. Their collective efforts provide ADA members with an all-in-one resource designed for quick and easy access.

This issue has been organized to address questions regarding the current state of knowledge-what we still must learn and how we seek that knowledge. Reading these articles and keeping this publication for future reference will allow dentists to respond with both facts and reason to questions stemming from the public's preoccupation with dental risk. ∎

# Emotion and science

*Originally published in JADA 1991 122: 10-11*

Concern? Anxiety? Fear? Panic? Absolutely. One reported cluster of HIV infection involving one dentist and five patients, and the nation responds as if health care workers were eager to inoculate their patients with the AIDS virus.

Consider these developments:

■ A U.S. senator proposes legislation that would imprison HIV-infected health care workers for up to 10 years, if they fail to share their health status with their patients. The legislation passes the Senate—with Republicans and even liberal Democrats voting yes.

■ A bipartisan group of senators passes legislation requiring the states to adopt Centers for Disease Control guidelines for HIV-infected workers or lose their federal funding.

■ Federal and state legislation would require mandatory testing of health care workers as a condition for licensure and relicensure.

All this legislative activity occurs despite the fact that during the entire decade of HIV case reporting, with some five billion dental visits and an almost uncountable number of medical encounters, just one instance of doctor-to-patient transmission has been noted.

So why the public outcry for mandatory testing of health professionals? Any testing program would contain a number of false negatives (health care workers infected but not yet detected) as well as false positives, a situation that could destroy an individual's professional and personal life.

Why the outcry? Because AIDS is an ugly disease that destroys the body and mind insidiously; because it can strike the young and old, even the newborn; because it still carries a negative social connotation for those who contract it. And above all, because there is no known cure.

The ADA trustees understand their public and professional responsibility. After considerable debate, they have placed for discussion at the forthcoming House of Delegates meeting in Seattle a resolution that opposes any federal or state laws or regulations requiring mandatory testing of health care workers or patients. The resolution states that there are times when it is desirable that the HIV serostatus of the worker be known. In that regard, the trustees propose policy stating that dentists who perform exposure-prone procedures or believe they are at risk of HIV infection should know their HIV status.

Depending on subsequent interpretations of "exposure-prone procedures," this policy calls for "voluntary" testing of only a few dentists or includes almost the entire profession. Considering the limitations of testing, are these proposed policies appropriate?

Perhaps. They surely provide answers to those who question what the profession is doing to prevent further dentist-to-patient HIV transmissions. Personally, I believe these policies ignore what science tells us. Present epidemiology of HIV indicates a disease of limited infectivity. Barrier techniques, not testing, should be the mechanism to prevent HIV transmissions.

Furthermore, the false security generated by a massive HIV testing program of health professionals would soon evaporate as occasional transmissions from supposed HIV-negative health care workers became known. Nevertheless, the public is demanding some demonstration of action by the health professions.

This can be achieved by adopting the trustees' proposals, but only after special attention is given to interpreting the term "exposure prone." If broadly defined, it could encompass almost every dental procedure—resulting in a de facto mandatory testing program. However, by acknowledging past scientific accomplishments in the area of infec-

> **Present epidemiology of HIV indicates a disease of limited infectivity. Barrier techniques, not testing, should be the mechanism to prevent HIV transmissions.**

tion control and then factoring them into the assessment process, few dental procedures should fall into the "exposure-prone" category.

Presently, the dental profession, in consort with other health professions, has initiated preliminary discussions to define "exposure prone" procedures. Let's proceed on the basis of science, not public pressure. ■

# The amalgam restoration— worth its weight in gold

*Originally published in JADA 1991 122: 6-8*

**W**ell, maybe not gold, but for decades general practitioners have agreed that dental amalgam is an outstanding restorative material that is interchangeable with gold in most cases.

With its superior properties of strength, durability and ease of placement, only its color has prevented it from being used universally throughout the mouth. These factors, coupled with its reasonable cost, have made dental amalgam the restorative material of choice for many patients. Estimates indicate that more than 150 million amalgam restorations are placed yearly in the United States.

Because of amalgam's color incompatibility, there have been continuous attempts to find an adequate substitute. Composite resin, amalgam's most successful competitor, does contain the desired esthetic properties. Unfortunately, it does not demonstrate the required durability or ease of placement. While research continues to strive for that "perfect" restorative material, none appears ready to replace the old standard.

Considering these facts, it is understandable that the profession showed concern when those who attribute adverse health effects from mercury derived from dental amalgam found a national forum for their views. Television's slanted expose of the dangers of dental amalgam reached over 20 million viewers.

You know what followed—upset patients, concerned parents, severely handicapped individuals reaching out for any help, then public demand for a government investigation into the safety of amalgam.

To date, two such reviews have been conducted.

In March, the FDA held hearings on possible adverse effects of amalgam. Its assessment, after extensive testimony, indicated no need to alter amalgam's present Class III status-but it recommended more research to alleviate patient concerns. In late August, the National Institute of Dental Research held a consensus conference on the safety of dental restorative materials. Its expert panel concluded:

"Virtually all restorative materials have components with potential health risks. However, there is no scientific evidence that currently used restorative materials cause significant side effects, ... it must be recognized that the supporting data are incomplete."

What course of action should the profession take until the "definitive" research report gives dental amalgam an unqualified approval rating? Should the dentist "play it safe" and use composite resin even if its properties are lacking? I think not.

The NIDR report presents convincing evidence for continued use of dental amalgam. Its conclusions should give dentists the necessary confidence to use amalgam restorations when indicated. If questions arise about the release of mercury vapor— especially during early stages of amalgam placement—the use of rubber dam and high-volume suction may help alleviate those concerns.

Dentists may even wish to cover the newly placed amalgam with sealants. A recently published clinical research report notes statistically significant reductions in mercury vapor using this technique.[1]

Whatever your chosen course of action, remember: amalgam may not be worth its weight in gold, but for the foreseeable future it remains the preferred material for most dental patients. ∎

> **The NIDR report presents convincing evidence for continued use of dental amalgam. Its conclusions should give dentists the necessary confidence to use amalgam restorations when indicated.**

1. Ahmads R, Stannard JG. Mercury release from amalgam: a study in vitro and in vivo. Oper Dent 1990,15:207-16.

# Doctors, dentists and other health professionals

*Originally published in JADA 1991 122: 8-10*

Recently the section on Lawmakers contained a reference to "doctors, dentists and other health professionals, ..." a common enough error, but not one you would expect to see in the premier professional dental journal.[1]

After decades of striving for public and professional recognition as doctors, as healers, as learned men and women, you would think every dentist, and every person working with dentists, would correctly reference physicians and dentists-after all, we're both "doctors." And yet, inadvertent as it was, the passage slipped through.

This slight to the profession, our profession, could be counted among the most observable errors we could make. It's bad enough when the lay press reserves the term "doctor" for physicians but for our publication to do so is unforgivable... or is it?

Surprisingly, the telephone lines were not jammed. Extra trucks were not required to deliver the mail. Pickets did not march at 211 E. Chicago Ave.

The response? Only one letter. Dr. Richard D. Williams of Southfield, Mich., wrote: "I expect it from the public media but not in our publication!! And in a report from an ADA department yet. No! No! No!

Why did only one of our over 130,000 members react? I can think of at least four reasons:

■ No one except Dr. Williams read the JADA Lawmakers report.

■ Those who read the Lawmakers report and were offended by the terminology distinguishing between "doctors" and dentists were simply not inclined to comment publicly.

■ Those who read the report do not believe this is an issue of importance. Thus they give credence to the public distinction that reserves the title Dr. "as a formal title before the name of an individual who holds a doctor of medicine degree."[2]

■ Those who read the report have grown apathetic, have lost their sense of pride in their profession. Or, even worse, perhaps some do not see themselves sufficiently skilled in the healing arts to warrant the title "doctor."

I have no basis to either accept or reject the first two explanations.

I reject the third because it totally ignores the holistic commitment of the dental profession to treat oral conditions as integral components of the entire human system. While the technical excellence of American dentists is unparalleled, it does not occur in a vacuum.

Whether the procedure be the placement of a Class II amalgam restoration, the surgical alteration of a Class III malocclusion or the preparation of the maxilla for an eventual implant, our dental "doctors" realize that the success of these procedures depends on a positive response by the tissue and organ systems of the human body.

I reject the final explanation because I see dentists as integral members of the health care team possessing skills and knowledge mastered by only a minute fraction of humanity. They are active participants in the legal, ethical and political arenas of modern life. They are civic leaders, philanthropists, scholars. Above all else they are healers. Truly, by any definition, they are deserving of the term "doctor."

Physicians and dentists—of course!

Doctors and dentists—absolutely not!

Do you agree? ■

> **I see dentists as integral members of the health care team possessing skills and knowledge mastered by only a minute fraction of humanity.**

1. American Dental Association Department of State Government Affairs. Medicaid: how it relates to dental care. JADA 1991; 122(6);83-4.
2. The Associated Press. The Associated Press stylebook and libel manual. New York: The Associated Press; 1988:65.

# Where the women are or where are the women?

*Originally published in JADA 1991 122: 8-10*

Women may soon comprise the majority of entering U.S. dental freshman. Constituting just over 3 percent of dental freshmen enrolled in 1971, women entering dental school increased to 38 percent in 1990. These gains, coupled with increased retirements of predominantly older male dentists, should push the percentage of practicing female dentists to approximately 20 percent by the year 2000.

Considering these increases, it is predictable that women dentists will become increasingly visible in all aspects of dentistry, including dental politics. The selection of Dr. Geraldine Morrow as the first woman president of the American Dental Association is evidence of this change. With this precedent established, no longer will important leadership positions in dentistry be reserved for males. Or will they?

With females now constituting 6.3 percent of all ADA members, it would be expected to note a similar percentage holding ADA offices. This, however, is not reflected in present membership records, which show the percentage of women officers at 4.3 percent. In some ADA offices, the proportion of females falls far below the expected value.

For example, just 2 percent of the 1991 House of Delegates that welcomed incoming President Morrow were female. Furthermore, none of the present trustees and only one state president are female. The component societies are more representative, with 6 percent of the president and secretary positions held by female members.

How about the various councils and commissions? These are appointed positions. Nine of the 161 places are filled by women, with the Commission of the Young Professional and the Council on Dental Research accounting for the majority of the appointees. Half of the 14 councils and commissions do not have a single female member.

We now know where the women leaders are, but where are the rest of the women dentists who should be seeking leadership roles? Like so many situations, there is not always one answer that characterizes all members of the group. In this instance, information obtained from ADA membership records is helpful.

Records show that 2 percent of male and 1.4 percent of female dentists are politically active—a 30 percent difference. This disparity is accentuated when the younger dentists are compared: 40 percent fewer women than men under age 39 are active. With two-thirds of all women dentists clustered in this lower age bracket, continuation of their present low participation rate will ensure a dearth of future women trustee and presidential candidates. These latter opportunities come only after gaining experience in component and constituent positions.

For dentists 39 or older, there is no gender difference in the proportion of leadership activity. There are, however, major differences in level of positions held—very few are involved in national and state executive roles. Most are in component, council or commission offices.

Considering the large increases in the number of female dentists, lack of leadership participation, especially from those in the younger age category, should be of great concern to organized dentistry. Females already demonstrate a lower rate of membership in the ADA than their male counterparts.

The inability to observe females in leadership positions may make recruitment of new female dental graduates into the ADA even more difficult. It is conceivable that present women ADA members may not renew, believing that the under-

> **Considering the large increases in the number of female dentists, lack of leadership participation, especially from those in the younger age category, should be of great concern to organized dentistry.**

representation of women in leadership positions is an indication of indifference and continued male dominance.

What should the profession do?

While I do not advocate a quota system, believing rather that individuals should be selected on merit and not on what proportion of an organization they represent, I do strongly suggest that our present ADA leadership make extraordinary efforts to recruit females for political office. This will not be easy.

Why?

We have no information that ascertains interest levels of female ADA members in seeking leadership roles. Nor do we know what their perceptions of opportunity are. Through written and personal communication, it appears that there are factors specific to female dentists that might impact on their seeking leadership roles.

For example, 30 percent of all female dentists are married to another dentist.1 Usually only one will be active in ADA politics. Exceptions notwithstanding, the wife will more often opt for "being with the family," while the husband takes on extracurricular professional duties. Furthermore, the frugal dual dental career family may purchase just one membership in the ADA.

If this occurs, it is more often the male who joins. Childrearing also occupies the "flexible" time of many female dentists—restricting their ability to take on structured ADA political activities. Finally, the lack of female leadership role models may discourage potentially interested females from even considering participation.

Overcoming these barriers requires that all present officers in the ADA, especially those in component positions, identify potential female leaders. Special attention must then be directed to involving these women in activities that fit their tight schedules.

Whenever possible, women should be considered for appointed positions including those on councils and commissions. Finally, the assumption of a role by present dental leaders may provide the most valuable contribution. None of these activities will be of value unless our female membership accepts the responsibility of leadership when offered.

Success in these endeavors is critical if we do not want to disenfranchise this important and growing segment of the dental profession. ∎

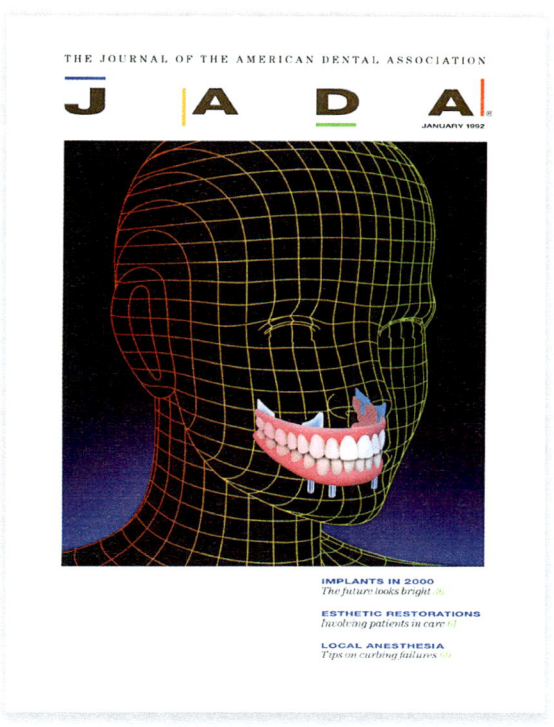

# 1992

"Dentistry's mandate as a health profession
is to advance the public's oral health status.
As the sole purveyors of dental care,
dentistry has the obligation to continually seek
new knowledge that will enhance its mission."

# It's time for action on licensure

*Originally published in JADA 1992 123: 8-10*

On Nov. 2, 1926, 250,000 Colorado residents cast their yea or nay on Amendment six, or the Parker amendment as it was more commonly called. At stake was the ability of the dental profession to restrict who could practice dentistry in Colorado-could the dental board continue to test dentists who wished to practice in Colorado even if they held a dental license in another state?

Dental organizations throughout the country anxiously awaited results. If the voters passed the amendment, similar legislation could be expected in their states.

## WHAT LED TO THIS CRISIS?

Painless Parker, an entrepreneur the likes of P.T. Barnum, had achieved his goal as America's premier advertising dentist. Not content with 30 successful "advertising" dental practices established throughout the Western states and Canada, Dr. Parker set his sights on the lucrative Colorado market.

Without a dental license in Colorado, Parker employed as many Colorado licensed practitioners as he could. Demand for his "low-cost services" quickly outstripped his supply of dental practitioners.

The only way for Dr. Parker to expand was to hire dentists from other states. But they would have to pass the Colorado board, and Parker knew that the fringe dentists that would work for an advertiser would not have the skills to pass the dental license exam. Thus his attempt to force the issue through a public vote.

## THE ISSUES

Section 4574 of the Parker amendment was intended to allow licensing of dentists without examination if the dentists were graduates of a reputable dental college, of good moral character and licensed by the board of dental examiners of any state in the United States. Passage of this legislation would allow Parker to continue to expand this advertising empire in Colorado.

The Colorado Dental Association contended that approval of the amendment would make it possible for anyone licensed in any other state, for the fee of $10, to practice in Colorado. Concern for this proposed "licensure by credential" was based on the lack of uniform educational standards for dental training institutions and the knowledge that dentists could often "buy" a license from some political appointee on a dental board who wanted to make an extra dollar or two.

Painless Parker spent more than $100,000 in his attempt to break the "Dental Trust," the term he used for ethical dental organizations. The Colorado Dental Association's appeal was based on its mandate to protect the health of the public. Organized dentistry prevailed, and the Parker amendment was defeated by a 3 to 1 margin. Ramification of this decisive vote still remains.

Currently, Louisiana has become the most recent state to enact legislation granting authority to state dental boards to license by credential. Thirty states, plus the District of Columbia, have enacted this legislation. Only 24 states and D.C. have actually exercised that authority. The remaining states still require performance exams for all dentists that desire licensure. That policy is questionable considering the major changes that have taken place in our profession since the days of Painless Parker.

Are our dental training institutions today still unregulated, graduating students of questionable skill? Hardly! For years, the ADA, working with the Commission on Dental Accreditation, has established standards that ensure the highest quality dental training in the world.

Furthermore, the American Association of Dental Examiners has promoted regional licensure exams with standardized components. Dentists success-

> **The time has come for the remaining states to consider establishing a mechanism for "licensure by credential."**

fully examined in one state should be able to practice in other states by credential examination.

The days when the Painless Parkers could undermine the dental care system are gone. Professional quality can be ascertained from credentials. The time has come for the remaining states to consider establishing a mechanism for "licensure by credential."

Failure to do so could bring federal intervention—an initiative that could only compromise the profession's ability to control its future. We have already noted attempts to accomplish this.

Now is the time for discussion, debate and action! ■

# Too much OSHA

*Originally published in JADA 1992 123: 8-10*

For many dentists any OSHA is too much. The U.S. Occupational Safety and Health Administration's intrusion into the dental office with regulations and visits and even fines for non-compliance has placed the organization high on the list of concerns among dentists.

Thus, Assistant Secretary of Labor Gerard Scannell's proposed new OSHA regulations (Dec. 2, 1991) to protect the health of "millions of American workers who are occupationally exposed to blood-borne diseases such as those caused by Hepatitis B and AIDS virus" has generated scant enthusiasm among dental professionals.

Not that dentists aren't concerned with the health of their employees. They are, but they would argue that these new OSHA standards will do little to accomplish that goal. Instead, they may actually inhibit future access to needed dental care by patients fearing that they might contract a serious disease while visiting the dental office. The dentist-patient relationship may also suffer from these regulations.

### IMAGINE

Children-even adults-observing the appearance of fully masked, gloved and gowned dentists and auxiliaries, could easily become fearful, potentially eroding the confidence they have developed in their dentist. This would be especially true if the visit was for a routine checkup or some minor non-surgical procedure. Additionally, those paying out of pocket for dental services might be forced to defer needed dental care because of higher dental fees resulting from compliance with the new OSHA regulations.

These facts notwithstanding, the dental profession would never object to the institution of any valid procedure or regulation that prevented harm to dental team members. Many critical components of the new OSHA regulations, however, lack a scientific basis for incorporation into the regular regimen of most dental practices. Once again the "plague" mentality incited by the presence of AIDS has resulted in capricious and hasty rule-making.

For example, where is the science that HIV is actually spread through dental aerosols? Or even better, where is the evidence that HIV, if spread through dental aerosols, has ever caused a single infection? I have not been able to find any reference that would answer either of these questions. Neither have my associates engaged in HIV research.

This skepticism should not be interpreted as a call for abandonment of any of the established barrier techniques now employed in dental offices. Absolutely not! Gloves do make a difference-so does protecting the eyes and using masks.

But why the need for additional recordkeeping that can only compound the complexities of simple dental procedures? For example, the detail in dental records now requested by OSHA after any post-exposure incident does not appear to be rational. In addition, the proposed clothing restrictions for dental personnel need to be further denned.

Some parts of the new OSHA regulations do make sense. Few professionals would object to the requirement that all health workers have the opportunity to be inoculated against HBV. The handwashing practices advocated by OSHA have been part of dentists' customary infection control procedures for decades. Unfortunately, many other proposed regulations seem more appropriate for hospitals and industry. Their introduction into dental practice would only add to the cost of providing dental services.

In that regard, OSHA's estimates of the economic impact of its regulations are ludicrous—consider an annual expenditure of $97 for sterile gloves. That's for a year—not a month-but a year. Other expenses are similarly understated. For example, OSHA's estimate of less than $900 per year for a dental office

> **Many critical components of the new OSHA regulations, however, lack a scientific basis for incorporation into the regular regimen of most dental practices.**

to institute these regulations is so far from reality that it adds credence to those who question the credentials of the regulation developers.

What can be done about this latest intrusion into dental practice?

Efforts by the American Dental Association are under way to return the regulation of dental practice to the dentists. The privilege of licensure that permits the dentist to determine which procedures should be used in a particular situation must be maintained. We hope our judicial and legislative systems will agree. ∎

# Expanding the scope of dental practice

*Originally published in JADA 1992 123: 8-10*

Should dentists conduct screening tests in their dental offices for diseases such as diabetes? How about routine administration of electrocardiograms? Two recent dental publications say yes.

One report cited evidence that 4 percent of patients screened in a dental setting had arrhythmias of sufficient magnitude to warrant further medical evaluation. Based on this finding, it was suggested that all patients be tested before invasive dental procedures are performed. To support their conclusions, the authors indicated that tested patients viewed the EKG as a valuable service and were not concerned with the dental setting for the procedure.

Similar conclusions were noted by a group of investigators who evaluated the use of the fasting capillary blood glucose test for patients who had "no consultative relationship with a physician."

Does the appearance of these reports signify a new effort to incorporate previous "physician only" tests into routine dental procedure? Why not? Supporters of additional in-office testing would argue, suggesting that skeptics look at the list of "medical" tests already incorporated into routine dental practice. For example, blood pressure cuffs, rare a decade ago, now are standard equipment in many dental offices.

While I'm personally unaware of general dental practitioners offering WBC, hemoglobin, clotting time and other blood tests to their patients—surely some oral and maxillofacial surgeons and periodontists must. In fact, considering the invasiveness of many surgical dental procedures, would physicians perform this type of surgery without these basic tests?

Is there any reason to question the actions of those dentists who wish to expand the scope of dental practice by including additional medical proce-

dures in their everyday practice regime?

Dentistry's mandate as a health profession is to advance the public's oral health status. As the sole purveyors of dental care, dentistry has the obligation to continually seek new knowledge that will enhance its mission. If offering medical tests, previously in the domain of other health professionals, assists in accomplishing this goal, then arguments against such procedures are spurious. If, however, the evidence for inclusion of such testing indicates potential harm-even to a few patients-the legitimacy of the procedure(s) must be questioned.

For example, in the instance of fasting capillary blood glucose test, is the dental office the appropriate site for such testing? How many dental patients would be willing to fast for 10 hours before their dental appointment? Compliance issues aside, for elderly patients heavily involved in a regime of polypharmacy, how safe is it for them to refrain from following their normal prescription schedule prior to invasive dental procedures? Can the dentist perform the procedure at a level of competency consistent with other medical settings? What about false positives and negatives? Do they occur at a greater rate in the dental office?

> **As the sole purveyors of dental care, dentistry has the obligation to continually seek new knowledge that will enhance its mission.**

Other questions must be addressed. Is the dentist trained in the interpretation of these tests? What will the dentist do with the test results? How will these procedures be paid for? Medical insurance? Highly unlikely. Dental insurance? Even less so.

If payment for testing is out of pocket, will dental patients be willing to obligate themselves for the additional costs? Will this affect their use of dental services?

Each dental practitioner must answer these questions satisfactorily before accepting new medical procedures as "standard of care" in his or her dental office. There will be no universal answer. Many dentists will reject increased activity, others will participate at different levels.

As dentists assess their personal interest and competence, the precept "do no harm" should be the basis for the judgment process. ∎

# Dental office visits: high-risk behavior?

*Originally published in JADA 1992 123: 8-10*

One of our fellow dentists has been threatened with a lawsuit by a patient. "Unfortunate," you might say, "but surely not an unusual happening in these days of our litigious society."

But this lawsuit is different. It doesn't involve an alleged "ill-fitting denture," a cut or laceration of the mouth or supposed failure to diagnose periodontal disease. Nor does it involve potential fines levied against the dentist by OSHA or other federal agencies.

Different, according to an op-ed column in the Fort Lauderdale, Fla. Sun-Sentinel, because this threatened legal action alleges that a Mr. James Charles Sharpe Jr. became infected with the AIDS virus in a dental office. Not from the dentist, he contends, but rather through improperly sterilized dental equipment. This appears to be the first threat of a legal challenge of this type. Unfortunately, it will not be the last for the "plague mentality" response to HIV, which has placed dentistry at center stage.

The column indicated no evidence that the office environment of Mr. Sharpe's dentist held any greater risk of HIV transmission than any other dental office. The dentist himself, having tested negative for HIV 10 months after the plaintiffs visit, could not be the source.

Evidently Mr. Sharpe bases his complaint on a patient-to-patient transmission caused by inadequate infection control.

The dentist maintains that his infection control procedures incorporated all accepted methods to prevent HIV transmission.

This was not a high-risk practice in regard to the patient population. But according to the plaintiff, the office was located in an area that contained large numbers of IV drug users. The author of the Sun-Sentinel story quotes the dentist as denying any activity that might have put Mr. Sharpe at risk; denied treating any known HIV patients during that period; and, after examining his infection control procedure, could not identify any procedures that would compromise the patients' safety.

So why is Mr. Sharpe suing the dentist? Because he contends he has none of the risk factors associated with HIV infection. The newspaper article states that "Sharpe is not gay nor has he ever had sex with a man. He has never used intravenous drugs." No extramarital affairs, wife is HIV negative, etc., etc., etc. The only "high-risk behavior" identified by Mr. Sharpe was a dental visit—to a dental office located in an area the plaintiff maintains has a large number of drug users.

One instance of dentist-patient HIV infectivity (Acer) and now a dental office visit becomes classified as high-risk behavior for HIV infection. No scientific evidence whatsoever to support dental patient-to-patient spread of HIV through contaminated instruments—yet Mr. Sharpe contends that's how he was infected.

Consider the accused dentist. He apparently follows all presently known infection control procedures, yet he faces a lawsuit. Most likely he will be legally exonerated, but what about his good name, his future dental practice, his family of patients? Won't some of them wonder, even a little—could Mr. Sharpe have possibly become infected in their dentist's office? Maybe, just maybe, they should change dentists—just to be on the "safe" side.

What about all the dental consumers who read about this legal activity? The Sun-Sentinel column has been reprinted in at least one other newspaper. I'm sure others will carry this story because of its

> **No scientific evidence whatsoever to support dental patient-to-patient spread of HIV through contaminated instruments—yet (the patient) contends that's how he was infected.**

sensational appeal.

Will these "other" dental consumers become susceptible to the plague mentality and restrict dental visits? If there is a quick judicial response that indicates no basis for the suit, lawyers will be less inclined to take on a case with little chance for success and financial gain.

Conversely, if the court will actually give credence to these allegations with attendant national publicity, then the plaque mentality may grow into panic. ∎

# Dental care for the elderly
# A call for affordable service

*Originally published in JADA 1992 123: 5: 008-010*

Unprecedented drops in interest rates have left many Americans concerned about their future. Those on fixed incomes, predominantly the elderly, are particularly affected. Concerned, they are reducing expenditures, maintaining their previous spending patterns only for necessities, often foregoing out-of-pocket expenses for dental care. Is the dental profession concerned? Probably not. Should it be? Absolutely.

For a multitude of reasons, the dental profession has not recognized the impact of growing numbers of elderly on expenditures for dental care. Even though they number more than 31 million (14 percent of our population) they generate little enthusiasm as a viable market for comprehensive dental care.

Most dentists remain convinced that older adults are underusers of dental services, cannot afford regular dental care and make dental visits only for emergency treatment, palliative care or denture adjustments. That dental insurance rarely extends into retirement age and Medicare does not cover routine dental services only enhance this view.

Until 1983, little evidence existed to convince the profession otherwise. Those aged 65-plus had user rates significantly below any other age group. Between 1983 and 1986, that discrepancy disappeared. A 40 percent increase in dental visits by this group positioned them as significant consumers of dental services.

Presently, they are making more dental visits than would be expected, based on their representation in the population. For example, in Florida the elderly represent 17.6 percent of the population—but they were responsible for 26 percent of all dental visits. Remarkably, they also spent more on dental treatment annually than patients under 65. Yet, only 10 percent of elderly spending was assisted by private dental insurance. Eighty percent was out of-pocket-the remainder from public or donated service.

## HOW COULD THE ELDERLY AFFORD THIS DENTAL CARE?

Those between 65 and 74 have the greatest amount of discretionary income available compared to other age groups. Furthermore, in the last 15 years, real income has increased in the 65 and older age group by 18 percent vs. just 2 percent for the remainder of the population. And more is forthcoming.

The next group of older adults, those 55-64, have the greatest net worth of any age group. Those 50 and older represent 70 percent of the nation's wealth. Given present trends in dental expenditures and visits, spending for dental care will increase by 20 percent in the next 10 years solely as a result of the changing demography of an aging America.

Furthermore, demand for care should increase as the numbers of edentulous individuals—presently low utilizers of dental care are succeeded by dentate older adults who have a history of comprehensive dental care.

A "golden" opportunity for dentistry indeed, but only if the demand for services can be underwritten by sufficient out-of-pocket resources. Until the dramatic drop in interest rates, it appeared that both motivation and finances were available.

With serious reductions in monies generated from interest, however, future use of dental services by many elderly may be jeopardized. If low rates prevail for an extended period, the negative impact on dental spending could be massive, as millions of new 65-year-olds retire and lose their dental insurance.

> **Greater support for accessible and affordable dental service must be offered to our elderly, ensuring that the oral health gains of the past decades not be lost.**

## WHAT CAN BE DONE TO ENSURE THAT THE ELDERLY WILL BE ABLE TO RECEIVE COMPREHENSIVE DENTAL SERVICES?

There will be no Denticare program in the foreseeable future. The country cannot afford it, and the politics of extending dental insurance into retirement will require the dental profession and industry, not government, to offer assistance. This will be difficult as reductions in benefits, not increases, are being sought by industry. There are possible solutions.

Many benefit plans allow the individual to choose their benefits from a menu. Perhaps an inexpensive prepaid dental plan—subsidizing dental services during the retirement years—could be developed and offered to the employee. This might prove to be an attractive choice for those 10 to 15 years from retirement and who place a high value on dental health.

Another option that might provide prepaid dental care would be post-retirement dental insurance offered by the American Association of Retired Persons. To date, this organization has shown little interest in this type of membership benefit. AARP should be encouraged to investigate this important benefit.

Innovation is critical. Greater support for accessible and affordable dental service must be offered to our elderly, ensuring that the oral health gains of the past decades not be lost. The dental profession must give this issue high priority. ∎

# Non-maleficence: do no harm!

*Originally published in JADA 1992 123: 8-10*

**D**ental hygiene, or at least the American Dental Hygienists" Association, wants out. It wants out from under organized dentistry's "control," its "grasp."

About two years ago, the ADHA House of Delegates advocated promotion of "self-regulation of dental hygiene education, licensure and practice."

What rationale does dental hygiene use to justify severing its 75-year link with the dental profession? Organized hygiene's answer is that it wishes to become an autonomous health care profession, and self-regulation is basic to that goal.

Hygiene's original arguments in support of unsupervised practice focused on improving access and reducing costs. Hygiene said it would provide access to dental care for those unable to reach dental services: nursing home residents, the poor, those in rural areas. It pledged to provide these services at costs lower than those that would be charged by dentists.

Wrong!

In Colorado, the dental practice act has allowed hygienists to practice unsupervised in nursing homes and at industrial sites since 1979. Not more than a handful have availed themselves of this opportunity. So much for improving access.

On the cost issue (and again using Colorado as the example) less than 1 percent of registered hygienists have attempted to establish independent practices since state law gave them that right in 1986. Why? Because it's not cost effective. Office overhead, labor costs, insurance and other expenses make it impossible to offer hygiene services at a fee equal to or less than what a dentist would charge. And those costs will escalate when government-required infection control measures are added to the overhead.

So the ADHA's arguments on cost and access have proved specious, rendering invalid its claim that self-regulation would be good for the public's dental health. On the contrary, because of their limited training and knowledge, hygienists practicing without supervision conceivably could cause great harm to the public, which would constitute a breech of professional ethics.

The codes of conduct and ethics for both medicine and dentistry call on health professionals to use their skills, knowledge and abilities to benefit patients (beneficence). The codes also require professionals to "do no harm" (non-maleficence). Ethicists typically declare that when there is a conflict between beneficence and non-maleficence, the latter takes precedence.

ADHA take note. In your reach for self-regulation, you have not demonstrated beneficence: lower cost, improved access. You have instead undermined dentistry's greatest contribution to patient care: the ability of the general practitioners to provide continuous care to their patients.

By wedging your ambition between patients and dentists, you jeopardize a unique relationship. You also risk creating detrimental, even life-threatening situations. In a self-regulated, unsupervised dental hygiene practice, you alone would decide if your patient should be referred to a dentist. That decision necessarily involves diagnosis, a process reserved only for those who have been trained and licensed as dentists. Are you capable of making a diagnosis? You say YES.

*"I'm saying that, yes, that [patient referral] in fact involves diagnosis, and that dental hygiene, as a licensed profession, is responsible and accountable."*

—Virginia Woodward,
ADHA president
April 6 ADA News

Dental educators would say NO. Contrary to statements often made by hygienists seeking self-regulation, dental hygiene students do not receive

> **Is organized hygiene so determined to sever its long relationship with organized dentistry that it would compromise the health and well-being of the American people?**

the same clinical training as dental students. They do not take the same basic science curriculum. They are not trained to handle emergency procedures or diagnose oral cancer. They are not trained to prescribe drugs and so on.

To attempt diagnosis without appropriate training must be classified as maleficence. Is organized hygiene so determined to sever its long relationship with organized dentistry that it would compromise the health and well-being of the American people?

Let the clear thinkers prevail. ∎

# A matter of trust

*Originally published in JADA 1992 123: 8-10*

**D**entistry is very precise. No matter what you do, sometimes things just don't go right. One of the big diseases dentists have is stress. If you're not satisfied when you've completed your work, nobody else knows, but you do. You're your own worst critic. If you do a good job, damn it, you're proud of it and you want other people to appreciate it. I don't think a patient knows whether you're a good dentist or a bad one."

—A dentist interviewed by author Studs Terkel for his book "Working," 1972

Do you enjoy the practice of dentistry? Is it still personally and professionally stimulating? Do you look forward to getting up in the morning and going to the office? Would you leave dentistry for another career if the situation permitted?

Twenty or 30 years ago, most dentists would have answered yes to all but the last question, citing as their rationale personal satisfaction, economic enrichment and the importance of belonging to a health profession held in high esteem by the public.

Today, this professional satisfaction is being tested by recurring media events that continue to focus on the dental profession and its members. Look at the issues!

Awaiting the government's forthcoming report on amalgam, we have not forgotten about:
- the implied dangers of amalgam;
- the possibility of cancer caused by fluoride;
- unannounced visits from OSHA;
- HIV-infected dentist and patients;
- HIV testing of health professionals.

And then the latest: the media indictment of dental handpieces as the supposed vehicle for HIV transmissions from patient to patient.

Individually, each of these items is a problem. Collectively, it would appear that someone is ganging up on dentistry, shredding its professional im-

> **As the profession fights to maintain public trust, it must ameliorate the constant pressure and stress now being placed on its constituents.**

munity, destroying its public trust. And public trust is what it's all about.

The public has been extremely loyal to its dentists. Few patients, as Terkel's dentist points out, can judge the quality of their dentist's performance. Rather, these patients have an unspoken confidence that the dentists will act only in their best interests.

But the media broadcast that a visit to the dentist may be unsafe, that the dentist may not be protecting the patient's interests because he or she doesn't sterilize but only disinfects dental handpieces. The fact that investigators at the federal Centers for Disease Control are not aware of any studies that confirm the transmission of a blood-borne pathogen through contaminated dental equipment appears to have had little influence on television reports.

The well-publicized regulations of the Occupational Safety and Health Administration—with the attendant threat of unscheduled dental office appearances for infection control violations—further contribute to the fears of those considering their next dental appointment.

What's more, TV pictures of Kimberly Bergalis just before her death do nothing to assuage mounting dental patient concerns. Add to this equation last year's national expose on amalgam and it becomes obvious that the profession, and each individual dentist, must work constantly to restore and preserve public trust. And just when success appears imminent, a new cataclysmic event takes place, further challenging professional stamina and perseverance.

How much can the individual dentist withstand before "stress marks" appear? Will we soon note earlier and earlier retirement ages for dentists? Or perhaps a switch to other endeavors for those in mid-career? Will the best and brightest students be turned off to what was once considered a shining career opportunity?

As the profession fights to maintain public trust, it must ameliorate the constant pressure and stress now being placed on its constituents. The ADA should consider offering innovative health education programming that promotes recognition and alleviation of this "internal" stress.

Course content might include stress manage-ment, how to cope with and respond to media attacks, responses to patient questions generated by the media and methods of achieving self-fulfillment in difficult times.

These interactive sessions, developed for all levels of dental participation, should be offered as a membership benefit. By addressing this issue, the ADA may be initiating a critical component of its proactive response to a troubled environment. ∎

# The next revolution: it's here

*Originally published in JADA 1992 123: 8-10*

In the '60s, American dentistry witnessed a revolution unparalleled in the history of the health professions. Two technical and scientific developments did more to alter the nature of dental health care delivery than any other innovation before or since.

The first was the high-speed handpiece; the second, community water fluoridation. The first doubled or tripled the speed at which restorations could be completed. The second represented a quantum leap in preventive dentistry, dramatically reducing the number of restorations that would be needed by future dental patients.

Today we stand on the verge of a new revolution. This revolution, based on another technological development, will alter the way we manage our practices day to day. It will change the way we practice and provide services, and alter the services we are able to provide. Some visionaries might suggest that dentistry will be transformed to an even greater degree than occurred in the '60s.

The first salvo in this revolution was fired in the early '80s with the introduction of the personal computer. Many dental practices today are using powerful desktop computers to perform billing and accounts management, word processing, patient tracking, claims processing and newsletter publishing. These services, significant as they are, represent only the tip of the technological iceberg. Many more sophisticated and exciting computer aids to dentistry already exist for today's practitioner.

Visualize yourself in the dental operatory performing an oral exam. Only you and the patient are present. Into a small microphone you record the patient's oral condition. As the computer screen chronicles your clinical observations, the observations also are verified by a voice response from the computer.

Science fiction? Absolutely not. You are using a voice-activated system to record the patient's oral exam. These systems allow caries and periodontal

**Many more sophisticated and exciting computer aids to dentistry already exist for today's practitioner.**

measurements to be recorded automatically recorded and displayed visually on terminals-and can act as a new medium for case presentations. Patients will be able to monitor their own progress before, during and after therapy.

Manual periodontal probing will give way to computerized probes that will locate gingival margins and attachment losses much more accurately and sensitively. Radiographic film will soon become a museum relic: filmless, computer-controlled intraoral sensors now reduce radiation by 90 percent and eliminate the need for darkroom processing. Images can be stored on optical or hard disks, transmitted over phone lines to insurance companies or colleagues, and submitted to more sophisticated analyses than were available in the past.

Stereo-photography and laser-diode scanners are used in computer-assisted design/computer-assisted manufacturing of dental restorations. Current systems can produce an MOD porcelain inlay (from the time of activity preparation) in less than 90 minutes. Computer imaging, using topographic mapping and three-dimensional simulations, allow dentists to present patients with visible alternative treatment options in cosmetic and rehabilitative surgery.

Tomorrow's practice will have access to literally dozens of innovations ushered in by computer technology.

The real question is: will tomorrow's dentists be ready, willing and able to take advantage of the new technology?

Most dentists readily accept the application of computers to office management functions. As for other advancements, many dismiss them as too much gadgetry. Often their caution or quick dismissal stems from lack of computer literacy. They suffer from understandable discomfort, believing that there's simply no way for the ordinary dentist to have access to these technologic marvels, let alone have the opportunity to learn how to use them.

Because of the sophisticated technology and high cost of these innovations, organized dentistry, in concert with industry, should consider providing its members with a number of regional advanced dental technology demonstration centers. There, new technologies could be introduced to the profession, tested by prospective purchasers and evaluated by patients.

As a new model for "continuing education," these proposed centers could provide basic training and "hands-on" experience for those dentists who want to be active participants in dentistry's next revolution. ∎

# The dental hygiene story
# One more chapter

*Originally published in JADA 1992 123: 8-10*

**W**anted—Dental Hygienist. Appearing in newspapers throughout the United States, the frequency of these ads underscores the frustration of thousands of dentists unable to attract one of today's scarcest health worker. For many, especially those in rural areas, the situation has become untenable. Despite the offering of many incentives by some practitioners, months, even years have passed, without hiring success. Solutions are needed! Demanded!

Considering the well-documented shortage of dental hygienists, large-scale activities to increase the number of graduates from existing education programs would be expected. So would newly developed education programs especially created to serve the workforce needs of rural dentists.

Incentives to encourage the present workforce to continue their employment coupled with hygienist re-entry programs should abound. Development and implementation of these programs should be the result of cooperative efforts between dental and dental hygiene leaders.

Expected perhaps, but surely not observed!

Rather than working toward solutions, a schism has developed over the appropriate practice role for dental hygienists. At issue, from the perspective of organized dentistry, is dental hygiene's nationwide campaign to create a "new" and "unneeded" self-regulated independent profession—offering services directly to the public. These services, duplicating those offered by the dentist, are to be delivered by individuals who have not undergone the rigorous training and accountability required of the licensed dentist.

Without documented public need for this "new" profession, it can only be surmised that dental hygiene's thrust results from frustration with a delivery system offering them little opportunity for upward mobility. Locked into a perceived dead end, they seek to create new opportunities for themselves.

To address this issue, consider the merit of the following proposals:

■ Dental educators should develop innovative programs and financing that facilitate the entrance of practicing dental hygienists into specially tailored D.D.S./D.M.D. training curriculums. Guaranteed placement, with advanced standing, before completing selected prerequisites, might motivate dental hygienists who are frustrated by the treatment limits of their profession. Hygienists able to select this option should find sufficient challenge to allow them to achieve their potential.

■ For dental hygienists unable to enter formal D.D.S. program but wishing to expand their scope of services, perhaps the Physician's Assistant program might serve as a model. These practitioners, working under the direct supervision of a physician, deliver a wider scope of services than do the independently practicing nurse practitioners. Perhaps self-regulation and independence will not provide anticipated opportunities.

As potential solutions to the shortage of dental hygienists, organized dentistry might contemplate the following action items:

■ To increase the availability of dental hygienists, the profession should actively participate in the expansion of the two-year dental hygiene training programs. This can be assisted through active support and lobbying for increased program funding.

■ Professional activities should also be directed to encourage dental hygienists who have previously left the workforce to return. Retraining programs tailored to family and work schedules need to be developed and widely publicized. Financial incentives supplied by dentists to those who enter retraining

> **It can only be surmised that dental hygiene's thrust results from frustration with a delivery system offering them little opportunity for upward mobility.**

might alleviate concerns of program affordabilty.

For the rural dentist (and those in urban areas demonstrating long-term need), the following action is suggested:

■ For those areas defined by state boards of dentistry as "hygiene shortage areas," registered dental assistants who have successfully completed formal advanced training in scaling and polishing would be allowed to provide this treatment under the direct supervision of the dentist.

Actions that address the present shortage of dental hygienists have been proposed. Individually, each would assist in alleviating a void that has left many dental teams unable to function at their desired level. Collectively, they offer opportunities to all who have a vested interest in seeking positive closure on an issue of critical importance.

Any additional thoughts? ■

# It's not over yet!

*Originally published in JADA 1992 123: 8-10*

**D**ental care in the U.S. has achieved a hallmark of success that continues to elude most areas of medical practice-economic stagnation, even decline, because of preventive measures that decisively reduce the need for many services.

Editorial, The Lancet, Aug. 8, 1992

The ultimate goal of any health profession should be its dissolution. Heady words, more attuned to discussions by students in a philosophy class than a discussion item among dentists. That is, until late July when the National Institute of Dental Research announced that Americans "saved nearly $100 billion dollars in dental bills during the 1980s because of improvements in oral health."

Referencing economic statistics from the U.S. Commerce Department, these researchers indicated that the nation's dental bill increased just 1 percent annually from 1979 to 1989—contrasted to a 5 percent yearly average rise in previous years.

The NIDR report attributed major "improvement in oral health" as THE factor in holding down expenditures. Citing reductions in refined sugars, increased use of fluoride and better oral hygiene practice, the institute's economists were able to calculate a $99.1 billion savings for consumers over the 11-year period.

Assessing the economic impact of increased population growth, greater insurance coverage and larger disposable income, this finding is all the more striking. Impressed, many in the health community interpreted this as a signal that U.S. dental needs had been satisfied.

While accolades are called for, the dental profession should not allow the NIDR report to serve as the basis for diminishing its renowned service, education and research programs. To do so would ignore current documented need for continued progress in arresting and preventing dental disease.

> **This is not the time to contemplate closing dental schools, shutting or reducing dental practices or seeking alternative employment for the dental work force.**

This is not the time to contemplate closing dental schools, shutting or reducing dental practices or seeking alternative employment for the dental work force. No, there is still much to be accomplished before dentistry can even consider the lofty philosophic goal of its own dissolution.

Consider the following:

■ A nationwide evaluation of the clinical condition of lower left first molars of 35- to 39-year-olds counted 4 percent decayed, 29 percent missing and 58 percent filled—hardly a remarkable dental health status for an age group considered to have had favorable access to preventive and restorative care. v For the 18- to 24-year-olds, nurtured in an era characterized by fluoride and prevention, the same study indicated that one of 10 young adults had already lost that lower first molar. Additionally, 70 percent of those molars showed clinical evidence of restoration or active decay.

■ In 1987, more than 50 percent of children between the ages of 5 to 17 had no decay in their permanent teeth. Yet, by age 19, only 7 percent were caries-free. That percentage dropped below 2 percent by age 35. Obviously, dental caries had not been eradicated.

■ Due solely to the increasing number of older adults, dental visits and expenditures for dental care will increase by 20 percent by the end of this decade. The present group of elderly has already demonstrated more visits and higher expenditures than earlier cohorts and should continue to do so as they attempt to maintain high levels of oral health throughout their lifetime. As dentistry positions itself to treat the needs of these individuals, it will require more—not less—dental resources and energy.

■ Successful preventive efforts do not necessarily mean less dental need. While dramatic reductions in complete edentulism will occur in the future, the remaining teeth will require extensive dental attention. Complex re-restoration procedures combined with single and multiple implants will demand the full attention of dental practitioners.

Also: Oral cancer. Pain control. TMD. Facial abnormalities. Periodontal disease. Too many to list. All will require continuing research and treatment. It's not over yet. Not even close. ∎

# Health care reform: taking charge

*Originally published in JADA 1992 123: 8-10*

**W**ith health care reform a major presidential issue in this month's national election, many states are calling for congressional action to reform the health care system. Some states aren't waiting.

The Minnesota law does not allow the new tax to be itemized on dental bills, but reality dictates that some or all of the 2 percent dental contribution will be passed on to the dentist's current family of patients. Conceivably any increase in fees could drive away those patients who are marginally able to afford dental care. Furthermore, we can seriously question whether HealthRight will increase access or merely restructure the payment system for individuals already receiving care under public assistance.

We must also consider potential loss of substantial free or contributed dental care currently supplied by dental practitioners. Motivation to continue these charitable efforts could be severely limited after the implementation of HealthRight benefits.

Economic benefits from HealthRight could accrue from fees generated from dental copayments. These fees would increase total dental spending if the payment came from new users of dental care. Offsetting this potential increase would be the dentist's need to produce more dentistry to generate the same income—a result of their increased percentage of gross income derived from the lower medical assistance fees.

Regardless of these caveats, public opinion will demand that this month's political champion offer some type of health reform. Both parties are searching for models, and Minnesota's HealthRight with its medical and dental programs has all the ingredients to be a top contender.

Dentistry, take note. Aside from Oregon and Minnesota, Hawaii, Massachusetts and Vermont have also enacted universal health insurance programs. Health care reform is no longer a cause looking for a champion, an idea waiting to be born. There will be no escaping involvement in these future health programs with:

- Medicaid programs pushing states to the financial breaking point;
- health insurance premiums rising dramatically;
- more citizens finding themselves uninsured.

Albeit a minor component of most health plans, dentistry is already being buffeted about as new initiatives are formatted. Programs like HealthRight must be scrutinized, analyzed and evaluated. Even more important, our dental leadership must preemptively introduce its own initiatives that address legitimate public needs while preserving professional integrity and independence.

Demonstrating a vision that recognizes the present and anticipates the future, leadership should advance dental health care programs created by dental societies, not state or federal bureaucrats. Tax credits, not gross earnings taxes, should fund these programs. Choice, not managed care, should govern their access. Professional control is essential. To ensure this outcome requires dentistry's proactive engagement in the design of any health care program that could affect its future. ∎

> **Public opinion will demand that this month's political champion offer some type of health reform.**

# The nation's top schools are...

*Originally published in JADA 1992 123: 8-10*

Your school. My school. My associate's school. Every dentist's school. Ask practicing dentists how they would rank their dental school—from a clinical perspective—and almost without exception they would place their dental alma mater in the country's top five. This being the case, the dental universe must be comprised of 55 dental schools resembling atoms in constant motion—all have a momentary place in the winner's circle—before being replaced by the next best dental school.

Does this then mean the notion of the best dental schools is meaningless? Perhaps. After all, what dentist would admit that his or her dental clinical training wasn't received at one of the nation's best. The truth is that in an era where everyone and everything claims to be the best—the best pizza, hot dog, hamburger, toothpaste, college, business or engineering school—we are in danger of embracing mediocrity with every stroke of the marketing consultant's pen.

Should we ever try to speak of the best dental schools?

Yes, if you're a dental educator.

Yes, if you're a prospective dental student.

Yes, if you're one of the "wet-gloved dentists" interested in improving the profession's educational base.

Yes, if you're a dental consumer who must depend on these professionals to ensure the quality of their future dental care.

Decidedly, the answer is yes. However, our dental accreditation process uses standards that represent only the "minimum requirements expected from a dental education program." At present, the accreditation process acknowledges deficiencies, not excellence. The Conditional or Provisional accreditation rankings (that is, less than acceptable) provide a stimulus to improve only to the minimum level. With no mechanism to describe programs with superior qualities, dental education programs of excellence cannot expect to receive appropriate public acknowledgment.

Does this mean that all dental schools, save the few on probation, are of similar quality with none being better or best? Is it easier to enumerate deficiencies than it is to quantify excellence? Are there objective criteria that could be used to distinguish better and best, just as we've done with sorting the poor from the acceptable? And if criteria for excellence exit, what can be done to utilize them?

The Fourth Trustee District recently submitted a resolution to the ADA House of Delegates that supports the concept of providing educationally beneficial information and data from programs that "substantially exceed minimal standards" to the minimal standard education programs. The ADA Board of Trustees, while supporting this resolution, was concerned that such procedures might breech the confidentiality of the accreditation process and seeks further information to clarify this subject.

But some dental schools that believe they have exemplary programs aren't waiting for the go-ahead. Many distribute brochures, directed to potential students, emphasizing their uniqueness and excellence. One dental school touts its revolutionary problem-based curriculum in the basic and clinical sciences. Another institution states that its strong basic science program gives their graduates a 21st century background in physical diagnosis and medicine. One Western school has built a seven-month general practice residency into its four-year curriculum—maintaining that its graduates will have a head start as they enter practice.

Dental schools with small class sizes proclaim their educational and social benefits, and the high cost of dental education has been uniquely addressed by one institution which offers a compre-

> **It should be obvious that many of our dental schools are exceeding, not just meeting minimal standards. Educational innovation abounds!**

hensive D.D.S. program requiring just three years of study. In contrast, students desiring a research experience may select still another dental school, which adds a fifth year to their curriculum in order to achieve that goal.

Perhaps the boldest institution is the University of Minnesota which recently announced its Guarantee of Quality Undergraduate D.D.S. Program. This program offered to 1993 and succeeding graduates warrants the student's knowledge base and clinical competency for 18 months after graduation. Eligible graduates will be offered unlimited free access to continued education programs plus the ability to enroll in any undergraduate didactic or preclinical courses with tuition paid by the school.

It should be obvious that many of our dental schools are exceeding, not just meeting minimal standards. Educational innovation abounds! We need to modify dental school accreditation so that excellence, not substandard performance, drives the process. Assuming a green light on the confidentiality issue, dental education should revamp the thrust of its accreditation process.

Formal recognition of excellence will serve as declaration of what can be achieved, motivate less regarded programs to become better, reduce complacency among the minimally accredited and provide an objective means for prospective dental students to choose the program that best meets their needs. ∎

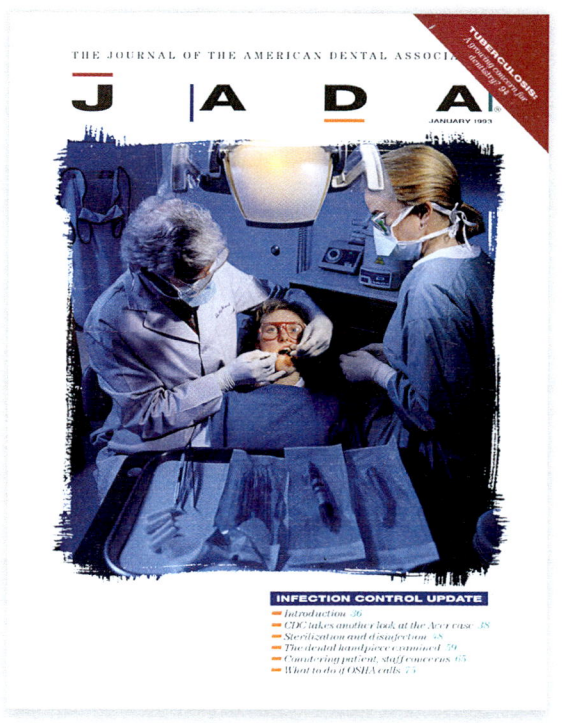

# 1993

"Obviously, dentistry, having fulfilled the
mandate required of health professionals
'to place the public's need above your own,'
truly warrants public acclaim as a significant
contributor to the nation's health."

# No laughing matter

*Originally published in JADA 1993 124: 8-10*

Dancing wildly from the effect of the inhaled "gas," the gentleman stumbled, jamming his leg so hard as to draw blood. Miraculously he felt no pain. Only later, as the effect of the "gas" diminished, did he realize how much damage he had done to himself.

This incident, observed by Connecticut dentist Horace Wells, led to the celebrated first removal of a tooth by nitrous oxide inhalation, or "laughing gas." Just four years later, embroiled in a vicious controversy with others who also claimed initial discovery of inhalation anesthesia, Wells took his life.

Twenty years later, the fledging ADA credited Wells with the discovery that revolutionized dentistry. Before Wells' discovery, dental extractions were performed with little pain control. Only the skill of the surgeon plus whiskey and occasionally cocaine were available to minimize the inescapable pain.

For 150 years dentists have relied on Dr. Wells' method to alleviate pain. Today at least 60,000 dental offices report the ability to deliver nitrous oxide inhalation anesthesia. Most dentists believe it to be the safest technique available for outpatient use. While it is impossible to accurately measure how many patients receive nitrous oxide yearly, conservative estimates would place the number in the millions. Adverse reactions are rare. Serious concerns are being raised, however, about its use.

Since the mid-1970s, scientific reports have cast suspicion that nitrous oxide might have potential side effects for those involved in its frequent administration. Birth defects, higher frequencies of spontaneous abortion, renal, hepatic and neurological disorders have all been associated with chronic low-level exposure. Acute neurological symptoms have been noted when nitrous oxide is used for recreational purposes—similar findings have been noted in practitioners exposed to high levels of the gas for prolonged periods.

A well-designed study published in JADA in 1980 surveyed more than 30,000 dentists and an equal number of dental assistants. Results were startling. A 1.7- to 2.3-fold increase in the rate of spontaneous abortions and a 1.5-fold increase in the rate of congenital malformations were noted in female chairside assistants working in offices where nitrous inhalation was used. Increased risk for cancer was also noted in this group.

Liver, kidney and neurological diseases also were significantly elevated in male dentists and female chairside assistants. Surprisingly, a 50 percent increase in the incidence of spontaneous abortion was noted among wives of male dentists.

A recent study in the New England Journal of Medicine extended the scope of the previous study by examining the fertility patterns of female health workers exposed to nitrous oxide in the dental office. Women not exposed took 6.4 menstrual cycles to become pregnant—compared to 32 months for women who worked in offices using five or more hours of unscavenged nitrous oxide per week. Significantly, women similarly exposed but working in offices using a scavenger took no longer to become pregnant than those who had no nitrous exposure.

These results present solid evidence that the levels of ambient nitrous oxide left after scavenging are unlikely to effect the fertility of dental workers. These findings must be directed to the attention of the National Institute for Occupational Safety and Health, which for years has suggested permissible exposure levels of no more than 25 ppm nitrous oxide in the dental operatory.

Scientists working in this area consider the 25 ppm unusually arbitrary, citing a lack of scientific data to substantiate the NIOSH recommendation.

> **Minimize nitrous oxide ambient by all available means, including daily and weekly inspections for leakage or damage to the nitrous oxide system.**

Nevertheless, some officials are likely to press the issue even though it would be virtually impossible to achieve that level even with present state-of-the-art scavenger devices. A capricious limit should be discouraged. Instead, further studies to determine "safe" levels of nitrous oxide need to be supported.

What can be done in the meantime? Minimize ambient nitrous oxide by all available means, including daily and weekly inspections for leakage or damage to the nitrous oxide system. Checks for pressure loss as well as adequacy of ventilation systems should be carried out routinely. Above all, an updated scavenger device must be used.

The 1991 ADA Survey of Dental Practice found that 58 percent of general and specialty practitioners report nitrous oxide capability. One-third have no scavenger. Do they use nitrous oxide? If so, how often? Considering the results of the New England Journal of Medicine report, we hope the answer is rarely or not at all. ∎

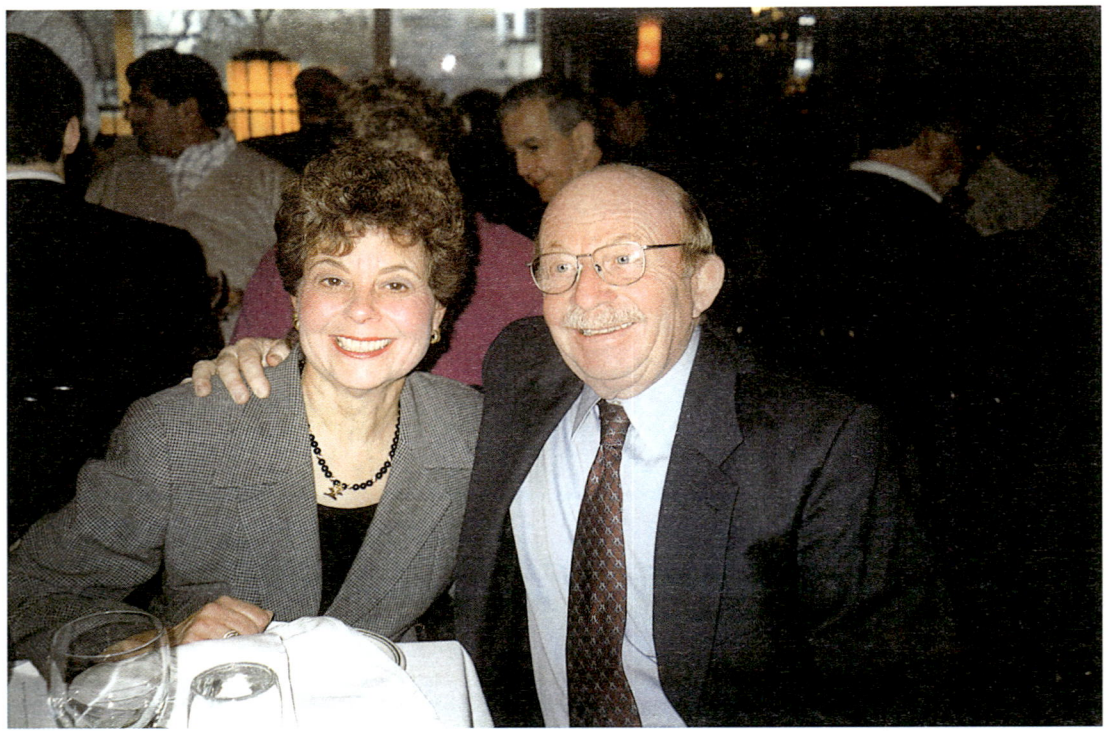

Dr. Larry Meskin and his wife, Estelle, at a Board of Trustees function in the mid-1990s. The two were married for 48 years and had a son, Scott, a physician; and a daughter, Sarah, an architect.

# Is there life after dentistry?

*Originally published in JADA 1993 124: 8-10*

A colleague called recently to talk about a decision he was wrestling with: retirement. He explained that at age 63 he was beginning to tire at the end of particularly busy days. Also, the sudden death of an older brother made him stop and think about how he wanted to spend his remaining years. He realized he was still young, in good health and financially able to retire. The problem, he confided, was fear. "I'm scared," he said, "because I honestly don't know what I'd do all day. Dentistry has been such an important part of my life."

This is a question faced by several thousand dentists every year, although dentists appear to put the decision off longer than many others. Nationally, the average retirement age for males is 62; for dentists, the age is 66. Data on retirement of female dentists is sparse. Most dentists choose to phase out of practice gradually, often practicing on a part-time basis for two or more years after they "retire." It's not unheard of to find a 70-year-old or even an 80-year-old dentist still practicing a few hours each week.

Comparatively little has been written about the retired or retiring dentist. We do know that personal health, financial concern and feeling productive are among the chief concerns of those moving into retirement. Worries about premature death after retirement are largely unfounded. Most deaths occurring close to the date of retirement result from conditions that existed before retirement and often precipitated retirement.

There are other issues, which are often less apparent, and thus less effectively addressed by most dentists. At the most fundamental level, the critical issue is the individual's sense of identity.

> **Retirement need not be something to fear. It presents an opportunity for renewal and broadened perspective.**

Among those for whom dentistry has played a dominant role in defining who they are, retirement can be extremely threatening, necessitating the need to reestablish one's sense of identity. A second critical issue for married dentists is the marital readjustment, the redefining of roles which must inevitably occur when a major life change takes place. Yet a third issue involves the loss of centrality that many dentists feel as their professional role diminishes: the staff whose lives revolve around you, the patients who seek your advice and treatment, the colleagues who respect your skills and opinions.

There are a host of other matters to be dealt with as well: how and when to dispose of one's professional practice, how to transfer patients to another colleague and whether to relocate to a retirement community. Often, the most difficult challenge can be the one of finding meaning and purpose, of filling the hours after the first few "honeymoon retirement months" of fishing and golf have passed.

Counselors who work with retiring professionals suggest that those who start their psychological planning early are the ones most likely to have happy, successful retirements. Activities and relationships that have the potential to affirm "self-worth" should be identified and cultivated early in a dentist's career.

Clearly, regardless of the dentist's commitment to his or her profession, career pursuits must be kept in perspective. Dentistry is but one facet of life. It should not be allowed to become one's total universe. Those dentists who succeed in broadening their perspectives will find that life after dentistry can be as enjoyable—perhaps even more so—as dentistry itself. ∎

# Proposed: the ADA National Service Award

*Originally published in JADA 1993 124: 10-12*

Imagine graduating from dental school with an obligation to repay educational loans totaling $147,919. Or "only" $103,000. Inconceivable? Overwhelming?

Yet, these are actual values representing the highest and mean amounts of educational indebtedness accrued by last year's graduating seniors at a private dental school. Educational debt, of course, is not confined to private dental school students. For all 1992 dental degree candidates, 48 percent owed more than $50,000 at graduation.

How stressful this must be for the young professional faced with monthly $1,500-2,000 debt payments that are not tax deductible. And be sure to include in this financial equation the young dentist's family obligations.

Professional options traditionally available to the new dental graduate may be limited or constrained by the urgency to initiate repayment of these educational debts. In their need for immediate income, these youthful high debtors may become unwilling candidates to staff storefront advertising clinics or managed care operations.

Six-figure education debt should spur our professional concern, as increasing numbers of low-income students turn away from a dental career. Dentistry's well-deserved reputation as an upwardly mobile profession could end abruptly if only those with significant economic means are able to pursue a dental education.

If you're still not concerned, consider who will buy your practice when you retire. A sizable portion of a dentist's retirement income is based on revenues realized from the practice sale. With future security in mind, how many dentists will risk selling their most valuable asset to a young profes-

> **The awards program would present striking evidence to the American public and government that the dental profession is resolved to assist people who traditionally have had less access to dental services, while also assisting those who would have been otherwise unable to afford a dental education.**

sional already encumbered with huge debts?

Solutions to this problem require bold untested initiatives. Dental schools, responding to university-imposed budget reductions, have become significantly leaner. Recent tuition increases barely approached inflation. Major reductions in educational costs will likely result with the development of educationally acceptable "patient simulations" to replace the present, high-cost, manpower intensive, clinical instruction systems. Until that time, however, only small cost reductions can be expected from dental schools.

At a meeting of dental deans and ADA trustees, Dr. Arthur Dugoni, dean of the University of the Pacific School of Dentistry and former ADA president, called on the Association to "establish a long-range goal to create a national endowment for dental education of $1 billion over the next 25 years." With the ADA playing a major role, Dr. Dugoni suggested that funds for student scholarships and low-interest loans be solicited from "the profession, the dental industry, corporations, foundations, insurance companies, consulting firms and the public."

Yes, Art, let's do it. But not over the next 25 years. Financial assistance for dental education needs to begin now.

Let me suggest that in order to address the growing need for all segments of society to access health care, the ADA and its industrial associates establish a student grant award program. Titled the "American Dental Association National Service Award," it would grant up to $10,000 yearly, with a maximum of $40,000, to students whose financial needs significantly exceed the average loan indebtedness of current dental graduates.

The number of awards would be limited to 2 percent of the entering freshman class, or a maximum of 80 students each year. Upon graduation, each award recipient would be required to give one year of service to a dentally under-served area designated by the ADA in consultation with its constituent and component societies. Unlike the National Service Corps, after which this program is modeled, it would be professional dentistry, not government, setting the criteria for placing ADA National Service Award dentists.

The awards program would present striking evidence to the American public and government that the dental profession is resolved to assist people who traditionally have had less access to dental services, while also assisting those who would have been otherwise unable to afford a dental education.

Yes, there is a cost. About $8 million would be needed each year after the fourth year of the program. If half that amount could be raised from industry, the annual cost to each ADA member would be $25—a relatively small amount considering what past public relations campaigns have cost.

And this award would provide great public relations! ∎

# Might does not equal right

*Originally published in JADA 1993 124: 10-12*

Promising radical changes in our health care system, President Clinton and his advisers are "floating" various mechanisms that could offset the costs of providing health care benefits for millions of uninsured Americans.

Special priority has been given to proposals that would tax employer-paid health benefits. Such a tax might raise necessary revenues, and it might help make consumers more informed and wiser. These measures might even help constrain mushrooming medical costs. These measures are not, however, right for dentistry!

Consider the long-term effects of taxing dental benefits:
- the number of people covered by dental benefits will decline;
- a reduction in the number of people receiving preventive services will result in increased disease and treatment costs;
- consumer delays in seeking treatment will compound severity of disease and raise ultimate costs.

These effects are all contradictory to the goals of health care reform. Taxing dental health benefits will destroy a health care delivery system that should be the model for other health care providers.

Few citizens question the development of programs that will give all Americans access to health care. None, however, should favor attaining that goal at the expense of an essential component of that system: dental care.

Regardless of who ultimately pays the health benefit tax, the deleterious impact on dentistry remains the same. Denying all or part of the tax deduction allowed businesses for health care plans will almost certainly result in the elimination of some employee benefits. Dentistry, often the last added, could be the first to go.

Equally damaging is the Clinton proposal to re-

> **Taxing dental health benefits will destroy a health care delivery system that should be the model for other health care providers.**

gard the value of employee health benefits as taxable income. Presently, all health benefits are exempted from taxation. The sales pitch for this proposal features the suggestion that some component of "basic medical services" would not be taxed, but thus far, dentistry appears to have been excluded from any exempt status.

If the Clinton proposals, as they presently stand, are enacted, comprehensive dental services will shrink or disappear as employers restructure their benefit packages. Workers, faced with taxation of their dental plan will elect dental options only if they anticipate substantial future need for dental care. These adverse selection factors will only escalate the cost of dental premiums, and as a consequence, depress the percentage of the work force willing or able to pay taxes on their dental plans.

The administration's taxing "suggestions" do not have popular support. Two recent polls showed that 70 to 90 percent of Americans oppose taxes on their employer-sponsored benefits. Sixty percent of them voiced the opinion that this action would break the Clinton pledge not to tax the middle class. Business, labor unions and the insurance industry are also on record opposing any form of benefit taxation. Your Association has actively opposed such taxes since 1969.

The proposed health benefit tax is unacceptable. Immediate action from the dental community is required. Actively oppose these administration proposals. Educate yourselves, your patients and your community. Contact and influence the actions of key political decision makers.

This debate must not be lost!

The consequences of failure are too great. Without your involvement the dental profession and its patients will become the first casualties of health care reform. ∎

1 9 9 3

# Speaking out for dentistry

*Originally published in JADA 1993 124: 8-10*

America's most influential financial monthly recently advised readers that, if forced to pay taxes on their health care benefits, they should drop rarely used health services.

Dental care was named a prime candidate for exclusion.

Since 60 percent of current dental spending revenues involve third-party financing, the effect of excluding dentistry from employer benefit plans would be devastating for our profession and the public's dental health.

Under pressure from labor and industry, this approach has been abandoned, at least for the time being. In its place the President's Health Care Task Force continues to explore the use of financial disincentives to coerce employers to modify their present health packages.

Proposals that would tax employers who offered more than a limited health package would certainly foster the introduction of "cafeteria style" choice plans for the newly excluded services.

Dentistry would suffer under this system since less than 15 percent of those currently covered would be expected to re-enroll for dental coverage. The result could easily be a reduction in dental spending that approaches $9 billion—a 25 percent decrease in total expenditures for dental care.

Any government suggestion that employers should alter their employee health benefit packages to help finance the Clinton health care reforms must be vigorously opposed. If the administration wishes to limit present tax incentives to consumers of health care, it should eliminate the personal income tax deduction for health services.

The present $3.3 billion yearly tax exclusion could be used to support new health initiatives. While no tax benefit that assists health consumers in financing health services should be capriciously eliminated, removing this deduction would be far less detrimental to providers and consumers of dental care than any present proposal.

Also of concern to the practicing dentist will be Health Care Task Force proposals to control, quickly, the double-digit inflation of health care costs. The administration realizes that no plan for health care reform can be successful until the inflationary spiral of employee medical benefit costs, rising at a rate of 18.9 percent each year since 1989, is addressed.

Stopgap measures, such as "temporarily" freezing health care costs at their 1993 levels, are being considered by some administrative officials. Other measures would either freeze or limit increases in health insurance premiums to general inflationary levels.

Discussions also focus on extending current Medicare payment restrictions to all services delivered in the private sector. Finally, some policy "gurus" are even advocating a national gross earnings income tax on all health providers similar to the tax recently instituted in Minnesota.

Regardless of the mechanism used, financial controls directed only at health providers will fail. Dentists who practiced in the 1970s will recall that price controls were an unmitigated disaster. While wages and dental material costs rose, dental fees remained fixed. Opportunities for practice efficiencies soon dwindled.

Substituting alternative dental materials and reducing the office labor force challenged dentistry's ability to deliver quality care. There were no winners. All who survived vowed "never again."

And we must not forget that vow.

Dentistry—determinedly fighting to control

> **Dentistry—determinedly fighting to control costs—has held its inflationary increases to 5 percent less than the Consumer Price Index during the last two decades. We should be emulated, not punished.**

costs—has held its inflationary increases to 5 percent less than the Consumer Price Index during the last two decades. We should be emulated, not punished for our fiscal responsibility.

If America is serious about health care reform, serious about providing health care for all, why not consider implementing a nationwide consumption tax? Most European countries did so years ago.

The tax could be made less regressive by exempting housing, food and health care. If needed, selectively higher "sin" taxes or higher rates on certain luxury items could be added.

With all Americans participating, this approach could go a long way toward providing a universal good for all citizens. ■

# Dentistry's voice unheard

*Originally published in JADA 1993 124: 10-12*

Former U.S. Surgeon General C. Everett Koop established a new standard for federal health leaders. His flamboyant, outspoken style—coupled with his single-minded dedication to the health of the American people—brought national attention to each of his pronouncements.

People didn't necessarily always agree with him, but no national health leader in recent decades has done more to bring critical health issues into the sharp focus of public debate than Dr. Koop. To paraphrase E.F. Hutton, "When Koop spoke . . . people listened."

People listened to Dr. Koop because he was highly respected, articulate and he had the strength of conviction to speak his mind regardless of whether his superiors and colleagues agreed with him. His effectiveness in bringing critical health issues into public awareness showed that strong leaders who are willing to speak forcefully and who can present complex issues to the public will be heard. Our complex societal interactions demand that policy development be promoted by acknowledged leaders in their respective fields-dentistry and its constituents not excepted.

National events over the last three years now dictate that a highly informed and universally respected cadre of dental leaders emerge as national opinion and policy leaders-the C. Everett Koops of dentistry. Are there dental leaders whose interests supersede a particular subject-whose thoughts are global rather than singular, whose presence evokes respect both from within and outside the profession, who are capable and willing to guide dentistry into the 21st century?

In all but one constituency, Yes! The ADA, AADS, NIDR, expert clinicians and members of our science community provide the profession with a significant number of highly regarded opinion leaders. Only in the executive branch of federal government is dentistry's voice absent. A generation of governmental retrenchments and organizational realignments have left dentistry without noticeable representation. As a profession, we are invisible, unheard.

But there's still a chief dental officer, you might argue.

True.

Dr. Robert J. Collins holds that title, but only in conjunction with his major responsibility as director of the Indian Health Services dental program. Aside from what he can garner from his own IHS budget, he has no staff lines, no support budget and no venue for the office of chief dental officer. Dentistry's voice in government affairs has been effectively silenced, leaving us vulnerable to any federal official who chooses to sacrifice the public's dental health interests in favor of his or her own agenda.

Some might argue that we don't need centralized federal dental leadership. Federal regulations are suffocating us as it is, they'd say. Not so! Consider how much more favorable our position might be if a respected and outspoken federal dental leader had voiced professional opposition to OSHA's irrational proposals.

With no need to consult dentistry's equivalent of Dr. Koop, OSHA could dismiss ADA's views as parochial self-interest and throw their regulatory steamrollers into gear.

Five years ago. Congress, aware of dentistry's lack of voice, called on the DHHS secretary to establish an interim study committee to review the department's dental programs. The committee was to "consider appropriate organizational and administrative arrangements for achieving maximum coordination and effectiveness of dental health

> **Dentistry's voice in government affairs has been effectively silenced, leaving us vulnerable to any federal official who chooses to sacrifice the public's dental health interests in favor of his or her own agenda.**

activities within the department."

Three recommendations resulted:

- establish a focus for oral health activities in DHHS with clearly visible administrative and policy responsibility;
- call for a strong, clearly identified oral health presence in any DHHS agency which conducts oral health activities;
- advise the chief dental officer through a formally chartered external committee that reports annually to Congress.

To date, not one recommendation has been implemented. With a new ADA executive director and Washington office chief, both of whom are skilled politicians, now is the time to press Congress to act on these recommendations.

Dentistry must regain its voice in the halls of government. Too much is happening in the public policy arena for us to remain silenced. ∎

# Dentistry may be hazardous to your health

*Originally published in JADA 1993 124: 10-12*

**N**ew missiles launched by the anti-amalgamists claim that mercury from dental fillings contribute to the development of antibiotic-resistant bacteria in humans. On another front, our public image has been compromised by the confirmation of a sixth HIV transmission in the same dental office. The profession responded, providing scientific evidence once again, that the public's risks are minimal.

So is dentistry hazardous to your health? Not if you're a dental patient. But if you happen to be a dentist, a dental team member or even a member of a dentist's family, you may be at risk.

While some practitioners might agree that dentistry is a high-risk profession, most would probably scoff at the thought that their dental license should carry a Surgeon General's statement:

**Warning: the practice of dentistry may be hazardous to your health. Prolonged exposure to dental patients and the environment of the dental office could result in a compromised health state and, on occasion, even death.**

But if dentists don't think that practicing dentistry places them at high risk, they should ask their spouses, children and significant others. Many would confess concern for the personal safety of a loved one engaged in patient care.

Consider the following:

Every patient must be treated as though he or she is HIV positive. Despite all appropriate and recommended precautions, needlesticks and instrument punctures do take place. The risk is small, but it is still a risk.

The hepatitis B virus once was a major threat to dental team members. The disease itself can be life-threatening. Even worse, a carrier state exists, and a dentist so infected might not be able to practice again. Some dentists and team members have not availed themselves of the vaccine. There is no

reason for HBV to become hazardous to your health.

Recent studies have shown that long-term exposure to nitrous oxide in the dental office not only affected the dental team, but team members' families as well. Significant reductions in fertility were observed in those practices where ambient exposure wasn't controlled. Roughly, a third of dental offices with nitrous oxide capacity may still be operating without an appropriate scavenger system.

Office water supplies and instrument water lines may become contaminated with one or more of the various strains of *Legionella*. Aerosolization of the water could proliferate the spread of these bacteria. Positive antibodies to *Legionella* noted in 50 percent of dentists and 38 percent of dental assistants validate this observation. Dentists who were constantly exposed to aerosols generated by high-speed hand-pieces had the highest prevalence of antibodies. Although there have been no reports of clinical *Legionella* in dentists caused by contaminated water supplies, care must be taken to minimize repeated inhalation of these aerosols.

The resurgence of tuberculosis, especially antibiotic-resistant TB, may soon become a threat to the dental team member. Detailed federal protocols required to treat known drug-resistant TB patients underscore how dangerous the bacteria can be. Some of the infected will not be aware of their status. Dentists will have to take precautions to protect themselves and office personnel from this serious condition.

Then, of course, there are the "normal" hazards of dental practice like carpal tunnel syndrome, latex allergies, handpiece-induced hearing loss, lower back problems and psychological stress.

There should be no question that the practice of dentistry can be hazardous to your health. Surprisingly, there has been no exodus of dentists leaving

> **There should be no question that the practice of dentistry can be hazardous to your health. Surprisingly, there has been no exodus of dentists leaving the profession.**

the profession. Just the opposite. Student applications to dental schools have risen over the past three years.

Obviously, dentistry, having fulfilled the mandate required of health professionals "to place the public's need above your own" truly warrants public acclaim as a significant contributor to the nation's health. ∎

# One house of dentistry

*Originally published in JADA 1993 124: 10-12*

Dentistry's educational leaders are seeking advice from the highly prestigious Institute of Medicine, hoping to strengthen themselves as they move toward the 21st century. How successfully dental education addresses the public need over the next quarter century may well depend on the IOM'S interpretation of future oral health status, demographic trends, anticipated technological and scientific discoveries, and funding priorities for health education institutions. Considering the reputation of the IOM, its forthcoming recommendations could reform the future composition of the dental profession.

While educators might focus only on those portions of the forthcoming report that concern them directly, it would be the myopic individual who fails to appreciate the inextricable links between education and dental practice—one doesn't change without the other. Nor can predictions regarding dentistry's future have value without input from both groups. Fortunately this input is being provided.

Although the IOM project was initiated by leaders of the American Association of Dental Schools, these individuals understood the importance of including dental practitioners in the IOM deliberations. Three practicing dentists were named to the study panel. Desiring even more involvement, the ADA supported a recent meeting of active dental practitioners with IOM panel members. The agenda included the opportunity to share their views on what's right and wrong with today's dental education process.

**What's right about today's dental education?**

The ADA practitioners had the following comments:

"The dental participants applauded the dental schools' record of training a majority of their students for careers in general practice. The pitfalls of medicine's highly specialized workforce had been avoided. Students were considered to be well-trained in diagnostic skills. Diversity of the student body has increased, with women constituting almost half of new dental school entrants. Minorities continue to increase, albeit at a slower pace. Foremost, the schools are considered the loci of new information—information pertinent to clinical practice."

**What's wrong with today's dental education?**

"Some of the dental practitioners stated that some dental schools may be taking in substandard students in order to meet budgets—thus, the quality of the applicant pool is not what it used to be.

> The education and practice communities have failed each other—failed to effectively communicate their concerns.

Also cited was a lack of ethics training in the dental curriculum. Practitioner concern that students need to learn more about the real world of dental practice evoked support for increased amounts of practice management in the dental program."

"Another dental concern was the insufficient emphasis on developing a scientific background for students-graduates are 'just' clinicians. A few participants remarked that schools should start patient contact with students earlier in their training and that dental students should have more interaction with auxiliaries. Many of the dentists held the opinion that professors don't know how to teach and don't respect students. Additional critiques included the following points. The patient pool is not sufficient to build or promote competence in all dental procedures. The dental curriculum is too crammed. There is too much emphasis on research.

Continued education programs are inadequate to meet the needs of today's practitioners."

While isolated examples of the "what's wrong" issues do exist, the last two decades have witnessed an explosion of creative and innovative changes in all aspects of dental education. Most dental faculty have access to educational psychologists who assist them in teaching methodology. Today, increased instruction in ethics finds attentive listeners. It may be easier to learn how to cut a MOD than to explain to a needy patient and her children that you can't backdate their insurance.

Oral biology programs dedicated to integrating science with clinical practice abound and to those who question the qualifications of the present student body, high-quality applicants to dental schools have increased significantly in the last three years. While it may vary by region or by specific school, gaining a position in a first-year dental class is exceedingly competitive.

Yes, dental education has changed dramati-cally. From many of the comments offered by dental leaders to IOM panelists, however, it might be construed otherwise.

**Why?**

To a concerned observer the answer is clear. The education and practice communities have failed each other. Failed to effectively communicate their concerns—to share their innovations-to understand each other's problems—to visit each other in their respective domains. The forthcoming Institute of Medicine recommendations will challenge the preconceptions of both educator and practitioner. Let these two dental communities build consensus in an atmosphere of mutual trust.

Let their final response emanate from "one house of dentistry." ■

# Much ado about nothing?

*Originally published in JADA 1993 124: 10-14*

Sell by Oct. 1, 1993" and "Best if used by Oct. 1, 1993"—two consumer advisories. Together, they provide a semantic illustration of how shaded meanings can influence behavior.

As a shopper on Sept. 30, 1993, which product would you most likely purchase? Probably most of you would dismiss the "Sell by ..." product as being too close to its expiration date. Although the "Best if used by ..." label actually means the same thing, consumers selecting that product would likely feel more confident that they were getting fresher goods.

In our professional settings, we often banter words about with little thought as to how our patients may be interpreting them. Examining a few common dental terms may disclose interpretations that detract from, not enhance public perception of our profession.

Consider, for example, the fact that American dentists earn either a D.D.S. or D.M.D. degree. Few of us give much thought to the existence of two doctoral degrees granted for identical dental training. Yes, the occasional dentist will write a letter to The Journal complaining that holders of the D.M.D. may have an economic advantage over those with the D.D.S. Other than that, it hardly seems to be an issue.

Most dentists are unaware that the D.D.S. degree was first awarded by the Baltimore College of Dental Surgery in 1846. Even fewer will know that Harvard offered the first D.M.D. in 1869, but only after first rejecting a proposal to create a Doctor of Dental Science degree because dentistry was not considered a proper science. The Harvard faculty fully expected its D.M.D. to become the profession's standard. While this never happened, 18 dental schools presently grant the D.M.D., accounting for 28 percent of current dental graduates.

Educational programs offering either degree have the same accreditation requirements, and regulatory bodies do not differentiate between the two. Nevertheless, while most dental professionals appear unconcerned about the separate existence of these dental degrees, consumers of dental care may not share their indifference.

Often confused by the different designations, many question whether the dentist with a D.M.D. has more or different training than the D.D.S. dentist. Still others think that the holder of a D.M.D. has degrees in both medicine and dentistry.

The American Association of Dental Schools, state boards and professional dental groups are virtually silent on this issue.

> **Often confused by the different designations, many question whether the dentist with a D.M.D. has more or different training than the D.D.S. dentist.**

Denied a professional explanation, potential purchasers of dental care often seek clarification from dental care advertisements appearing in newspapers or other media.

The following advertisement from an Eastern newspaper vividly highlights this issue. Two dentists are depicted, with prominent attention given to the D.M.D. credentials. The caption under their picture boasts that, "Beside having a dental practice here in [.... ...], Drs. [...] and [... ] hold memberships in many respected medical associations, and are instructors for the American Heart Association."

Are these dentists deliberately misleading the consumer by innuendo, creating the impression that they are physician-dentists? Or is the caption a truthful rendition of their professional affiliations? The correct answer to this advertising narrative is unimportant. What is of consequence is how easily the two degree designations can be misconstrued and lead to abuse of the public's trust-actions that ultimately undermine our professional credibility.

Since the D.D.S. and the D.M.D. degrees represent identical standards of academic rigor and training, the profession should act responsibly by using one nomenclature. Selecting one degree should eliminate ambiguity and maximize public understanding. The final decision should be based on which degree designation will yield the highest level of public confidence in the dental profession. ∎

# Expanding the bubble

*Originally published in JADA 1993 124: 10-12*

First-time wilderness hikers and campers often find it difficult to believe a "crystal clear" stream is actually contaminated. While they soon learn caution, the long-standing, rigidly enforced U.S. potable water standards continue to create a false sense of security.

Most people assume any water supply that looks, tastes and smells OK is healthy. And our dental unit water supplies (DUWS) are no exception. After all, if the water source meets U.S. standards, why be concerned?

One reason is that research spanning 30 years uniformly describes high levels of microbes exiting the dental unit as aerosolized water sprays or through the unit's water syringe.

The culprit is a biofilm that forms on the walls of narrow-bore tubing or connections and valves in the DUWS system. Just like dental plaque, biofilms become a matrix for the reproduction of microbes. Often the flow of water over these biofilms will dislodge microorganisms that then may be aerosolized or sprayed into the oral cavity. Organisms found in these biofilms, while generally non-pathogenic, may include microbes such as *Pseudomonas aeruginosa* and *Legionella pneumophila,* both having the potential for disease production.

No clinical cases of Legionnaires' disease have ever been associated with dental procedures. But researchers have found antibodies to *Legionella* strains ranging as high as 50 percent in practicing dentists. Also, two cases of local oral infections have been traced to *P. aeruginosa.*

Without clearcut evidence that contamination of DUWS presents a disease threat to patient or dentist, why should professional policymakers and researchers give priority to this subject? After all, the problem is not confined to dentistry. Similar biofilm contamination has been noted in hospitals, restaurants and even home water supplies.

Perhaps in an earlier—pre-HIV—era, these findings would have been shrugged off. The oral cavity is far from a sterile environment, so why worry about the possible addition of a few more "bugs"? With the infection control bubble in dentistry constantly expanding, the driving objective today appears to be zero risk for our patients.

At least two focal points for action have been identified. First, ensure that the water supply servicing both the handpiece and water syringe is potable at the point of use. Second, do not allow "suck-back" to contaminate the sterile water supply.

Researchers agree that bio-films and water line contamination cannot be completely eliminated in current dental units. Flushing the waterline systems between patients reduces—but does not eliminate—microbial contamination. Similarly, even with the best anti-retraction system, some passive suck-back will occur.

With the average daily consumption of water for each dental unit approximating just 1 liter, the use of a replaceable sterile water mechanism for each unit would be a feasible first step in initiating a sterile chain for water supply delivery.

However, even this type of system would not be foolproof if suck-back was not completely eliminated, as microbial contamination would eventually involve the new waterlines and the mechanical components of the sterile water supply components. This is a physical problem that must be overcome if this type of system is to work.

One potential solution would be to use a sterile disposable water system for each patient. The cost/benefit of such a device would have to be weighed against future innovations, such as chemical purging, disposable filtration devices or heat sterilization of waterlines. Until a satisfactory solu-

> **With the infection control bubble in dentistry constantly expanding, the driving objective today appears to be zero risk for our patients.**

tion is found, research into the effectiveness of a post-procedural mouthrinse might be indicated. It could be a worthwhile adjunct to lessen microbial proliferation.

Should the ADA give priority and devote resources to this issue? The Association's scientific staff thinks so. To attack this problem, a meeting of industrial, government, ADA and community scientists was held in August under ADA auspices. From this gathering, specific work and research assignments were initiated. Future meetings are anticipated.

Some dentists may believe there isn't enough in-formation to warrant a proactive initiative—that such an initiative might boost practice costs, with little or no benefit to patient or practitioner. This is an unacceptable argument. To serve the public and its constituents effectively, the ADA must continually scan the dental environment, gather appropriate information and develop appropriate action plans to avoid possible crises.

The approach to this issue taken by the ADA's Division of Scientific Affairs should be applauded. It's an excellent example of your dues dollars at work. ∎

# An issue of dental necessity

*Originally published in JADA 1993 124: 10-12*

LAW 198: If someone injures the eye of an inferior, he is fined a mina of silver.
LAW 201: If someone knocks out the tooth of an inferior, he is fined a third of a mina of silver.

These laws, set down more than 3,700 years ago by Hammurabi, the ruler of Babylon, characterize the importance this early civilization placed on the retention of teeth. The early Hebrews placed even greater value on teeth, for their laws read that if someone knocked out the tooth of a servant, the servant was given his or her freedom.

Times have changed!

President Clinton's recent televised pronouncements, launching his highly touted health care reform package, appeared to contain little of the importance the ancients placed on the health of teeth. The president made no reference to dentists or dental health—just to "doctors, nurses, pharmacists and mental health workers." Some dentists, worried that the president's proposals might irretrievably jeopardize the high standards and quality of dental practice, may have been relieved that dental care was not mentioned.

Doctor, the president's omission of dentistry gives no reason to rejoice.

While the debate on health care reform has just begun and no one of sound mind would dare to predict the outcome, the preliminary working draft of the president's proposal does include a "basic preventive dental package" for children younger than 18 plus a timetable to include restorative dentistry for children and adults by the year 2001.

The most disturbing elements of President Clinton's proposed "dental package" for children is the apparent failure of his task force to understand the basics of dental treatment. It's irrational to recommend preventive service without an accompanying treatment component.

Imagine completing a pediatric oral examination, cleaning the teeth, establishing a treatment plan, applying fluoride, placing sealants, giving oral hygiene instruction and then dismissing the patient with six untreated carious lesions.

And to make matters worse, the president's plan would remove the restorative benefits currently provided children under Medicaid—a program destined for the scrapheap under Mr. Clinton's proposals.

The architects of the Clinton dental plan have clearly ignored dentistry's many contributions to public health. Of all the health professions, dentistry has done more to demonstrate that prevention is the best and most economical approach to health care. Moreover, the dental profession has championed the health promotion movement by encouraging and instructing people to take responsibility for their own dental health. By instituting prevention, participation and cost containment in its dental insurance programs, dentists have already established the essential framework of the Clinton proposal.

> While dentistry has done a good job promoting sound health principles, it must now challenge its undeserved reputation as an "expendable" health service.

The failure of the Clinton administration's health task force to design an acceptable children's dental health program also reflects dentistry's failure to convey to the public what must be accomplished if all children are to achieve optimum oral health.

A new initiative is urgently needed. The "public's" elected leaders, at both state and federal levels, must be convinced that access to comprehensive dental care is a necessary health service, not a luxury. They must understand that there will be additional costs, costs that must be given equal priority with other essential health services even in the face of competing needs.

The dental professional must be willing to develop and support ways to implement this concept. While dentistry has done a good job promoting sound health principles, it must now challenge its undeserved reputation as an "expendable" health service.

Frustrating as it may appear, a renewed and more targeted effort by all those involved in health care reform will be necessary if dentistry is to become a meaningful participant. ■

# Truth or consequence

*Originally published in JADA 1993 124: 10-12*

The right to search for truth implies also a duty. One must not conceal any part of what one has recognized to be true.
—Albert Einstein

Located in the garden surrounding the National Science Foundation's office in Washington, D.C., is a sculptured bust of Albert Einstein. Each section of that sculpture's four-cornered base contains a quote attributed to the world-renowned scientist. With just four opportunities to communicate Einstein's philosophic genius, each quote takes on added meaning.

Yet, without knowing the context of when or to whom this statement was made, its meaning is open to conjecture. Was he implying that some scientific researchers were not reporting everything they had observed? Or perhaps was Einstein concerned that all facets of a scientific discovery had not been disclosed? In either case, whether purposeful or by negligence, those who might have benefited from a particular scientific inquiry would have been short-changed.

Few dentists are aware that The Journal of the American Dental Association uses a "peer" review process to fulfill its obligation to print only what can be objectively substantiated as truth. After an initial screening for their suitability for the general dental practitioner, submitted manuscripts are sent to a minimum of three subject experts. Those individuals are requested to examine the manuscripts for accuracy as evaluated against known information.

Assuming that new manuscripts are considered as valuable to JADA readers, the authors are then required to respond to the reviewers' written critiques—altering their earlier submission if necessary. Re-review, by the same or different peers, if successful, is followed by publication. With more than 300 manuscripts received yearly by JADA editors, less than a third survive this extensive procedure.

Occasionally, potential conflicts of interest among contributing authors may cloud the review process. All submitters of manuscripts are required to disclose any vested interests in the subject being reported.

While financial interests do not preclude publication, JADA believes it is in readers' interest to note such relationships and let the readers draw their own conclusions.

Peer reviewers work under additional constraints. To guard against reviewer bias, all manuscripts sent to reviewers have all author identification removed. While this ensures a confidential appraisal, it prohibits face-to-face opportunities between author and reviewer in which direct questions could be posed.

At times, further critiques appear after publication-this time supplied by readers questioning the authors' paper. The interesting exchange between authors and readers in JADA's Letters To The Editor offers an additional peer group comment.

This involved review process is followed by virtually all of the major scientific journals. Many local and state dental journals and most commercial publications, whose pages are primarily concerned with advertised products, are not peer reviewed. Articles in these latter publications often are staff written.

Does this mean that the editorial information contained in these publications should be questioned? Not necessarily—just remember that it has not been subjected to the watchful oversight of scientific experts.

What about Einstein's concern that there be full disclosure of results? Does the peer review process guarantee that what is printed is the whole truth?

> **Reviewers have ensured that researchers seeking JADA audiences for their discoveries were allowed to report information only after extensive professional scrutiny.**

Unfortunately the peer reviewers do not have access to the original data on which submitted manuscripts are based. They conduct their review assuming that the material is truthful—examining the manuscripts for accuracy as evaluated against existing standards.

It is an honor to be asked to be a peer reviewer.

With no compensation offered for their efforts, the 297 JADA reviewers in 1992 must be content with a published thank you.

But they know that they have ensured that researchers seeking JADA audiences for their discoveries were allowed to report information only after extensive professional scrutiny. ∎

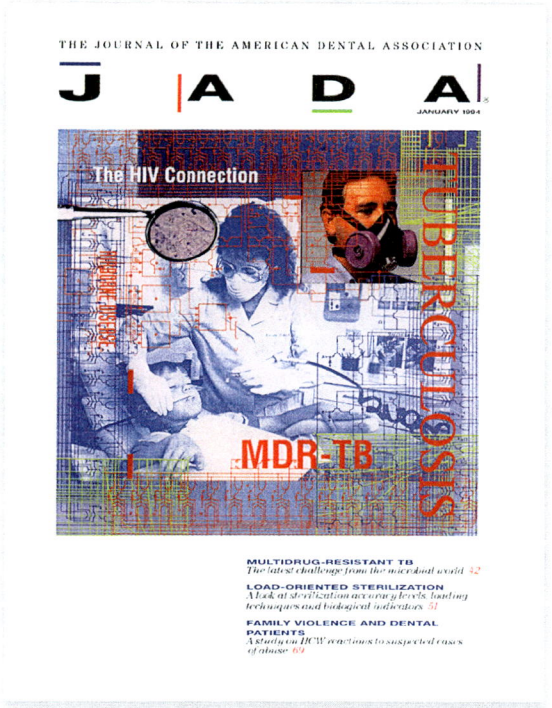

THE JOURNAL OF THE AMERICAN DENTAL ASSOCIATION

JADA

JANUARY 1994

The HIV Connection

TUBERCULOSIS

MDR-TB

MULTIDRUG-RESISTANT TB
The latest challenge from the microbial world 42

LOAD-ORIENTED STERILIZATION
A look at sterilization accuracy levels, loading
techniques and biological indicators 51

FAMILY VIOLENCE AND DENTAL
PATIENTS
A study on HCW reactions to suspected cases
of abuse 69

# 1994

"The critical factor is quality. Not technical quality, for few dental consumers are capable of assessing the quality of dental service. Rather, it is the patient's perception of quality that will influence choice. At issue is the quality of service offered by you and your dental team."

# If not us, then who?

*Originally published in JADA 1994 125: 10-12*

Violence sweeps through our society sparing neither the rural nor the urban resident. While the high-profile terrorism of urban gangs, drugs and guns dominate the nightly news, it represents only a small fraction of attacks against our citizenry.

Rather, it is the insidious, highly pervasive, events of family abuse that account for the greatest number of violent encounters. Consider these facts:

■ The National Committee for the Prevention of Child Abuse estimates that almost 3 million children were reported to social or child protective services for suspected abuse in 1992. That's 45 of every 1,000 children in the United States. And that figure represents an 8 percent gain over the previous year.

■ Battering of adult females appears to be even more pervasive. U.S. statistics indicate that every 7.4 seconds a woman is battered by her mate. Domestic violence is considered one of the most frequent causes of injuries to women contacting health care providers. Researchers have found that in families where women have been abused, 54 percent have associated cases of child abuse.

■ The elderly are also vulnerable to this violence. A congressional report indicates up to 2 million older adults are abused annually. An incidence rate of 26/1,000 has been estimated. With the elderly representing the fastest growing population group, further increases in abuse can be expected.

Most states have legislation requiring the health professional to report suspected incidents of child abuse. Mandatory reporting requirements for abused women or elders are not as prevalent.

Health professionals may be reluctant to report cases of child abuse, fearing possible misdiagnosis or retribution from the abuser. They should be aware, however, that protection is provided by laws that exempt the health professional from either civil or criminal actions for reporting child abuse. Some states are beginning to adopt similar protections for reporting other types of abuse.

Discomfort in reporting suspected cases of abuse must be overcome, since hesitation may only provide encouragement for more serious violent behavior by the abuser.

Reluctance to report suspected abuse aside, health professionals may occasionally fail to detect signs and symptoms of abuse because of lack of diagnostic training.

Dentists, as the first and perhaps only health service contact for many of the abused, often represent the sole opportunity for abused individuals to escape the cycle of violence. Because a large proportion of abusive injuries occur in body regions open to direct observation, dentists should ensure they are competent to recognize the most subtle signs of abuse.

> **Dentists, as the first and perhaps only health service contact for many of the abused, often represent the sole opportunity for abused individuals to escape the cycle of violence.**

For example, 68 percent of battered women's injuries will involve the face, 45 percent the eyes arid 12 percent the neck. Frequently the extremities also will show signs of abusive actions. While some of these abusive injuries are overt and easily diagnosed, others may require additional diagnostic training.

Recognizing the importance of the dentist in breaking the chain of violence, the 1993 ADA House of Delegates amended the ADA Principles of Ethics to state that "dentists shall be obliged to become familiar with the perioral signs of child abuse and to report suspected cases to the proper authorities."

A 1993 House resolution extended the scope of the dentists' observations for abuse to include "all physical signs of child abuse that are observable in the normal course of a dental visit." Additionally, it called for the "ADA and its constituents and components to make training courses available to its members."

These resolutions clarify the responsibility of dentists with regard to suspected abusive behavior to children. The ADA should consider submitting future resolutions that would acknowledge the dentist's responsibility in the diagnosis, treatment and reporting of other victims of domestic violence—battered women, the elderly and disabled.

The new ADA resolution stresses the importance of enhancing the dentist's diagnostic acuity in recognizing abusive insults. A few states require the completion of a continued education course dedicated to the recognition and referral of abuse as a precondition for licensure renewal.

Those course participants agree that the training was invaluable—that without this additional instruction they would be unable to detect many signs and symptoms of abuse.

In that regard, the American College of Dentists and the International College of Dentists, as a public service initiative, should consider sponsoring a nationwide no-fee continued education program for the dental team on the subject of abuse.

Serious and timely consideration should be given to these suggestions. As the point of first contact for many victims of abuse, if not us, then who? ∎

# Conventional wisdom

*Originally published in JADA 1994 125: 122-124*

Friends and patients hint that your recent trip to the ADA annual session in San Francisco probably wasn't overly taxing—implying that your attendance was primarily an IRS-subsidized vacation. But don't be unduly sensitive—you'll have an opportunity I to counter. Chances are your critics will be off to their own convention in the not-too-distant future.

Attending business and professional conventions has become a regular activity for a large segment of the American work force. For many, it's considered a major employment benefit. And while the benefit can't compare dollarwise with health care, it's still big business.

The yearly revenue associated with conventions—travel, hotel, meals—generates $75 billion and provides a direct employment augmentation of 1.5 million jobs. As an industry, conventions rank 17th among private sector contributions to the GNP. With airlines and hotels respectively reporting 22 percent and 36 percent of their sales linked to conventions, both would experience significant economic loss from any downturn in conventional activities.

Considering these facts, why does the American public still associate convention attendance with derogatory terms such as "junket," "boondoggle" or "IRS-subsidized vacations?"

Surely the media must shoulder some of the blame. It makes I good copy to expose conventioneers' late-night reveling in the streets of New Orleans, sunning on a Caribbean beach or attending lavish dinner parties,

But do these descriptions represent the real world of a conventioneer? Aren't there more meaningful reasons for coming together?

Perhaps America's Constitutional Convention, held in Philadelphia beginning on May 14, 1787, can provide a model by which today's conventions can be assessed. Those attending the Philadelphia gathering were skilled statesmen who, although of diverse interests and backgrounds, were committed to a greater good—the welfare of their new nation. Through intense debate they were able to create a document that has guided our nation for more than 200 years.

While the issues are dissimilar, analogies can be drawn between our present dental conventions and this illustrious example. Dentists, through their covenant with the public, have a professional mandate to provide oral health care for all Americans. To satisfy this obligation, dentists must remain continuous students. By keeping current and staying abreast of our rapidly evolving profession, dentists will be better able to fulfill their public responsibility.

> **For dental practitioners seeking additional professional interactions and networking, the dental convention provides an appropriate venue.**

Attendance at dental conventions has become critical to attaining this goal. By providing participants with a centralized forum to listen to and view the offerings of the nation's most knowledgeable clinicians, opportunities for professional growth in a highly cost-efficient manner are ensured. As an illustration, 59,000 bar-coded registration slips, each signifying an individual's completion of a continued education course, were recorded at the 1993 ADA annual session.

What tourist would go to Boston in January, Chicago in February or New York in early December? Few, I'm sure, unless snow, sleet and cold are major attractions. Yet this year, more than 100,000 dentists and their associated personnel will register for the Yankee in Boston, the Chicago Midwinter and the Greater New York dental conventions. Why? Because these conventions, like the ADA'S, offer exposure to world-class clinicians—often at no fee to their membership.

And registrations at dental conventions continue to grow. The 135th ADA annual session in San Francisco drew 54,000, 15,000 of them dentists-a new record. Last year's Greater New York meeting noted 13,368 dentists among their 33,500 attendees. The smaller regional and state conventions are observing similar increases.

Citing a major restructuring, designed to increase the caliber of its speakers, the Metropolitan Denver Dental Society's Winter Regional Meeting has shown a 50 percent increase in registrants during the last five years. With 32 states actively mandating continued education as a prerequisite for relicensure, convention attendance can be expected to increase.

Dental conventions provide more than educational opportunities. For those who have become active participants in dentistry's policy and politics, conventions provide a gathering place, not unlike the Philadelphia Constitutional Convention, where future leadership and professional policy are debated, voted and instituted.

Dentistry, with its dependence on technology and material science, needs a venue where practitioners can test new advances in their field. The dental convention, with hundreds of trade exhibits in one central area, facilitates practitioner decision-making.

By working in hospital settings, physicians are constantly exposed to professional interaction and feedback. In contrast, dentists' professional contacts are often limited to their dental staff. For dental practitioners seeking additional professional interactions and networking, the dental convention provides an appropriate venue.

Yes, friends, neighbors and patients of dentists, and yes, general critics of all convention-goers, dentists do go to conventions—in ever-increasing numbers.

Conventional wisdom says: with good reason. ∎

# 'Royal Mineral Succedaneum' revisited

*Originally published in JADA 1994 125: 234-236*

Controversy surrounding dental restorative materials is not new. Recall the restrictive patents related to the use of Vulcanite, Taggert's attempt to control the lost wax casting process and the Amalgam Wars that followed the 1833 introduction of "Royal Mineral Succedaneum."

You remember that story. A silver/mercury paste was cleverly promoted by two French dentists, who more often than not placed the filling material over carious areas—without removing the decay. More than a few patients responded poorly to this procedure, and many dentists sought to ban its use.

The furor caused by the scandal fragmented the young dental profession and destroyed its newly founded American Society of Dental Surgeons. Fortunately, those dentists who recognized the potential of this restorative material prevailed, and "silver" amalgam became the profession's restorative mainstay for the next 150 years.

Today, amalgam alloys are again at the center of a dispute. This time it's a federal court action testing an interpretation of California's Proposition 65—a law mandating businesses with 10 or more employees to warn their customers about chemicals used in their operations that "cause birth defects or other reproductive harm."

Citing the mercury found in amalgam as one of these chemicals, California's Environmental Law Foundation requests that all dental offices display this sign:

"WARNING. This office uses amalgam filling materials which contain and expose you to mercury, a chemical known to the state of California to cause birth defects and other reproductive harm. Please consult your dentist for more information."

Their demand is an insult to the profession. If amalgam were truly linked to birth defects or reproductive harm, no dentist would ethically offer the material to anyone of reproductive age.

No signs would be needed!

Meanwhile, although mercury is on California's chemical hit list, the state's chief deputy attorney, after extensive investigation, found "no conclusive evidence of the reproductivity toxicity of mercury and no established level at which mercury has been determined to cause productive harm."

Even with this knowledge, one amalgam manufacturer already has caved in to the demands of ELF. But it's hoped the preemptive lawsuit instituted by 10 dental manufacturers will terminate Proposition 65's required warnings.

Unfortunately, legal success in California will not end the continued attacks on dental amalgam. Despite repeated scientific affirmation of amalgam safety, every new research report on amalgam is open to misinterpretation by amalgam's vocal critics.

As an example, consider the recent report linking occupational exposure to mercury vapor and reduced fertility of female dental assistants.[1] Readers seeking to incriminate dental amalgam will interpret the findings incorrectly; that is, by directly associating amalgam use with decreased fecund-ability (probability of conception each menstrual cycle) in dental assistants and extending that assumption to infer that any woman who has amalgam restorations will also demonstrate reduced fecundability.

They couldn't be in greater error. The study demonstrated no relationship between the number of amalgam restorations in the teeth of dental assistants and reduced fecundability—and no association between high exposure to amalgam and fecundability if good mercury hygiene was maintained.

Only those assistants who reported high frequency of poor mercury hygiene (for example, frequent hand contact with mercury, not using

> **The future of dental amalgam is too important to be left to haphazard research agendas. Definitive answers will come only from well-designed prospective research studies.**

pre-capsulated amalgam or not wearing gloves when preparing amalgam) suffered any adverse effects. Interestingly, dental assistants who practiced good mercury hygiene had increased fertility.

Regardless of this assurance, dental amalgam will continue to be the subject of investigative concern. Present efforts to limit waste water containing mercury from dental offices as well as environmental concerns for mercury released from fillings during cremation support this contention.

Some fear the dental profession eventually may become unable or unwilling to provide proof for the "innocence of amalgam"—that dental leadership might downgrade its present acceptance of the risk/benefit of amalgam alloy. It's imperative that an acceptable restorative substitute be identified before that possibility ever becomes a probability.

The restorative value of dental amalgam cannot be overemphasized. Discarding it would cause worldwide repercussions. Amalgam's ease of manipulation, durability and low cost has made restorative dentistry affordable to millions who otherwise would be offered only extractions. And a suitable substitute is not on the immediate horizon.

Composite is a potential successor, but although as wear resistant and clinically functional as amalgam, it requires placement under the most rigorous and exacting conditions. Placement in posterior teeth may require twice the time as amalgam, necessitating significant increases in patient cost.

Furthermore, we still don't have information regarding the safety of composite. The presence of excess monomer after curing and the possibility of inhalation of filler particles during composite finishing require further study.

The future of dental amalgam is too important to be left to haphazard research agendas. Definitive answers will come only from well-designed prospective research studies. The urgency to initiate these studies must be conveyed to organized dentistry, government and industry.

A concurrent priority for research into new restorative materials that are economical, biocompatible and free of environmental contaminants must also be articulated. More resources should be directed to the ADA's Paffenbarger Research Center, where research is already under way to find a mercury-free alloy. University research laboratories also could become major research sites if supported in their efforts to address this issue.

The necessity for immediate action is not overstated. Already one of Europe and Canada's major manufacturers of dental amalgam alloy recently ceased amalgam production—citing as its rationale a recent European publication linking the number of maternal amalgam restorations to elevated levels of mercury in newborns. ∎

1. Rowland AS, Baird DD, Weinberg CR, Shore DL, Shy CM, Wilcox AJ. The effect of occupational exposure to mercury vapor on the fertility of female dental assistants. Occup Environ Med 1994;51:28-34.

# 'Do you know a good dentist?'

*Originally published in JADA 1994 125: 352-354*

As a dentist working with a large number of non-health related professionals, I often find myself serving as their impromptu dental consultant. Aside from specifics regarding dental procedures, the question I am asked most often is, "I need a dentist, do you know a good one?" For them, selecting a new dentist often proves difficult and time-consuming, leaving them susceptible to commercial dental solicitations.

What is a "good" dentist? If asked, people typically say "one who is … experienced, personable, reasonable, efficient, accessible, explains procedures and although not altogether painless, painless whenever possible." These qualities, they say, make up the fabric of the dentist they are seeking.

But are there "bad" dentists? Dentists that do harm? Dentists to be avoided? If so, how many? And what criteria are used to make this determination?

Concern that all dentists are not equally competent—that some might be "bad" enough that they should not practice dentistry—gave birth to state dental practice acts. Originally designed to prevent unscrupulous or questionably trained dentists from harming the public, these acts continue virtually unchanged. Today's dental profession scrutinizes the abilities of its new trainees using written and patient-based clinical examinations to determine suitability for licensure.

But what about the remaining 30 or more years of professional life? Is the knowledge base of dentistry so static that testing skills at entry is sufficient to verify competency for the rest of one's professional life?

If not, is it enough to rely on the dentist's self-assessment to fulfill his or her professional obligation to continually pursue new information pertinent to

> **A computerized group of standardized simulation case examinations can be designed to evaluate practitioners on their medical and dental history assessment skills, diagnostic capabilities, and, yes, even clinical acumen.**

dental practice? Or is some form of periodic testing necessary to ensure compliance?

Developing and implementing a continued competency evaluation system could be costly and time-consuming. Because only a small fraction of dentists (perhaps less than 1 percent at any time) are involved in disciplinary or malpractice actions, those who advocate mandatory assessment of continued competency must convince others that public safety is at significant risk. They must explain why present methods of complaint investigations should be replaced with costly and threatening evaluation requirements.

The "push" for competency exams comes from pre-emptive actions by the certifying boards of two dental specialty groups, the American Association of Dental Examiners and the federal government. The Oral and Maxillofacial Surgery certifying board has already implemented requirements for re-certification and will use a written exam good for 10 years. Pediatric dentistry's certifying board also will be implementing a 10-year time-limited certificate requirement involving periodic re-examination.

The American Association of Dental Examiners is seeking continued competency programs that will assist it in fulfilling its mandate to protect the health, safety and welfare of the public. Federal government interest appears to arise from its investigations of state licensure practice for out of state dentists. Apparently it has become concerned about the minimal standards states currently use to assess the continued competency of their dentists. Additionally, expect health care reform proposals to stress practitioner competency as a means of assisting consumer choice.

Attempts to implement continued competency evaluations that satisfy all interested parties will be fraught with difficulty. Assuming that a valid assessment mechanism can be developed, it must minimally be non-punitive, non-threatening and reasonably priced. It must be objective, valid and reliable. Furthermore, practitioners who fail to meet the competency standards should be able to remediate without economic hardship and/or practice interruption.

Clinical examinations such as those now used to determine entry level competence would not fulfill these criteria—nor will fiscally prohibitive, potentially subjective, in-office assessments of daily procedures, case presentations, record audits and clinical patients. Fortunately, the computer age does offer a non-threatening way to satisfy professional and public interests.

A computerized group of standardized simulation case examinations can be designed to evaluate practitioners on their medical and dental history assessment skills, diagnostic capabilities, and, yes, even clinical acumen. The objective simulation exam, administered in the privacy of one's office or home, can incorporate motion, sound, 3-D and graphic data.

In position to develop this type of system is the Dental Interactive Simulation Corporation, a nonprofit organization sponsored by the American Association of Dental Examiners, the American Association of Dental Schools, the American Dental Association and four regional dental examining boards representing 38 states. If continued practitioner competency is judged important to the future of the dental profession, DISC, with a solid nationwide organization in place, is ready to assist.

What should the ADA's position be? Out in front—providing the logistic support necessary to ensure that all who seek a "good" dentist will be successful. ∎

# Don't bank here

*Originally published in JADA 1994 125: 488-490*

The National Practitioner Data Bank, an Orwellian creation of unsurpassed magnitude, promises to exceed any previous "Big Brother" initiative if the public is allowed access to its files. And President Clinton's health care reform initiative proposes to do exactly that.

By amending the Health Care Quality Improvement Act of 1986, individuals seeking to enroll in health plans under the new Health Security Act may obtain information directly from the data bank on physicians and other licensed health care practitioners.

A strong supporter of consumers' rights to select health care providers on the basis of their "needs" and the providers' "merits," Rep. Ron Wyden (D-Ore.) held hearings last year on the role of consumer choice in improving the quality of health care. Three panels of witnesses gave testimony: patients who had experienced difficulties with the present health care system, entrepreneurs who collect information on health care organizations, and access and consumer advocate groups. All strongly supported Chairman Wyden's goal to allow public access to the data bank.

To discount the importance of this public support for the data bank would be politically naive. Bureaucrats love this program. If legislation increases public access to its records, it will be difficult, perhaps impossible, to modify them. The prolonged and difficult struggle by the ADA'S legal staff to force the data bank to back off on listing refunds to patients as malpractice actions attests to this fact.

With dentists already accounting for more than 16 percent of the data bank's malpractice and adverse action reports, the issue of unrestricted public access to data bank files demands immediate professional attention.

At risk is the confidentiality of information in the data bank coupled with the concern that the data in their present form can easily lead to erroneous conclusions and inappropriate actions by data bank users.

Regarding confidentiality, can the bank be trusted not to share information with unauthorized individuals or organizations? An unbiased and highly reliable source says no. As recently as last summer the Government Accounting Office, which audits all federal programs, reported "continuing concerns about the management of the bank." Its conclusions fueled questions regarding the continued existence of an organization that has been cited repeatedly for mistaken release of sensitive data, poor monitoring of operations, insufficient attention to user needs as well as slow response time to legitimate queries.

As professionals committed to improving the health and welfare of Americans, dentists could hardly object to the concept of a National Practitioner Data Bank, whose stated purpose is to identify health practitioners who might harm their patients. But knowledgeable individuals will surely protest the existence of an organization whose actions may cause harm rather than good- whose inept administration and data collection could easily undermine the practice of ethical health care providers.

The data bank receives reports on adverse actions taken against dentists by licensing boards, hospitals or professional societies. In no case does the data bank make a judgment about provider competence. But you can be assured that the public will- just the fact that your name is listed in the bank's registry may prejudice consumers or health care entities as they select health providers.

And how wrong they might be! Your name could be added to the data bank list simply by deciding that you no longer wish to maintain your dental license in one or more states. By not paying your yearly fee, your license would be revoked. That action would be entered into the data bank as an ad-

> **Dentists—indeed, all health professionals—are at risk of being misjudged without benefit of immediate recourse.**

verse action. Drop your license in two states—two adverse actions on your data bank record!

And it only gets worse. If you apply to a hospital for privileges and are turned down because they do not have an opening, the denial of privileges would be reported to the bank as an adverse action.

As a further example, what if one of your patients claims you have not delivered a contracted dental service. You disagree and the patient sues. Adamant about the correctness of your position, you demand a trial even at risk of personal loss of practice income. The insurance company, without your consent, pays the patient $500 as a nuisance claim settlement—and the data bank registers a malpractice action against you.

Remember the data bank only registers data—it makes no judgments about competence.

Three adverse actions plus a malpractice citation. What will patients, considering you as their future dentist, think when they receive a data bank report with this information? Indeed, how would your present patients respond? Without any clarification of these negative entries, you can assume that most dental consumers will select dentists who have no data bank record.

Perhaps no government regulation or program holds the potential to be as intrusive and professionally damaging as does the National Practitioner Data Bank. Under its present format, the data it contains cannot be accurately interpreted by an inquiring consumer.

Dentists—indeed, all health professionals—are at risk of being misjudged without benefit of immediate recourse. Either the data bank must clean up its data—making them accurate and user friendly—or an entirely new format for reporting adverse actions of health professionals must be found.

Until that occurs, all health professionals must vociferously oppose public access to the present National Practitioner Data Bank. ∎

# The competitive edge

*Originally published in JADA 1994 125: 656-658*

**B**esieged, bothered and bewildered—appropriate terms to describe today's dentists as they attempt to sift through the proliferating numbers of delivery system alternatives. Either by innuendo or by hype, each proposal suggests that enrollment will ensure participants a continuing flow of patients. An outcome, they infer, that soon may not be available to non-participants.

Similar, but far less sophisticated alternative dental care financing schemes emerged in the late 1960s and '70s. Whether it was the economic climate or the programs' seemingly unethical approach in restricting practitioner access, most of these entrepreneurial offerings were soundly rejected by the profession.

Times have changed. Regardless of dentistry's past successes in containing costs, proposals to further manage dental fee schedules abound. Using the umbrella of "elective practitioner associations," previously unimagined financing and organizational plans crop up daily. And more activity can be expected as commercial purchasers of dental care gain power in their attempts to take control of the market.

Today, the commercial purchaser of dental care has an appetizing carrot: exclusive access to a restricted segment of the population.

The cost to practitioners: discounted fees, controlled utilization, lower income and potential loss of their present family of patients. The price to the profession: diminishing professional autonomy and declining ability to control its destiny.

With health system reform promising to accelerate this process, what advice should be given practitioners beleaguered by requests from patients asking that their dental records be transferred to another practice? "Sorry, Doc, you're not a preferred provider in my plan. ... I can't afford the difference between your fee and my plan's allowance for a non-participating dentist. Nothing personal."

In cases where the financial circumstances are such that the patient is truly unable to afford the difference, it's doubtful that any action on your part will dissuade the patient from leaving the practice.

For many of your patients, however, their decision will be "elastic." They'll stick with your practice if they can see some good reason for doing so. Here is where you and your office staff can really have an impact on the future of your practice.

The critical factor is quality. Not technical quality, for few dental consumers are capable of assessing the quality of dental service. Rather, it is the patient's perception of quality that will influence choice. At issue is the quality of service offered by you and your dental team.

The message is clear and unequivocal—enhance your commitment to service.

> **Practitioners who expect to survive today's marketplace revolution with their professional dignity intact will provide service that exceeds the professional norm.**

Practitioners who expect to survive today's marketplace revolution with their professional dignity intact will provide service that exceeds the professional norm. Their practices will demand that all staff members personalize every interaction with patients. They will provide services that assign the highest priority to minimizing logistic barriers, such as patient waiting time for appointments; service that defines a personalized after-hours communication system for patients in need; service that offers meaningful acknowledgments to loyal patients who refer friends and acquaintances; service that is innovative—such as providing transportation to the elderly or others who might have difficulty accessing the practice.

The realm of creative quality services is boundless, limited only by the creative energies and imagination of your dental team.

Do patients really respond to high-quality, personalized service? Check the cover story by Dr. Barbara Gerbert and others in the March 1994 JADA. Patients gave highest scores to dentists' caring attributes and professional competence.

Interestingly, the patients' beliefs about their dentist were more positive than the dentists' view of themselves. Major differences in scoring were noted between patients and dentists on the importance of the dentist "explaining dental procedures, offering reassurance, and being friendly and cheerful." Dentists rated these items 10 to 20 percent lower than patients. Dentists take heed: there is a not so hidden message in those responses.

What can the dental team do to reinforce its commitment to patient service? As an initial step, consider assessing the present quality of those services. Try a questionnaire to determine what patients do and don't like about your practice. You may even want to hold a series of focus groups bringing together a small group of patients over lunch or dinner and inviting them to be open and frank about their experiences in your office.

A useful initiative for the dental office might be to institute a Total Quality Management System. U.S. business and industry have successfully used this system to enhance their business operations and productivity. Some have characterized this system as the ultimate marketing tool. It is concerned with changing the organization by involving all members of the work force in a concerted effort to do things right the first rather than reactive manner.

In 1972, Studs Terkel published "Working," his description of the American worker. Included was a characterization of the dentist who was quoted as saying, "I've had some patients who did not stay with me. There are some people who are used to deference. This is not my way. ... Damn it, when they're in my office, I'm boss."

If Mr. Terkel's dentist intends to survive into the 21st century, someone must convince him or her that professional competence alone is not enough. To compete effectively in the dental marketplace of today and tomorrow, dental professionals must have an unwavering commitment to individualized patient service. ■

# Economic compression of the worst kind

*Originally published in JADA 1994 125: 776-782*

Sleepless nights may await the nation's dentists if reports of increasing dental overhead continue. Last month's ADA special report on the cost of infection control underscored the intense fiscal pressure on dentists brought on by additional bureaucratic overlays.

If you're an average practitioner with 2,700 yearly patient visits, infection control will cost you about $17 per patient or $45,718 annually. At 13.5 percent of total dental services, this is hardly an insignificant expense. OSHA requirements alone account for about $9 of the patient visits ($23,713 annually).

Additional overhead increases may be coming. OSHA is discussing new respiratory standards for the workplace and may consider work rules in the area of ergonomics. Other government regulators, like the EPA, have shown concern about waste water discharges from dental offices. Any of these issues translated into regulations could run up present overhead significantly.

With 60-70 percent of gross dental income already siphoned off for overhead, dental concerns intensify with each new government regulation. And well they should, since the mechanism for offsetting these increases through dental fee adjustments may no longer be viable.

Consider the basic formula of dental practice economics. Production (x) fees (-) office overhead (=) net income. By using this model, increases in overhead can be met by production increases, fee increases or reduction in overhead achieved through practice efficiencies.

Blocking these traditional avenues for addressing increases in dental overhead costs would severely compress dentistry's ability to function in an economically stable manner. Unfortunately, the components for this form of economic disequilibrium are already in place.

As part of today's health care environment, dentists are being pressured to hold or even reduce their fees. Managed care organizations are squeezing health professionals to join or be left out in the cold. Membership usually requires accepting a lower fee schedule—thus restricting the dentist's flexibility to account for increased overhead charges.

And it's not only the private organizations that are pressuring dentists. For instance, Tennessee, with its new TennCare program, is offering participating dentists 45 percent of their usual fee. It's hard to translate the combination of a 65 percent overhead and 45 percent of a normal fee into a profit situation—maybe this is the "new" math.

If fees can't be increased, except perhaps for some inflationary adjustments, then productivity must be increased either by increasing patient visits and/or making changes in the service mix. Physically, many dentists are at their limit—more hours at the chair would strain their ability to maintain quality.

Changing the service mix by boosting the numbers of more profitable services, although desirable, does not appear to be a workable solution for most dentists. Without fee augmentations or work hour increases, maintaining net income can only be achieved by overhead reductions.

Not a simple solution! Labor costs are difficult to reduce. Skilled dental team members cannot be replaced with lower-paid entrants without corresponding reductions in efficiency. Reductions in benefits affect both employer and employee and can destroy a harmonious work environment.

Trim supply and material costs? Perhaps, but many dentists already are buying through discount or buyers' cooperatives. And with the continued pressure on the use of amalgam, it can be expected that future substitutes will be more costly.

> **This litany of economic shocks—some already in place, others looming on the horizon—could thrust the entire dental delivery system into economic chaos.**

And then, add the potential for further economic compression if the outcome of the present health care debate results in the loss of tax deductibility of dental services. All practices would be affected. Besides reducing the absolute number of patients able to seek dental care, it surely would affect the present mix of dental service, especially in the prosthetic and preventive areas.

This litany of economic shocks—some already in place, others looming on the horizon- could thrust the entire dental delivery system into economic chaos. If they materialize, how will dentistry cope? Economists would suggest enlarging market share—increasing dental utilization by the non- or infrequent dental consumer.

At first glance, this appears to be sound advice for those dentists who can expand their treatment capacity. Closer scrutiny suggests that the mix of procedures required by this "utilization" group would require substantial financial underwriting by private or government sources. Any offered subsidization must be adequate. Otherwise, severely discounted fee schedules would only worsen dentistry's fiscal plight.

Presently, few signs of impending fiscal doom have appeared. Expected decreases in dental fees, reductions in net income, a drop in the number of those seeking a dental career and a general discontent with organized dentistry have not material-ized. Indeed, in 1992 real income gains for dentists more than tripled when compared to the previous five years. In 1994, the education sector witnessed an 18 percent increase in potential applicants to dental schools. And organized dentistry flourished, setting an all-time attendance record at the ADA convention in San Francisco.

What's missing from this picture? Has the case for economic compression been overstated? I think not.

More plausible is that dentistry is at a pre-symptomatic stage of a degenerative process. Solutions to how the profession can slow or even reverse this looming economic compression must be sought. Dental economists agree that to remain economically viable, dentistry must be able to respond to increased costs of doing business by instituting appropriate fee increases. Absent that opportunity, economists warn, dentistry as practiced today could cease to exist.

Is there any hope for turning the tide? Dentistry's message to Congress, "Health Care That Works," contains the social and political rationale to support the profession's need for economic flexibility.

Now is the time to lend your voice to ensure that the message is heard. Join the ADA'S grassroots campaign. Your participation can make a difference! ∎

# Oral cancer—the forgotten disease

*Originally published in JADA 1994 125: 1042-1164*

Seemingly lost in the constant attention to HIV and its regulatory baggage has been dentistry's "own" disease—oral cancer. Except for occasional reports citing incidence or prevalence statistics, the programmatic center stage, once reserved for oral cancer, is now occupied by infection control, OSHA and survival skills to meet the changing health care environment.

A most disturbing trend!

Not that dentists are any less conscientious in assessing the oral cancer status of their patients. More than 80 percent report including oral cancer detection as an essential component of the dental exam.

However, the almost total absence of public and professional notice relating to oral cancer detection and prevention points to oral cancer's lower priority among today's professional concerns. But with 30,000 new cases of oral cancer diagnosed each year, placing it on the back burner can cause real harm-especially since early diagnosis can result in permanent cures, and tobacco prevention programs can significantly lower the yearly incidence of oral cancer.

Health policy makers recognized oral cancer's impact on the nation's health and included it as a National Health Objective for the Year 2000: 40 percent of those 50 years or older will have received an oral cancer exam from a primary care provider during the preceding year. But without the assistance of a nationwide campaign, the worthy objective seems unreachable.

A 1992 National Cancer Control survey noted that less than 15 percent of all Americans could recollect ever having a cancer exam. Even correcting for those who had an oral cancer exam and did not realize it, that is a dismal percentage.

Regardless of this lack of progress and with 8,000 deaths resulting from oral cancer deaths an-

**As a health profession that contacts more than half the U.S. population at least once annually, dentistry is uniquely positioned for a central role in smoking cessation efforts.**

nually, the dental profession must intensify its commitment to detecting and preventing oral cancer. Public education programs headlining the importance of annual oral cancer exams, especially for those at high risk, should top the profession's public service priorities.

And with good reason: in a recent survey, only 25 percent of the U.S. public could name a single early sign of oral cancer. Just a third knew that increased exposure to sunlight was a risk factor in the development of oral cancer.

Even with a successful public campaign, many high-risk individuals do not have yearly checkups. They may, however, have contact with other primary care providers, who, with proper training, could conduct the oral cancer exam.

And training is needed. A recent survey noted that only 18 percent of M.D.s provided oral cancer exams on 50 percent or more of their patients. Forty-seven percent believed that their knowledge about oral cancer was not current. Considering that these primary care providers may be the sole contact for many high-risk individuals, organized dentistry needs to develop educational material specifically designed to assist M.D.s in conducting oral cancer examinations.

So much for the easy part. There is an even more urgent need to attack the use of an agent repeatedly associated with the development of oral cancer—tobacco.

Public health efforts continue to stress the importance of limiting tobacco use. With a half-million U.S. deaths traceable to smoking each year, health professionals must aggressively market intervention programs designed to modify or eliminate the smoking behavior of almost 50,000,000 Americans—many of whom would like to quit but require professional assistance.

As a health profession that contacts more than

half the U.S. population at least once annually, dentistry is uniquely positioned for a central role in smoking cessation efforts. With oral cancer rates among smokers ranging as high as 18 times those of non-smokers, no rationale for involvement should be needed.

So far the response has not been good. National Cancer Institute studies show dentists lagging far behind physicians in smoking cessation activities—only 48 percent of dentists attempt to counsel their patients compared to 94 percent of physicians. The difference may be ascribed to levels of competence.

Just a third of the dentists report feeling knowledgeable to counsel patients vs. 83 percent of their physician counterparts. This reported inadequacy may be responsible for dentistry's somewhat marginal interest in implementing office-based smoking cessation programs.

The initial lukewarm response by many dental state boards to the use of the transdermal nicotine patch did little to encourage dental participation. Fortunately, that myopic view is slowly giving way to recognizing that tobacco use and oral cancer are inextricably linked and that dentists should be involved in tobacco intervention activities.

Some already are. More should be. As demonstrated by a number of research reports, dentists can change smoking behaviors in patients who are interested in quitting.

Consider fluoride, sealants, oral hygiene instruction and nutritional counseling. Each is an essential preventive component of the dental treatment plan. All qualify for appropriate provider compensation.

Shouldn't programs directed to oral cancer elimination be added to this list? ∎

# In a fishing expedition, nibbles count

*Originally published in JADA 1994 125: 1162-1164*

Overt panic-mongering by British television and print journalists promises to further the cause of those seeking to ban dental amalgam. In a slick 30-minute TV presentation entitled "Poison in the Mouth," the British Broadcasting Corp. used data from an unpublished research report that claimed dentists are suffering neurologic damage from handling amalgam. The Reuters wire service covering the broadcast further linked "mercury from amalgam to brain damage in dentists and patients."

Reuters quotes the research report's principal author as saying, "The kind of things we have found are [dentist] losses in function, associated with the ability to move manually very small things with (their) hands, a manual dexterity problem." The quote continues, "Other kinds of really distinct functions are concentration—the inability to concentrate."

What makes this pseudo-expose so potentially damaging to the profession's stand on amalgam safety is its main source: the soon-to-be published, "Behavioral Effects of Low-Level Exposure to Mercury Among Dentists."

This report is based on observations of dentists participating in the ADA'S annual session health screening program. One of the coauthors is a world-recognized ADA scientist. Obviously, if the BBC and Reuters reports were accurate, this source of data would add credibility to the anti-amalgam arguments.

The critical fact is that this was a hypothesis-generating, not a hypothesis-testing, investigation. The authors were searching for relationships, not causality. And in that process, less rigorous statistical testing methods are employed.

The researchers did not expect their findings to lead to definitive conclusions but rather to the testing of future hypotheses—in a fishing expedition, nibbles count. You can be sure that the BBC and Reuters aren't interested in waiting for genuine conclusions. They have other fishing holes to explore.

Experience with past national TV revelations in which patients "throw away their crutches" after amalgam removal has left most dentists with a decidedly skeptical view of TV reporting. This program should be no exception. Once again dentistry has been victimized by unsubstantiated and inflammatory rhetoric.

This is not the way new information should be transferred. The normal progression starts with publication of the data, followed by a time for scientific assessment. Finally, critical responses are compiled and analyzed. Given the incomplete and pre-selected material supplied by the BBC and Reuters, this process cannot even begin.

But the media, feeding on the unquenchable public thirst for information that allegedly will enhance well-being, have their own ethic, and it doesn't include scientific verification. Nor does the press consider that a single research report may not accurately reflect the "real" truth.

Despite this study's preliminary nature, the profession and its scientists should look forward to its timely publication. As the first U.S. investigation linking elevated mercury levels to subclinical behavioral differences in dentists, it deserves special attention. To those who will examine the data, the ADA scientist who co-authored the research offers a series of caveats.

First, he cautions, the study was able to find only 19 dentists with mercury levels averaging 36 pigs/liter in urine. This number represents less than 3 percent of all dentists who participated in the screening, allowing a few dentists to have a large impact on the results.

Second, the researcher notes that the "urinary mercury levels were not significantly associated

> **Once again dentistry has been victimized by unsubstantiated and inflammatory rhetoric.**

with any of the individual cognitive or motor functions." He concludes that it was only the sum of ranked score measurements that suggested any mercury-induced effects.

Third, he cautions that the mercury levels reported for the sample dentists were seven to 10 times higher than the normal mercury levels noted in national surveys of dentists- and 15 times higher than mercury levels found in the general public. The BBC and Reuters failed to point this out, apparently content to infer that what was noted in a few dentists would also be noted in all those with silver fillings in their mouths.

These restrictions notwithstanding, certain elements of this investigation require immediate professional attention. For example, the excessively high urine mercury levels noted in the dentists studied should alert all of us to the hazards of poor mercury hygiene.

Are there dentists who still use squeeze cloths? Are some still not using pre-encapsulated amalgam? Or not wearing gloves when preparing amalgam? Are mercury spills more frequent than reported?

These are pertinent questions if you recall the recent research describing reduced fertility in those dental assistants whose mercury handling processes were inconsistent with ADA-advocated guidelines.

Urinary mercury concentrations in dental practitioners participating in the ADA health screening program have decreased more than fivefold in the last decade. With present technology there is no excuse for dentists to continue practices that may be harmful to themselves or their dental team members. ∎

# Dentistry has been good to me

*Originally published in JADA 1994 125: 1290-1292*

**A**re you ready to open your hearts—and your checkbooks—to help the ADA's newly expanded Health Foundation? Probably not, unless someone gives you a very good reason to support one more philanthropic organization.

After all, aren't dentists already major contributors to their churches, community charities, colleges and universities, their dental schools and countless other worthwhile causes and organizations? Why add a dental charity to the overcrowded list? And what happened to the American Fund For Dental Health? Isn't it dentistry's official fund-raising entity?

Good questions. The AFDH has indeed been the principal fund-raising entity for dental education and research for nearly 40 years. It is not, however, the ADA'S own foundation. The AFDH's goals, laudatory as they may be, have not always been able to meet the specific needs of the Association's constituencies.

A rapidly changing health-service environment demands an ADA foundation able to address the contemporary issues of dental education and research. Upgrading the Health Foundation to the status of dentistry's flagship charitable entity will provide this flexibility. The ADAHF's newly reshaped organization will allow it to apply its resources to finding answers to some of the most pressing questions facing dentistry today.

Through foundation partnerships with dental schools, researchers will be able to undertake applied research in education, clinical procedures, biotechnology and policy areas. The wide range of topics includes such nagging issues as dental amalgam, waste water, dental care delivery, ergonomics, dental care access, non-traditional auxiliary training and infectious disease transmission. With a new infusion

> **A rapidly changing health-service environment demands an ADA foundation able to address the contemporary issues of dental education and research. Upgrading the Health Foundation to the status of dentistry's flagship charitable entity will provide this flexibility.**

of funds, the ADA'S Paffenbarger Research Institute can accelerate its research into amalgam substitutes.

Just as research funding is likely to generate rich dividends for dentistry, so too will the Health Foundation's assistance in educating tomorrow's dentists.

Consider this potential agenda:

- The creation of a student loan program, allowing ADAHF to assist needy students by helping pay the interest on loans during their educational years. With per-student debt averaging more than $50,000, this kind of financial aid would improve the quality of dental student life, relieve stress and reduce the need for time-consuming extracurricular jobs.

- A foundation-supported grant program for dental practice start-up that could help new graduates get their practices off the ground.

- A National Dental Service Award, allowing selected students to pay back educational grants by providing dental care in under-served areas. Locations would be designated by the profession, not the federal government.

- Technology-transfer programs that would facilitate extension of educational services to individual dental practices using satellites, fiber-optics, computer networks and other state-of-the-art communication systems—an innovative approach to continuing dental education made possible through the Health Foundation.

These and other worthwhile programs have not been made available through other foundations or government agencies. The ADAHF agenda promises to be truly pioneering and exciting. But building a foundation portfolio of education and research programs capable of satisfying current needs will require a major infusion of funds.

While few dentists are actively seeking new charitable interests to support, the Health Foundation provides a direct route of contribution to those who believe: "Dentistry has been good to me. And now is the time for me to help dentistry."

The ADAHF is uniquely positioned to recognize and honor those interested in offering a gift. No donation is too small. A $25 contribution from just two-thirds of the ADA membership would generate more than $2.5 million—a substantial nest egg from which to initiate programming. State and local dental societies and related dental groups will find that cultivating relationships with the ADAHF can be mutually beneficial.

Dentistry also has been good to those who make their living manufacturing and selling dental products. We hope that those in the dental trades and manufacturing-and in supporting industries as well—will recognize the rewards they stand to gain by investing in dentistry's future.

If dentistry has been good to you, consider becoming an active contributor to the ADA Health Foundation. If the majority of us participate now, our efforts will help ensure that those who follow will also be able to say: "Dentistry has been good to me." ∎

# Time for a dental board checkup

*Originally published in JADA 1994 125: 1418-1420*

Something is radically wrong. Thousands of new dental graduates are failing their initial dental licensure exam. This summer the average failure rate on the Central Regional Dental Testing Service regional exam for its 10-member schools was 40 percent, a figure that, in itself, should be considered unacceptable.

But there's more: a shocking 80 percent or greater failure rate noted at two of the CRDTS examining schools. And these astronomical figures were not confined to CRDTS. Failures ranging from 50 percent to more than 80 percent were noted at certain exam sites in the Western, Southern and Northeastern regional boards.

Imagine the embarrassment of young dental graduates as they inform their prospective dental employers that they have flunked the dental board. No matter how excellent their previous academic records, a failing grade on the exam has to create questions in employers' minds about the skills of their new associates.

As for the "failed" new graduates, in addition to the practice time lost and the logistical costs of retaking the exam, their unacceptable performance does little to build professional confidence.

For the critics of initial licensure examinations, the high failure rates add credibility to their arguments. How, they ask, could 88 percent of a dental school's graduating class fail an exam if the test was valid? And why do almost all of these young graduates pass the exam at the first re-test, without any opportunity for interim clinical remediation?

In rebuttal, supporters of initial dental licensure exams point to the graduates' lack of success as either a failure of the dental education process or the admission and graduation of unqualified students.

For the record, the graduating dental class of 1994 entered dental school with grade point averages and dental aptitude scores equal to those of recent graduates. Assuming they were equally motivated and interested in their dental education, the reason(s) for their lack of success on the boards must be sought outside the students' inherent abilities.

Unquestionably, an analysis of this dismal board performance is in order. Each component needs dissecting. We know the students entered with acceptable pre-dental credentials. Could the fault lie with their professors? Did their teachers fail to apply the appropriate educational messages and techniques? Perhaps the failures could be linked to deficient exam construction or—for the exam's clinical portions—the reliability of the examiners.

What would a content analysis of each subject reveal? Does the didactic portion of the exam represent the universe of teaching in that subject area? Did the test credit alternative (but still acceptable) ways to treat a condition?

Variables such as the pressure of the exam need to be considered. With so much importance given to passing this single exam, the student's emotional state may be a factor. The contention that pressure is a way of life for the practicing dentist should not negate investigation of this variable.

The patient also may present an obstacle to examination success. Consider the impact of the patient who arrives late, who is generally uncooperative or who presents unusual clinical findings.

Recognizing what they believe are major deficiencies in present entry-level licensure examinations, the American Association of Dental Schools in 1991 adopted a long-term goal of eliminating state and regional entry-level exams. This policy would apply only to those who had graduated from programs ac-

> **The recent rejection, through the licensure exam, of more than 1,000 newly graduated dentists demands professional attention—not to undermine the states' right to protect their citizens' health and welfare, but rather to evaluate whether alternatives exist.**

credited by the Commission on Dental Accreditation and had passed the National Board Dental Examination.

To date the American Association of Dental Examiners has rejected any alternative pathways to licensure, "encouraging all state boards to continue to require an initial entry-level clinical licensure examination." This policy, although supported by the American Dental Association, has been tempered by the ADA's willingness to assess the ramifications of various alternate or optional pathways to licensure.

And well it should.

The recent rejection, through the licensure exam, of more than 1,000 newly graduated dentists demands professional attention-not to undermine the states' right to protect their citizens' health and welfare, but rather to evaluate whether alternatives exist.

Alternative suggestions are not lacking. For example, using the existing technology of interactive computer simulation, it would be possible to develop a highly sophisticated clinical decision-making exam. This new test, in conjunction with the Dental National Boards, Parts 1 and 2, would enhance our present testing by providing a comprehensive assessment of a student's didactic and clinical abilities.

Granting licensure without clinical examination to dentists who had passed these three National Didactic Exams and had also completed an approved general practice residency parallels the standards medicine uses to grant licensure to its emerging professionals. With a third of dental graduates enrolling yearly in residency programs, this mechanism could provide a reasonable alternative to today's testing methods.

A non-GPR option to granting licensure without involving a postgraduate Dental Board Exam could also be achieved by combining the proposed three National Didactic Exams with an "in-dental school" series of clinical examinations taken before graduation. The strength of this alternative: immediate and structured remediation for deficient students. Implementation would require close cooperation between dental educators and examiners.

More thought and some creative problem-solving should be focused on initial dental licensure. Dental students are anxious and concerned. They need and deserve our help. ∎

# A world without water fluoridation

*Originally published in JADA 1994 125: 1538-1540*

Colorado Springs, a tourist mecca and gateway to the Rocky Mountains, supports a large number of special-interest museums. One honors national figure-skating greats. Another honors cowboys, at the National Professional Rodeo Hall of Fame. But no museum—not even an exhibit—is dedicated to dentistry's monumental contribution to public health and the man who started it all.

In Chicago's affluent Gold Coast section, you will find a prominent statue of G.V. Black. And in Hartford, Conn.'s, Bushnell Park you can see the imposing figure of Horace Wells. But no where in Colorado Springs can you find a statue of this community's most famous dental citizen, Dr. Frederick S. McKay.

Having graduated from the University of Pennsylvania dental school, Dr. McKay arrived in Colorado Springs in 1901 and opened a dental practice.

He soon noticed that many of his patients had permanently stained or mottled teeth. His desire and relentless energy sustained an investigation that lasted 30 years and revealed the secret of the disfiguring mottled enamel called "Colorado Brown Stain."

Although occasionally joined in his research by local dentists and even once by the famous G.V. Black, Dr. McKay's search for the responsible agent was a singular one. He had very little assistance in his epidemiologic sleuthing. And just when financial support appeared to be on its way, Colorado Springs' newspapers, concerned that tourists reading about the "stain" might become fearful, failed to support his efforts. Undaunted, he continued the research with his own funds.

By 1915 it was agreed that something in the water was causing the brown stain. But test after test failed to identify the critical substance. Then

**In this day and age, when nearly everyone is speeding down the information highway, catching "sound bites" on the run, eyes focused on the future, it might serve us well to look back to our past, to reflect on the lives of those whose accomplishments have brought us to where we are today.**

in 1931, an ALCOA scientist wrote to Dr. McKay, suggesting that calcium fluoride might be the culprit. And so it was.

Dr. McKay often noted that people with the mottled enamel appeared to have less dental decay than others, but his interest was limited to identifying the causative agent. The next step belonged to the U.S. Public Health Service, which had been given the task of determining what level of fluoride caused mottled enamel. During this process, fluoride's decay-reducing properties were documented.

You know the rest of the saga. H. Trendley Dean's critical observation eventually led to the initiation of the first artificial water fluoridation project in Grand Rapids, Mich. The subsequent dramatic reduction in caries gave credibility to fluoride's powerful abilities as a preventive agent.

Today, more than 300 million people enjoy the benefits of fluoridated water. Reductions in pain and suffering associated with the carious process, plus the billions of dollars in personal health savings, vividly illustrate why health leaders consider water fluoridation one of the most successful public health measures ever instituted.

Next year, Grand Rapids, in conjunction with the West Michigan Dental Society, the Michigan Dental Association and with assistance from organized dentistry, dental education, the dental industry and government, will celebrate the 50th anniversary of this momentous event.

An international symposium underscoring the benefits of fluoride, coupled with the unveiling of a commemorative monument, will highlight the festivities. People from all over the world will attend.

In all this enthusiasm, let's not forget the contribution of Dr. McKay. After all, without his dedication and persistence, we might have a world without water fluoridation. I'm not suggesting a statue or a monument in downtown Colorado Springs. Rather, how about a continuing tribute to Dr. McKay's career, his intellectual curiosity, observation and information gathering—those qualities and actions that create new knowledge?

Every three years, the ADA, in cooperation with Chesebrough-Pond's USA Co., grants dentistry's highest research award to a deserving recipient. Each awardee receives a gold medal and a $25,000 prize.

Perhaps the ADA would be willing to co-sponsor with industry a new prestigious award carrying the name of Frederick S. McKay. Those honored with this citation would be chosen from the ranks of practicing dentists who, without major support from academia or industry, have made a significant contribution to the public well-being. Finding worthy recipients would not be difficult.

In this day and age, when nearly everyone is speeding down the information highway, catching "sound bites" on the run, eyes focused on the future, it might serve us well to look back to our past, to reflect on the lives of those whose accomplishments have brought us to where we are today.

Wouldn't it be appropriate to acknowledge the life's work of a dentist whose professional commitment resulted in one of the world's greatest public health successes? ■

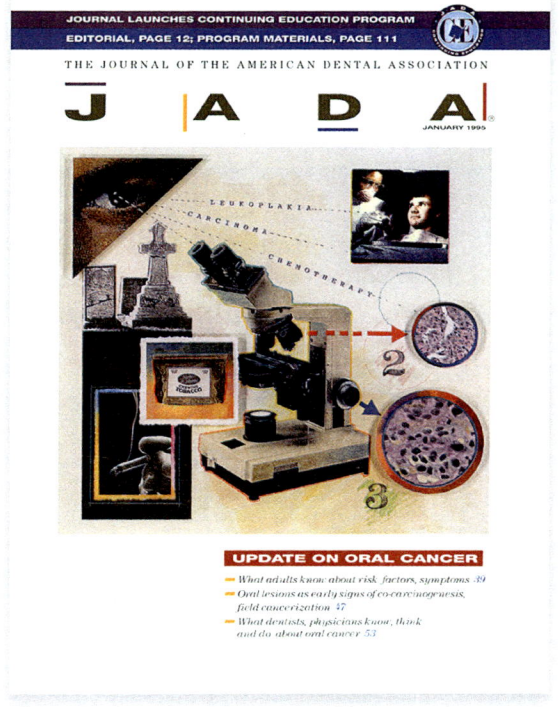

# 1995

"Dental schools face an extraordinary
opportunity. Despite naysayers, they must
change if they wish to remain viable.
New solutions to old problems must be
intertwined with visionary advancements
that challenge the present underpinnings
of dental education."

# For members only

*Originally published in JADA 1995 125: 12-13.*

Has the tight margin between office overhead and profit made your regular attendance at Continuing Dental Education (CDE) courses economically difficult? Have CDE tuition, travel and lodging costs dampened your enthusiasm for yet another continuing education course? Do you live in a remote area that requires excessive travel time to reach continuing education sites? Are you pressured to satisfy mandatory CDE requirements for relicensure?

If your answer is yes to any of these questions, consider attending a monthly continuing education course that won't take you out of your office, has no travel or lodging costs and charges minimal or no tuition. The only prerequisites are membership in the American Dental Association and reading specified articles in this and subsequent issues of The Journal of the American Dental Association.

For ADA members only, JADA now offers the opportunity to earn one credit hour of CDE per issue—up to 12 credits per year for those who participate each month.

Many of our readers will earn these credits doing exactly what they normally do—read the articles in JADA. To receive the monthly credit, you need only score 75 percent on 12 questions drawn from the contents of three clinical articles. The University of Colorado's Continuing Dental Education Division will administer this program and grant credit to participants.

A caveat to users: the number and type of CDE credits accepted by ensuing jurisdictions will vary. Some may limit the number of credit hours from this form of CDE instruction. Check with your state board for specific requirements.

You need not sign up for credit to benefit from this new CDE offering. JADA will publish the correct answers in subsequent issues to promote self-testing, which can reinforce learning.

> **Consider attending a monthly continuing education course that won't take you out of your office, has no travel or lodging costs and charges minimal or no tuition.**

The inclusion of CDE in JADA further exemplifies JADA's goal of enhancing the ability of practitioners to better serve their patients. The importance of promoting access to CDE as an ADA member benefit cannot be overstated.

The ADA Principles of Ethics and Code of Professional Conduct allows for no ambiguity when it addresses the issue of continuing education for members of the profession. It emphatically states that "the privilege of dentists to be accorded professional status rests primarily in the knowledge, skill and experience with which they serve their patients and society. All dentists, therefore, have the obligation of keeping their knowledge and skill current."

Until recently, the dental profession relied on self-assessment as the professional standard for meeting this educational mandate. No longer. Today a majority of the states want assurance that professionals are continuing learners–to protect the health and welfare of their citizens.

In 1969, Minnesota became the first state to require mandatory continuing education. While nine more states quickly followed Minnesota's lead, only recently has major growth been noted. Since 1990, 28 licensing jurisdictions have added mandatory CDE requirements. Now, almost 60 percent of all practicing dentists reside in areas mandating CDE. Other licensing bodies are contemplating similiar action.

Yet, the concept of mandating CDE for relicensure is not without its detractors. Some claim there is little evidence indicating a transfer of information from classroom to patient treatment. They further question the validity of dentists' submitting lists of completed CDE courses as evidence of professional growth.

"Dentists can just show up at a meeting and get credit," runs their line of thinking. "But as a minimum some testing should accompany any submission of credits." Examination, they believe, while not guaranteeing information retention or transfer, does indicate enhanced educational involvement by the participant.

Mandatory CDE proponents admit that data on the effectiveness of CDE are limited. The most extensive analysis to date reviewed all CDE evaluation studies and concluded that while "these studies do suggest that direct effects of CDE can be demonstrated under some conditions ... these effects do not appear strong and may not be those anticipated."

Nevertheless, with continuing pressure to ensure dental competence, recording CDE activity does provide some, albeit limited, objective evidence of practitioner involvement in a learning exercise.

JADA addresses the evaluation issue by testing knowledge gained from three selected readings. Its test questions highlight the important contributions of the articles. Each question is scrutinized by educational experts to reduce ambiguities.

The offering of CDE credits in JADA is a pilot project. Membership comments and suggestions are welcomed. It is expected that program modifications will be made. Those of us involved in developing this membership benefit will continue to tailor it to meet your CDE needs. We hope it will assist you in fulfilling your professional obligation. ∎

1. Bader JD. A review of evaluations of effectiveness in continuing dental education. Mobius 1987;7:39-48.

# If it's not broken...

*Originally published in JADA 1995 125: 140-141.*

"If it's not broken, don't fix it." This timeworn, oft-repeated maxim should have no place in the vocabulary of the enlightened dental professional. But sometimes, as a means of maintaining the frequently comfortable status quo, that attitude becomes a roadblock to continual assessment and measurement of outcomes evaluations that just might indicate that a dental procedure or office system needs improvement.

Dental history proves that continual reassessment often benefits patient and provider.

Compound impressions might still work—but poorly, compared to present-day impression materials. The first composite restorations initially were esthetically pleasing, but they did not compare in longevity and function to a well-placed amalgam. Yet today, in the hands of an experienced clinician, even posterior composites can be expected to give many years of excellent service.

The 2,000 RPM of dentistry's pre-high-speed turbine handpieces produced classic cavity and crown preparations, but at the expense of operator and patient fatigue. What practitioner today would ever conceive of using a slow-speed handpiece to prepare a tooth for a crown? All of these advances were produced by individuals who constantly assessed what they were doing and asked: Can it be improved?

That same attitude—a willingness to seek the proverbial "better mousetrap"—needs to be expanded to the major systems that support professional dentistry.

I offer as an example the dental education system. Too much time has elapsed without an in-depth evaluation of the system responsible for dentistry's future. It's been 34 years since Hollinshead published the Survey of Dentistry—a comprehensive report that had a major impact on how students were educated and how dental care was delivered. While four subsequent reports have added critical recommendations for dental education, there has been no assessment for at least the last decade.

Obviously, a review of dental education was warranted.

That need has been fulfilled. Under the auspices of the Institute of Medicine, with input from literally all of dentistry's constituents, a national report, "Dental Education at the Crossroads: Challenges and Change," has just been released. In this issue, we are pleased to present to our readers an abbreviated summary of that report specifically directed to dental practitioners' interests.

The report concludes that dental education, while not broken, will require fixing if the profession is to continue serving the oral health needs of U.S. citizens.

Among the changes called for in the report is an enhanced curriculum to meet the medical needs of an aging population. Many schools already have moved in that direction. One midwestern school, for example, soon will require all dental students to spend three months in a medicine clerkship working side by side with medical students.

While the report did not call for a single medical/dental profession, it did suggest that experimentation with different models of education was necessary. One such experiment with potential major ramifications for dental education may be getting under way in the near future. That program is based on the rationale that dentists of the future must transform themselves from oral health professionals into "oral physicians."

If implemented, this adventuresome proposal would train oral health professionals to competency levels warranting both D.M.D. and M.D. de-

> The IOM report concludes that dental education, while not "broken," will require "fixing" if the profession is to continue serving the oral health needs of U.S. citizens.

grees. To accomplish this, a five-year curriculum is suggested. The first three years would encompass all course work and clinical rotations in the standard medical curriculum. Two additional years would be devoted to dental subjects. The program would culminate with the awarding of dual degrees.

Many questions need to be addressed before this type of program gains wide acceptance by the educational community. Nevertheless, all types of research are needed; only through multiple investigative efforts will a significant body of knowledge become available for debate, discussion and eventual implementation.

The high cost of dental education, while not underscored in this abbreviated IOM/JADA presentation, was noted in the main document. It concluded that this was a problem requiring the attention of the entire professional community. With the costs of tuition, books, instruments and living expenses now exceeding $40,000 yearly at some private institutions, dental education soon may be accessible only to the sons and daughters of the very rich.

And public-supported universities may not be much cheaper. Under pressure from state legislatures, dental schools are being asked to assume more of their costs. Present mechanisms for increasing dental school revenues are student tuition and patient fees. Both components have limits, and those limits already may have been exceeded.

The IOM report recommends a year of postgraduate training for all students. Presently, these posi-tions go primarily to students who rank high in their classes. A universal requirement for a post-graduate year would upgrade the entry skill levels of emerging practitioners. But funding for this fifth year must not come from the student's pocket. Perhaps the innovative service programs previously suggested in this space could be used to fund this additional education.

One of the most important IOM recommendations relates to the number of dentists. Its study group found no rationale for increasing or decreasing the production of dentists. Rather, it stated, "If shortages in dental services should develop, responses should emphasize more productive use of allied personnel."

The IOM committee's recommendation has great merit. Today's dental practitioners claim excess capacity to deliver dental services. That potential should be tested to its upper limits before any increase in number of dentists is considered.

Other IOM recommendations, such as the development of new clinical education models and the need for dental schools to become integral partners in the university community, need immediate attention. Their implementation may mean survival!

Whatever the eventual outcome of the IOM recommendations, the dental profession must applaud the efforts of those who participated in this lengthy and difficult endeavor. They realize that for a profession to remain viable, it must constantly reassess what it is doing and ask: Can it be done better? ∎

# The marketplace will decide

*Originally published in JADA 1995 125: 274-278.*

Although last year's federal initiative for health system reform failed to garner any appreciable support, one of its major components, managed care, appears to be flourishing.

Substituting for government intervention are the health care insurers. These savvy entrepreneurs already have altered the medical delivery system for major segments of our population—using the rubric of managed care to gain fiscal control.

Dental care also has been targeted for inclusion in their managed care empire. But dental market penetration so far has been limited, compared to medical care. Recent data from an ADA survey indicate that just a third of dental practices participate in managed care programs. On average, only 8 percent of patients in U.S. dental practices are enrolled in managed care programs.

Despite this major lack of dental recruits to date, an aggressive strategy for enhanced market invasion has thrust the subject of managed care programs into the dental spotlight. Dentists want and expect information before deciding whether managed care participation is for them.

And well they should. Ill-informed dental practitioners, faced with various managed care opportunities, could make irrevocable and damaging economic practice decisions. Furthermore, because of inherent differences between medical and dental care delivery, dentistry could be even more vulnerable than medicine to the negative aspects of managed care programs.

Comprehending the reason for that requires an understanding of the medical care marketplace. In this economic arena, managed care is synonymous with managed costs. Those that finance medical care employ an industrial model that places production at the lowest cost level possible. For the delivery of medical care, this has been achieved successfully by cost shifting from specialists to generalists.

In many instances this policy makes sense. Why have a cardiologist monitor hypertensive patients if the same service can be accomplished by primary care physicians at lower cost? On the other hand, who wants a primary care physician performing angioplasty on them? No matter, in today's medical environment increasingly more medical treatment is being delivered by physicians who command lesser fees than specialists.

Compared to medicine, dentistry presents a totally different practitioner hierarchy for its delivery of dental services. Generalists, not specialists, dominate the profession. Unless a dental practice is heavily dependent on auxiliaries, attempts to cost-shift will not be productive.

Furthermore, cost efficiencies in providing dental care come mainly through reductions in fixed overhead expenses. And that won't be easily accomplished, since dentists already are paying increased sums for infection control, office materials and dental personnel. For those dentists considering managed care participation, increases in net income will depend heavily on new patient availability and the physical abilities of dentists to work longer hours.

Despite these caveats, don't expect dental managed care offerings to disappear. Managed care programs flourish on excess capacity, and dentists continue to indicate that they could absorb significant numbers of new patients.

In addition, present federal antitrust laws restrict the creation of new delivery systems that might allow dentists to offer competitive alterna-

> **Barring any outside interference, informed dental providers and consumers will determine whether managed care dental programs are worthy additions to the dental delivery system.**

tives to the managed care offerings of health insurers.

Conversely, don't expect managed care programs to gain a major market share of dental services. Successful growth of managed care programs requires that a majority of the population depends on insurers for financing care. Today, the number of dentally insured is just over 50 percent. That percentage has shown minimum growth—and, absent any major federal intervention, actually may decline in the future.

Other factors that might impede the expansion of managed care include a reluctance by dental patients to become part of a captive patient group— a major requirement for managed care success. Many dental patients, long accustomed to paying substantial deductibles, co-insurance and caps on certain dental procedures, may forgo participation in a managed care program if their present dentists are not participants.

The marriage of the art and science of dentistry to the business of dentistry has not always been a productive union. In the past, production costs and profit margins were terms reserved for industry, not as necessary components of dental fee calculations or of determining whether dentists should enter into contractual agreements with dental care insurers.

Still, the marketplace for dental services has changed. No longer can the business side of dentistry be regarded as a separate activity. Business and science must function in harmony if the dental professions' mandate to serve the oral health needs of the public is to be actualized.

The acceptance or rejection of new economic/ service programs should rest on marketplace judgments that evaluate cost and quality of service. In that regard, and barring any outside interference, informed dental providers and consumers will determine whether managed care dental programs are worthy additions to the dental delivery system. ∎

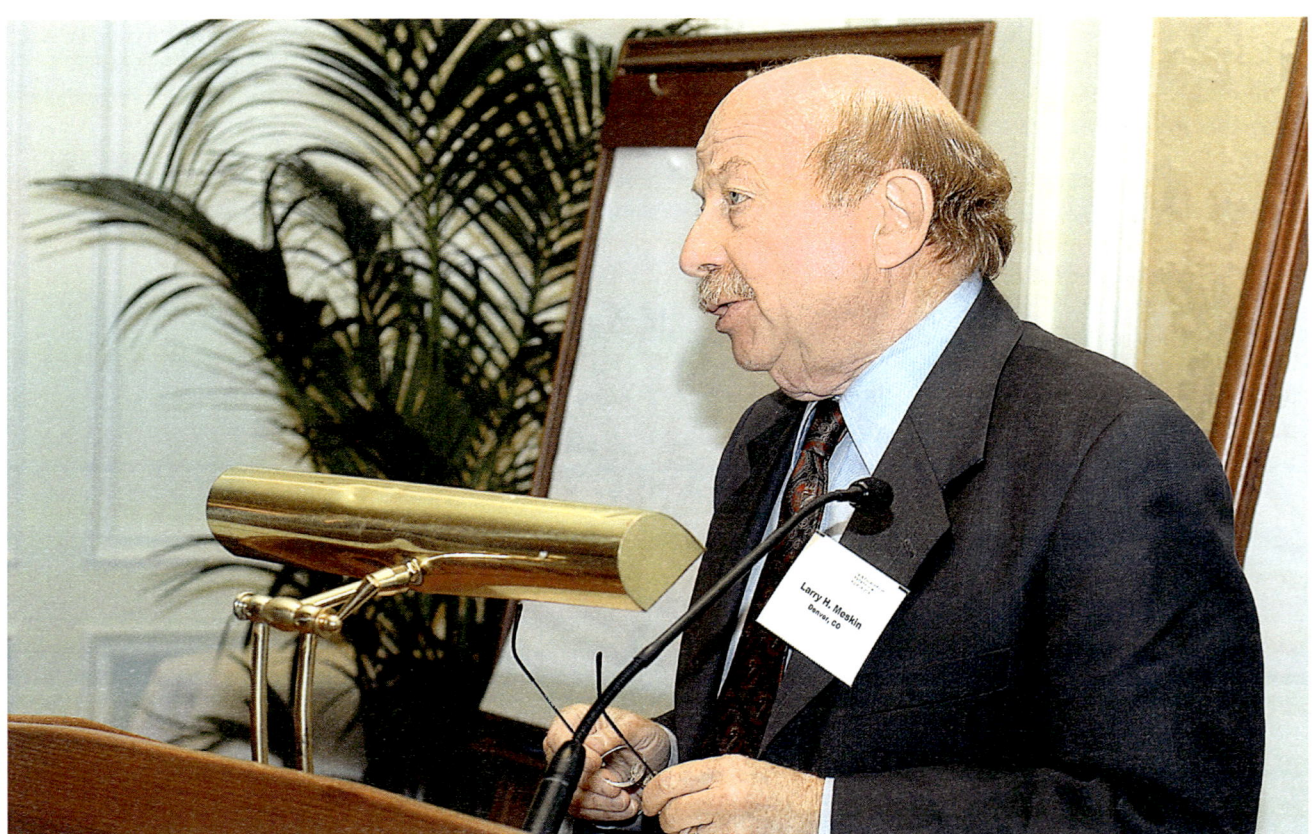

Dr. Meskin speaking at a dental meeting.

# If two's company, three may be a crowd

*Originally published in JADA 1995 125: 402-406.*

House Speaker Newt Gingrich and his Republicans aren't the only ones holding a "Contract with America." More than 100 years ago, the fledgling profession of dentistry adopted a social contract with the American people. Accepting responsibility for the oral health and well-being of Americans—and placing the importance of health above financial gain or other interests—the profession was granted a virtual monopoly as "sole provider" of those services.

To fulfill its part of the bargain, society has provided regulatory structures that prosecute unlicensed people who claim skills in treating dental disease. Dentistry has steadfastly kept its promise by actively promoting preventive solutions—water fluoridation, sealants and others—to dental diseases.

The success of this partnership centers on a dental delivery system based on the patient's free choice of a dentist and a fee-for-service payment mechanism. For years this system proved effective in providing U.S. citizens the highest level of dental care in the world.

It is with great concern, therefore, that we observe major organizational changes in the dental marketplace that threaten dentistry's ethical responsibility to promote patient welfare above all other considerations.

These changes began in the mid-1950s when the first dental capitation programs emerged. The philosophy behind capitation as a way to deliver dental care was commendable: give practitioners incentives to prevent disease, rather than treat it. Capitation proponents theorized that by treating patients' oral needs and monitoring their progress, more people could receive care. But this concept meant giving up free choice and abandoning fee for service. Not surprisingly, it attracted few converts and many critics.

The next test for dentistry's unique provider/

**Perhaps it is time to re-examine the role of the third party in the dental delivery system.**

patient relationship came in the 1960s with attempts to provide health services, including dentistry, through a national health insurance program. That initiative failed, but financial assistance for those needing dental care gained support. Labor unions and other organizations negotiating benefits packages started asking for dental benefits. By the 1980s, almost half the population had at least some of its dental care paid by a third party.

The results were dramatic: affordable, comprehensive dental care for millions of Americans—and full appointment books for dentists. But even positive changes carried a price. No longer was the relationship between dentist and patient purely one-to-one. Third parties with varying degrees of monetary authority now could affect a dentist's judgment or a patient's needs by denying payment for treatment.

Many dentists refused to accept third-party payments. But for the majority, the willingness of insurers to support fee for service and free choice of a dentist outweighed the negative effects of sharing patient care decisions with a third party.

Until recently, that is.

The chaotic marketplace dominating medical care services has started to spill over into dentistry, causing great concern and trepidation among many dentists. Dentistry uses a far simpler mechanism for delivering its services. It adjusts with difficulty to medical managed care models that reward and penalize according to rules that don't apply to dental care—rules that could lead to rationing of services or offering treatment plans that compromise quality.

That dentists are concerned is clear from their responses to a recent study[1] of the ethical problems they face in their everyday practices. Many respondents noted increased pressures to "join a PPO or similar organization to maintain patient flow."

They also expressed frustration with what they saw as inadequate payments from third parties that often placed them in conflict with patients.

The threat to the provider/patient relationship has prompted at least one state board to act. In 1994, the California Board of Dental Examiners added Section 1685 to the state dental practice act. This provision states that "it is unprofessional conduct for a person ... to require, either directly or through an office policy, or knowingly permit the delivery of dental care that discourages necessary treatment ... as determined by the standards of practice in the community."

Organized dentistry, acting through the ADA Council on Ethics, Bylaws and Judicial Affairs, also has addressed the ethical aspects of managed care. In a recent statement on the subject, the council concluded that while the method of health care delivery may change, "dentists must not allow these demands ... [managed care] to interfere with the patient's right to select a treatment option ... nor interfere with the free exercise of their [the dentist's] professional judgment ... or their duty to make appropriate referrals if indicated." The statement goes on to remind dentists that "contract obligations do not excuse them from their ethical duty to put their patient's welfare first."

These three examples of concern about the ethical implications of health market change serve as vivid reminders of the intense pressures being ex-erted on the dentist/patient relationship. The marketplace appears unrelenting—only more tension can be anticipated. There is growing urgency for action.

But what actions are appropriate? Legislation that ensures patient protection, coupled with antitrust relief, could help. But would that be sufficient?

Perhaps it is time to reexamine the role of the third party in the dental delivery system. Is there truly a benefit to their involvement? Or has that involvement become so intrusive as to compromise dentistry's own contract with society?

Dr. Jack Brown's article in this month's JADA uses a sophisticated simulation model to present "what-if" projections of the potential impact of society's losing 75 percent of its dental insurance. The prediction: a 5 percent to 7 percent reduction in dentists' gross income, plus minor reductions in U.S. oral health status.

Modern society would reject such outcomes. But that's now. If the future brings even greater challenges to dentistry's delivery system—if patient care is jeopardized—then perhaps it's time to affirm that if two's company, three may be a crowd. ∎

1. Kress GC, Hasegawa TK Jr. A survey of ethical dilemmas and practical problems encountered by practicing dentists. Final Report to American Fund for Dental Health. Chicago:American Dental Association; June 1994.

# Information, please

*Originally published in JADA 1995 125: 540-546.*

With the electronic revolution in full swing, it's striking how few dentists have sampled the high-speed lanes of the information superhighway.

In fact, most appear to be avoiding the highway altogether, presumably choosing the comfort and safety of previously traveled roads. As evidence, note their low utilization of Medline, the primary bibliographic data base for medical and dental information.

Medline can be easily and cheaply accessed from almost any modem-equipped computer. Yet, out of 100,000-plus subscribers, the Library of Medicine was able to identify only 852 dentists. This low enrollment is perplexing considering that of the 3,500 or so journals in the Medline data base, over 400 (12 percent) are dental or dental related.

Underscoring this lack of interest was the poor attendance of dental educators and researchers at a recent American Association for Dental Research (AADR) sponsored session on information retrieval. Fewer than 100 out of a possible 2,000 registrants showed up to hear the latest on information retrieval from the director of the National Medical Library.

What accounts for the low interest in computer-accessed information? Are dentists technically inept—unable to use their computers? Hardly! Besides, this lack of demand for research information is not confined to computerized data bases.

Consider the following:

From 10,000 invitations sent to dentists in a six-state region, only about 50 dentists chose to attend a symposium sponsored by the National Institute of Dental Research, the AADR and the ADA. Titled "Scientific Frontiers in Clinical Dentistry," this one-day educational offering included some of America's top dental researchers who translated their research discoveries into clinical practice applications. The tuition cost, subsidized by the organizations, was far below market.

The few who attended were treated to presentations in several permanent areas: pain management, new restorative materials, advances in periodontics, and when and how to use endosseous implants in children and adolescents. As in the previous example, symposium organizers were disappointed and puzzled by the paltry turnout of dental practitioners.

Why had dentists passed up this opportunity to enhance their knowledge? Was this poor response related in some way to the equally small number of dentists using the superhighway for information gathering?

Perhaps there is little new information to be gained. As the de facto world leader for dentistry, U.S. dental practice sets the standards. When at the pinnacle, why bother to change or alter a good thing?

Such an attitude would be professionally unacceptable. The ADA Principles of Ethics do not allow for status quo. Practitioners have an obligation to continually seek and assimilate information that might benefit their patients.

Besides, there is no lack of new information. Note a few highlights from the research abstracts presented at the 1995 AADR meeting:

- New methods to treat burning mouth syndrome;
- Fluoride exposure and osteosarcoma;
- Value of double gloving;
- Mercury release during ultrasonic scaling of amalgam;
- Relationship between price and quality of dental service;
- Incidence and consequences of tooth fracture;
- Three-year study of home bleaching.

When and how will this information reach the practitioner?

Dental leaders are concerned that the mecha-

> **Dental leaders are concerned that the mechanism to transfer scientific knowledge from researcher to practitioner is defective.**

nism to transfer scientific knowledge from researcher to practitioner is defective. All agree it needs immediate attention. Long delays in the transfer process are proving detrimental to patient treatment and health outcomes.

Practitioners generally do not know how to access new, clinically relevant research findings. Meanwhile, researchers concerned about peer review are not able to present their material in publications readily accessible or understandable to the average dental practitioner.

No wonder, then, that dental practitioners aren't breaking down the doors to enter information highways or even attend programs featuring researchers. Until the researcher/practitioner language barrier is eliminated, interpreters will be needed.

Research on how dentists become aware of new information is clear: the dental journal is their primary source. And national readership surveys indicate that JADA, the flagship publication of the ADA, is the most widely and well-read professional dental journal in America.

While this is heartening, it also imposes a continuing responsibility to find and evaluate hundreds of scholarly research contributions for potential clinical relevancy. Once identified, the science transfer process begins. Solicit, peer-review, edit and publish in a timely manner. Regardless of subject material, the overriding editorial philosophy remains to bring to JADA readers current articles of clinical interest in a readable format.

The recent establishment of a JADA advisory board consisting solely of practicing dentists is a further step toward ensuring science transfer. We expect that the board's clinical experience will provide meaningful assistance to the editorial staff in assessing and selecting scientific contributions.

Other potential JADA additions to enhance science transfer are under discussion. They include commentaries by noted clinicians preceding selected research articles; short clinical research briefs drawn from papers presented at research meetings; modifications in the abstract format that emphasize clinical implications; and, perhaps in the not-too-distant future, an electronic bulletin board that would allow personal communication between researcher and clinician.

Information, please? Turn to JADA. ■

# Dancing with regulators

*Originally published in JADA 1995 125: 706-708.*

If you believe in the tooth fairy, then maybe—just maybe—you can expect some relief from the onerous regulations that have plagued recent dental practice. The Republican Congress, especially the House of Representatives, is flexing its muscles, and the regulatory agencies are among its targets.

A $16 million reduction in the Occupational Safety and Health Administration's budget already has been approved. An additional $3.5 million cut could be forthcoming, owing to the remarks of a high-ranking OSHA official who publicly proposed that the agency could wait out any congressionally imposed regulatory freeze and then proceed with its rule making as it wishes.

This sort of attitude has undermined public support for regulatory activities. Regardless of how well-intentioned they may be, their compulsion to regulate every conceivable circumstance has overwhelmed their constituents.

The celebrated case of the tooth fairy's premature demise illustrated just how shell-shocked the "regulated" dentist had become. Although no regulation was ever instituted, existing OSHA rules were incorrectly interpreted by many dentists to mean that they could not return an extracted deciduous tooth to its owner. Fortunately for the children, OSHA and the ADA were able to set the record straight.

And there are thousands of other examples of bureaucrats, who, determined to cover all contingencies through explicit rules and regulations, have alienated many people and groups. Indeed, in a world consumed by bureaucracy and regulation, where we have committees for committees and supervising supervisors, it's no wonder that Philip Howard's national bestseller, "The Death Of Common Sense,"[1] has become required reading for those dissatisfied with the machinations of government regulations.

> **Until common sense prevails, financial and administrative support for Association efforts to rein in the regulators must continue.**

Mr. Howard describes an almost endless stream of regulations that impede rather than facilitate—and where attempts to apply common sense are simply dismissed. Although not cited in his book, dentistry has its own litany of bureaucratic rule making to parallel Mr. Howard's examples.

OSHA recently cited a dentist for several minor infractions, including failure to correctly label the X-ray developer and fixer bath. Instead of using the OSHA method, the dentist substituted color coding. Only after ADA lawyers demonstrated to OSHA that the dentist's staff could easily identify the substances did OSHA relent. A victory for the dentist, yes. But without legal assistance, the dentist would have been at a serious disadvantage. OSHA rarely is willing to withdraw a penalty.

With the scales tipped heavily in favor of regulation, the "gotcha" mentality of the enforcers can run amok—as a well-meaning dentist in Seattle found out. After scheduling a patient with HIV for a late afternoon appointment, the dentist was cited for noncompliance with the Rehabilitation Act of 1973. The dentist based his decision on the professional judgment that the appointed time would allow for the full effects of disinfectants on aerosols and provide for unlimited "downtime," as needed.

Rationalizing that all patients are to be assumed infectious, the Office of Civil Rights maintained that the afternoon scheduling was discriminatory. The patient should have been scheduled without consideration for his infectious state. No matter that the OCR commended the dentist for not denying services to persons with HIV.

Since dentistry's professional mandate is to offer access for all citizens, this citation becomes one more glaring example of how bureaucracy jeopardizes professional judgment. If the benefits outweigh the consequences, then the OCR commendation should have ended the matter.

The regulated are clamoring for change, and the politicians are responding. Even President Clinton appears supportive. He recently said, "We want a government that … shrinks bureaucracy. I think government can discard volume after volume of rules and instead set clear goals and challenge people to come up with their own ways to meet them."

The agencies are hearing the message. The ADA's Washington efforts have been rewarded by changes in OSHA policy. A new OSHA edict to cease conducting random visits to dental offices has been greeted as a solid indication of progress. OSHA's willingness to handle most complaints by "phone and fax" has drawn similar approval.

However, this is not the time to celebrate the demise of regulation. Looming on the horizon are proposed OSHA rules covering ergonomics in the dental office. OSHA estimates that the costs to small businesses (including dental practices) to comply with its proposals would not exceed $233 million.

Recalling the reliability of earlier OSHA cost estimates for infection control, don't bet on it.

And so the dance of the regulators and the regulated continues. It may be naive to view recent political events as evidence that understanding between the two might be achieved. But some rationality introduced into the pronouncements of regulators seeking absolute compliance certainly would be welcome.

Such agreements would not come easily. The regulatory system that President Clinton now characterizes as having "grown into a dense jungle of rules and regulations" drew its initial support from well-meaning reformers who wished to create a better society by offering regulations to cover every possible situation. Present members of regulatory agencies are not likely to willingly alter those earlier constructs.

Thus, until common sense prevails, financial and administrative support for Association efforts to rein in the regulators must continue. Success can be claimed only when the full range of professional decision making is returned to the dental practitioner. ∎

1. Howard PK. The death of common sense: how law is suffocating America. New York: Random House; 1995.

# MSAs: back to the future

*Originally published in JADA 1995 125: 820-822.*

A new concept to control health care costs is gaining momentum, and it could have major implications for dentistry. Modeled after the tax-exempt features of the individual retirement account, medical savings accounts, or MSAs, have caught the fancy of House Speaker Newt Gingrich and his associates. With that kind of support, congressional action is a distinct possibility.

Convinced that health care spending can be slowed only by introducing more competition in health care choices, MSA supporters see this mechanism as a way to put the patient back into the decision-making equation and to control costs at the same time.

They fault third-party health payers with pushing up the costs of care and cite studies showing that over the last three decades, out-of-pocket spending for health care, relative to personal income, did not increase, while total health care spending rose 300 percent. Rationalizing that "my insurance will cover it," the consumer has had few incentives to examine the cost of health care or demand spending accountability.

As proposed, MSAs would operate like IRAs: consumers deposit money in tax-exempt accounts and pay for health services directly out of those accounts. By returning control over health care spending to the consumer, any decisions to ration health services would take place at the doctor-patient level, free of the influences of for-profit corporations mainly concerned about a healthy bottom line.

Employees would benefit in the following manner. Employers would purchase high-deductibility insurance policies and place the savings from present health policy premiums into individual MSAs. Employees could then spend any amount of their MSA for health care until they reach the deductibility level of their health policy. At that point,

> **By returning control over health spending to the consumer, any decisions to ration health services would take place at the doctor-patient level.**

their insurance would be activated.

Unlike present flex plans, which send unused employee health withholdings back to the company coffers, the MSAs would roll over savings into employee-owned accounts. After a defined period of time, the employee could do one of two things with the savings:
- roll them into his or her IRA;
- purchase insurance for the future, either health care coverage for periods of unemployment or prepaid dental care for retirement.

Even without the tax incentives, a number of firms already applying the MSA concept report enthusiastic responses from their employees. When given the choice between the traditional health payment plans and the MSA program, employees have overwhelmingly chosen the MSAs. With no restrictions in choice of provider, employees have demonstrated their interest in cost and quality.

MSAs also can assist the self-employed. Right now they can deduct only 25 percent of their health insurance premiums. With a tax-exempt MSA, however, those in the lowest federal tax bracket would be able to deduct at least 35 percent of their health costs when Social Security and state and local taxes are considered. A higher-income self-employed worker could achieve tax deductions of 50 percent or greater—a significant offset if major medical or dental expenses are anticipated.

MSAs have their detractors. Managed care operators, HMOs and other large insurers see them as a roadblock to achieving dominance in the health field. Some politicians claim that the country cannot afford the loss of revenue resulting from MSA tax breaks. And some health policy types are worried that people might put off necessary care to build their MSA capital.

Considering that the MSA incentive is to save,

not spend, that last argument may have some validity for dental care. No one knows how consumers who make routine preventive visits under their traditional dental plan—especially those who believe they are in good dental health—will respond to MSA incentives. In order to save money, some might reduce their dental visits. This behavior could translate into higher dental insurance rates for those whose major dental needs are best served by maintaining their traditional dental insurance.

Since the potential for adverse selection is a distinct possibility, MSA supporters should qualify their endorsement until more experience with this concept is available. Conversely, MSA critics should take note that 50 percent of Americans have minimal or no dental insurance. If affordable dental care is made available to them through tax incentives, many out-of-pocket dental payers may be persuaded to seek more dental services.

The MSA concept is just starting to evolve as a way to control health care costs. Congressional debate is expected to focus on whether to grant MSA's the same tax exemptions presently enjoyed by traditional employee/employer health benefits. Meanwhile, seven states have already jump-started the process by granting MSAs a tax exemption.

Recent ADA policy endorses the MSA concept. If MSAs live up to their potential, they represent an opportunity for dentistry to return to a dental care delivery system in which doctor and patient, not a third party, decide treatment and fee. Few would object to such a development. ∎

# Abusive legislation

*Originally published in JADA 1995 125: 1080-1082.*

As the anti-regulation Republican juggernaut moves forward, dentists are reveling in its wake. And well they should. In just a few months the no-knock OSHA dental visits have been replaced by a more civilized phone and fax approach. Perhaps even more important, OSHA has dropped its initiative to promulgate ergonomic workplace regulations. Further easing of rules and regulations can be expected as efforts to reduce government influence continue.

Ah, finally the good life! But not for children who are or will be victims of abuse and neglect. The recent failure of the House to reauthorize the Child Abuse Prevention and Treatment Act, or CAPTA, may compromise the ability of dentists and other health providers to fulfill their mandated roles in reporting abuse and neglect of children.

The current law, scheduled to expire this September 30, requires health professionals to report suspected cases of child abuse and provides them with a statutory guarantee of immunity from prosecution, plus confidentiality of disclosure. While the new legislation still mandates reporting abuse, it strips away all of the existing protective clauses.

Substituted for the expiring CAPTA legislation is the recently passed welfare reform bill, H.R. 4. This all-encompassing welfare reform measure eliminates The National Center on Child Abuse and Neglect, placing future responsibility for child protection on the states.

Reformers believe that by returning authority and funds to states they will eliminate the massive federal red tape and place resources where they can best be utilized. While past experience with block grants to states has been equivocal, the crisis over the national debt justifies changing the way business is conducted.

But not for all programs!

> **By not including professional immunity and confidentiality of disclosure, H.R. 4 sends an ominous message to health professionals— report abuse and neglect, yes, but at your own risk.**

Well-intentioned efforts sometimes miss the mark, and that seems to be the case with H.R. 4. By not including professional immunity and confidentiality of disclosure, this legislation sends an ominous message to health professionals: report abuse and neglect, yes, but at your own risk.

Hardly an approach to encourage professional intervention. Those who defend this action point to state laws that presently offer immunity and disclosure provisions. But these laws also are being challenged. At least three states have introduced legislation to eliminate these clauses.

Supporting obstructions to professional involvement comes from such groups as Victims Of Child Abuse Laws, or VOCAL, which is upset by what it considers intrusions on the rights as parents. VOCAL argues that, unlike criminal law, where an individual is considered innocent until proven otherwise, child-abuse claims begin with an assumption of guilt. Although small in membership, VOCAL has become a major lobbying force.

In fact, the group appears to have captured some major new support. Federal legislation directed at further undermining the health professional's duty to report cases of abuse and neglect has been introduced in the House of Representatives. Titled the "Parental Rights and Responsibility Act," it purports to eliminate all state laws that grant immunity or confidentiality to professionals reporting cases of abuse. Its passage would impede the reporting process to the detriment of abused children.

To halt implementation of legislation that in itself is abusive will require a major lobbying effort from the ADA during Senate debate on the reauthorization of CAPTA. ADA attention should center on the conference committee, whose deliberations will shape the way professionals treat child abuse.

A positive legislative outcome will allow the ADA

to continue promoting its ethical mandate that requires dentists to detect and report incidences of child abuse and neglect.

And dentistry has been attentive to that goal, says PANDA (Prevent Abuse and Neglect through Dental Awareness), a highly successful voluntary education program designed by dentists and implemented in 24 states. PANDA notes that since its inception, dental reporting of child abuse has risen 60 percent while reporting of abuse by all professionals has risen only 6 percent.

If adverse legislation prevails, this commendable record could be dramatically altered. Research indicates that the fear of legal liability will have a negative impact on professional willingness to report suspected abuse and neglect.

The reporting process must be enhanced, not inhibited. National figures estimate that almost 3 million children were reported to social or protective services for suspected abuse in 1992. Up to 2,000 children, mostly under 4 years of age, die each year from abuse, and thousand are seriously injured.

Dr. Henry Kempe, the pediatrician who first described the battered-child syndrome, often said, "Abusive parents love their children very much but not very well."

These children and their parents need your help. Legislation that would inhibit the professional's ability to break the chain of child abuse is unacceptable. As I stated in an earlier editorial, "As the point of first contact for many victims of abuse, if not us, then whom?" ∎

# Invest now for the future

*Originally published in JADA 1995 125: 1200-1202.*

**M**illions of U.S. teens might be questioning the safety of going to dentists if the results of research reported in the Journal of the American Medical Association prove to be correct on a large scale. In an investigation designed to identify factors that affect adolescents' decisions to seek health care, the entire ninth grade student body of the Philadelphia public school system was surveyed.

Dentists should be disturbed by the students' responses.

The youngsters expressed major fears about the risk of contracting AIDS from their dentists. Their concerns, apparently stemming from the media coverage of the Kimberly Bergalis case, appear genuine. Ironically, they appear indifferent to the HIV risk of their own sexual encounters.

These teens must be shown that dental visits are safe and that dentists do not represent a threat to their well-being. After all, while not exactly listed in the "things to do this week" section of daily newspapers, a yearly visit to the dentist has become a common and safe activity for the majority of Americans.

Or at least it was regarded as safe until news of six patients, apparently all infected with their dentist's HIV, gave the public second thoughts about the safety of dental visits. The New York Times and television news magazines, some with audiences of more than 20 million, provided ongoing credibility to speculation that a visit to a dentist just might ... well, you know.

Rejection of nationwide HIV testing of health professionals on ethical and economic grounds did little to ease the concern of dental patients or those contemplating a dental visit.

Almost immediately, national surveys showed a drop in the numbers of individuals who considered a dental visit very safe. A professional media campaign explaining how dentists protected patients

> **We cannot permit teens to enter a parenting stage still concerned about dental office safety.**

from the remote chance of becoming infected by AIDS was needed, and the ADA responded.

Titled ADA C.A.R.E.S., the Association's nationwide education campaign provided the public with a list of infection control procedures that patients should look for during a dental visit. A second facet was directed to dentists to enhance their effectiveness in communicating infection control procedures to their patients.

It's doubtful if any ADA public education program has been more successful than ADA C.A.R.E.S. A multimedia blitz, starting with a "Good Morning, America" kickoff, immediately began rebuilding dentistry's credibility. The ADA message—"We (dentists) are not hiding anything; come visit us, and we will show you exactly how we are protecting you"—worked.

As revealed in a recent poll, six out of 10 adults now agree it is very safe to go to a dentist—an 11 percent jump from pre-C.A.R.E.S. campaign figures. At the same time, the percentage of concerned adults who thought the dental office visit would be only "somewhat safe" dropped 11 percentage points.

The ADA's C.A.R.E.S. program not only received accolades from a satisfied profession but also was bestowed a Silver Anvil award by the Public Relations Society of America. This honor, considered by members of the public relations community to be as prestigious as an Oscar, was a team effort involving members of ADA's Communications Division, the ADA Council on Communications and various other ADA volunteers and staff.

How sweet success is—well, not always. The ADA C.A.R.E.S. program targeted only adults. Now a similar effort, tailored to the needs of America's teens, should be mounted. The use of MTV and other visual and print media backed by specially crafted messages meaningful to these youngsters will be essential for success.

For content direction, communication experts should consider the ninth graders' list of concerns. Specifically, these young people want to observe whether the health providers wash their hands, wear gloves, remove instruments from sterile packages, maintain a clean office environment and present evidence that they are HIV-negative.

So when will the ADA develop a C.A.R.E.S. initiative for adolescents? ADA staff say they're willing, but special materials and programs tailored to adolescents cost money. Unfortunately, two programs that addressed the health education needs of adolescents were removed from the Communications Division's 1996 budget package—not due to lack of importance, but to strict attention to balancing the budget.

Unfortunately, this decision could have a permanent impact on the long-term dental behaviors of a generation that within a decade will be creating new family units. We cannot permit these teens to enter a parenting stage still concerned about dental office safety. Supplementary ADA funds need to be found to ensure that this doesn't happen.

Let's not look back in 10 years and say, "Why didn't we?" Now is the time to invest. Suggest a supplemental appropriation to your delegates to the 1995 House—or to your trustee. It will be money well spent. ∎

# A good deal for all

*Originally published in JADA 1995 125: 1330-1332.*

There is no such thing as "free" dental care. Eventually, someone pays—a fact often lost on health plan administrators. To them, a healthy bottom line, achieved through reduced fees and service limits, represents business as usual. Not so for more and more dentists who are finding themselves in the difficult position of having to treat patients without sufficient resources.

No wonder, then, that dentists yearn for a dental delivery system in which they and their patients, not a third party, decide how, when and where to treat.

Dentists need search no further. This dental oasis already exists. Through direct reimbursement, or DR, a small but growing number of employees and their dependents are receiving quality dental care from the dentists of their choice. They pay the dentist for services rendered and their company reimburses them.

Sound familiar? It should. Until the advent of dental indemnity plans, DR was the prevailing contract between dentists and patients. Now it's back as a professionally supported, viable alternative to the new cost-containment dental programs.

The appeal of DR to organized dentistry is understandable, but what about employers and their employees? Why should they change from their existing indemnity programs?

Employers would realize considerable savings by switching from traditional indemnity plans, with 19 to 29 percent overheads, to DR plans, which typically carry only a 3 to 6 percent administrative cost. Imagine a world in which dental insurance claims have been eliminated, patient records remain in the dental office, coordination of benefits is no longer an issue—and there's no one to fight with

> **Imagine a world in which dental insurance claims have been eliminated, patient records remain in the dental office, coordination of benefits is no longer an issue–and there's no one to fight with over denial of benefits. Can you think of a better medicine for reducing dental hypertension?**

over denial of benefits. Can you think of a better medicine for reducing dental hypertension?

DR offers all this and more. Employees choose their own dentists, know exactly how much they have available to spend for dental care, and, even more important, can direct their funds to areas of dental care need that have been denied in the past.

Testimonials from existing DR participants indicate high levels of satisfaction. The city of Greensboro's benefits manager stated, "Our employees are very pleased with the dental program. We've been able to apply the savings from DR and give our employees an even better benefit. ... Of all the employee benefit programs we offer, DR gets the fewest complaints."

Direct reimbursement appears, at least on paper, to be the universal antidote for dentistry's third-party problems. The question is: Why hasn't it gained greater acceptance?

It's true, DR's market share is minuscule when compared to the total pot of insured dental care: perhaps 1 to 2 percent and growing very slowly. The American Association of Orthodontics, one of the strongest active proponents of DR, claims that about 630,000 employees and their dependents enjoy DR as a result of AAO's promotions. The ADA has no way of placing numbers on its efforts, because most of its success has been in conjunction with constituent, component and other dental groups.

Both ADA and AAO work in the same manner, offering consultative services to dentists and dental societies who wish to promote DR. For example, the ADA supplies information to employers interested in DR programs. It offers a slide/tape presentation, IBM software, individualized employer actuarial data and on-going telephone assistance.

The AAO has made significant contributions to educate dentists in DR marketing techniques. It recently advanced a proposal to the ADA to initiate a joint venture between the ADA and the U.S. chambers of commerce to promote DR through the chamber networks across the country.

While these efforts are commendable, they haven't visibly affected the dental marketplace. And they probably won't if voluntary efforts by dentists continue to be the mainstay of the marketing campaign.

Dentists are trained to perform dentistry—not to sell employers on the advantages of dental care plans. Professional benefit consultants and brokers with a profit incentive need to be knocking at employers' doors.

Besides actively identifying and selling DR, benefit experts at the table will help address employer concerns, such as who watches over dental fees? Monitors treatment? Assesses quality? Dentists have the answers. But coming from them, those answers could appear self-serving.

Recognizing the need for a coordinated nationwide effort to market DR and other free-choice dental plans, a new entity, the Alliance for Dental Reimbursement Programs, is making its way onto the DR playing field. This non-profit group's membership includes dental practitioners, dental associations (including the ADA), the dental trades and employee benefit consultants.

The Alliance will place DR marketing in the hands of professionals where it belongs. Obviously there will be a charge, but by reducing the costly and burdensome administration of today's dental care programs, mutual gains for employer, employee and dentist will follow.

At a time when it seems we have become captives of third-party insurers, there appears to be a way out. Support DR. It's a good deal for all. ∎

# Follow the leader

*Originally published in JADA 1995 125: 1466-1470.*

Communications giant AT&T recently shocked the business world with its dramatic reorganization announcement. By deciding to conduct business in a totally different manner, AT&T has sent a wake-up call to its competitors: business as usual won't suffice in the changing world of telecommunications.

Dental education needs to heed that message.

Faced with a seemingly unending escalation in costs, dental education needs to bolster a system that has made past U.S. dental graduates the envy of the world's dental communities. With this year's graduates reporting an average debt of $60,000—ranging as high as $150,000—alternative funding sources must be found to lessen the heavy dependence on tuition.

Even with favorable interest rates, today's young professionals face an uncertain financial future as they attempt to balance new personal and professional costs while concurrently honoring their school debts. Future graduates will encounter even greater difficulties.

This is not a new issue. You probably have read and heard about it ad nauseam. But it has the potential to undermine our entire profession. We have already noted the susceptibility of debt-ridden young professionals to the siren songs of managed care operators. When they sign on, it places additional pressure on established dental practices.

And yes, you can expect a tougher time selling one of your key retirement assets—your dental practice. With a third fewer dental graduates, demand could tumble if potential buyers are unable to take on additional debt.

Most solutions to slow the skyrocketing student debt have focused on assisting students with scholarships and low-cost financial aid. But there never

> You can expect a tougher time selling one of your key retirement assets— your dental practice. With a third fewer dental graduates, demand could tumble if potential buyers are unable to take on additional debt.

seems to be enough support to help all students in need.

Dr. Art Dugoni, former ADA president and current dean of the University of the Pacific dental school, has suggested that dentists and the dental industry work together to create a billion- dollar scholarship fund over the next 25 years. The Dugoni plan calls for 150,000 dentists to give 73 cents a day for 25 years. Dr. Dugoni's heart is in the right place, but his well-meaning proposal will probably remain just that.

Action is needed now! The students can't wait. Neither can the dental schools, which are heavily dependent on tuition proceeds (47 percent of their total revenue).

In the recently released Institute of Medicine study, "Dental Education at the Crossroads," 87 percent of the dental deans mentioned "overall funding problems or specific funding problems related to over-reliance on tuition" as the most significant weakness of their schools.

The onus is on the schools to restructure their operating budgets to reduce dependence on tuition and state subsidies. Interestingly, the IOM report is conspicuously evasive on how to reduce the costs of education: "No grand solution to the financial problems of dental schools is on the horizon. ... rethinking requires more financial expertise and more detailed data than was feasible for this broadly focused study."

Let me suggest that "rethinking" dental administrators consider how most medical schools have managed to free themselves of the burdensome costs of owning and administering their own clinical operations.

Dental schools have long been accused by legislators or their universities of having the most expensive academic programs. At an average cost of more than $52,000 per student per year, they are indeed the most costly. A medical education prices out at a third less on average.

Yet, when you factor out the expense of operating the dental school's outpatient clinic, the costs for both programs are equivalent. Medical schools long ago relegated to affiliated hospitals most of the costs of clinically educating their students. Why can't dentistry follow that lead?

They can, and a number of schools already have. Unfortunately, many of these clinical programs are expensive to operate, basically reproducing dental school clinic costs in alternative settings. Also, they often are restricted to the most proficient students, thus denying needy students opportunities for professional mentoring.

One unique model that addresses these issues is located at the University of Colorado School of Dentistry. It requires all its students to spend at least six months of their predoctoral program in the clinics and offices of community dental practitioners. The student lives and works in the community, with living and travel costs supported by the University's SEARCH/AHEC program.

Do the students like it? You bet they do! Remember your dental school days? Wouldn't you have enjoyed working with a dental mentor in his or her office, unencumbered with the hassle of dental school red tape?

The dental school's community dental faculty members are also excited. Dr. Ron Johnson of Longmont, Colo., says he enjoys "picking a student's brain about new techniques and procedures." His involvement does not go unnoticed, as his patients are often complimentary of him for providing time and training to students.

As for the University of Colorado dental school, considering that faculty salaries represent about 55 percent of dental school budgets with auxiliaries accounting for another 20 percent, eliminating substantial dental school-based clinical activity should provide significant cost savings.

Colorado's off-site Advanced Clinical Training and Service Program represents a meaningful response for fiscal stability without educational compromise. Moving dental education into a community-based primary care environment gives new meaning to the relationship between dental education and health care delivery.

With the involvement of many community dental practitioners, the bond between the dental school and organized dentistry is strengthened. What's more, dental school expenditures are reduced, easing the pressure to increase tuition.

Dental schools face an extraordinary opportunity. Despite naysayers, they must change if they wish to remain viable. New solutions to old problems must be intertwined with visionary advancements that challenge the present underpinnings of dental education.

Business as usual won't suffice in the changing world of dental education. ∎

# Who will speak for dentistry?

*Originally published in JADA 1995 125: 1594-156.*

Threats turned into action this summer in the Academy of General Dentistry's House of Delegates. Rationalizing that additional initiatives should be instituted to attract new dentists, the ADA's longtime partner dropped ADA membership as a prerequisite for joining its organization. If criticism of this move by immediate past ADA President Richard D'Eustachio reflects the thoughts of ADA's leadership—and I believe it does—then AGD's capricious act will dramatically alter the more than 40-year-old relationship between the two organizations.

It appears that AGD, the premier organization for promoting professional continuing education, will broaden its mission and, in doing so, will become an ADA competitor. A look at AGD's most recent vision statement shows this organization laying claim to social, political and economic areas that have always been well-represented by the ADA.

AGD's conduct has drawn the ire of the professionally committed dentist who views the academy's separatist action as a major threat to the "one voice" that has served dentistry so well. The ADA's 73.5 percent market share of all practicing dentists is the envy of other professional organizations. Compare that with the American Medical Association's 45.5 percent, the American Bar Association's 38 percent and the American Dental Hygienists' Association's estimated 35 percent and you can understand why the ADA's membership enrollment has become the benchmark for other professional organizations.

Professional dentistry has realized enormous gains in its efforts to diminish the federal government's regulatory powers. A great deal of credit can be ascribed to ADA's efforts to present dentistry's perspectives through a well-developed lobbying campaign supported by an equally impressive

> **AGD's conduct has drawn the ire of the professionally committed dentist who views the academy's separatist action as a major threat to the "one voice" that has served dentistry so well.**

grassroots organization. You can be sure that legislators and their staffs are impressed that the ADA's message represents the views of the professional majority. To rephrase that popular TV ad, "When the ADA speaks, Government listens."

Why, then, the adverse action by one of the ADA's firmest allies? For years the ADA and the AGD have had a symbiotic relationship that has enhanced the professional lives of their more than 30,000 shared members.

Is it conceivable, as some have suggested, that AGD has higher aspirations—perhaps to supplant the ADA as the general practitioner's representative? Without insider information, I can only speculate that the academy's response is heavily linked to membership issues. For, as successful as both organizations appear, both the AGD and ADA are experiencing membership declines. AGD has a major retention problem with older dentists while the ADA struggles with recruitment of the newly graduated.

The ADA's excellent market share gets a big boost from its older members, but some recent graduating classes report membership levels as low as 55 percent. AGD presents the opposite scenario. Its market share of older dentists barely reaches 20 percent while 53 percent of the eligible 1992 graduates have signed on. (Remember, until now AGD's market has been confined to dentists holding ADA membership.)

Believing that recent dental graduates are most receptive of its message, the academy apparently will give high priority to new-dentist recruitment. With the "impediment" of ADA membership out of the way, AGD can argue that it represents the best value for the debt-strapped new professional.

This suggests that AGD will be in direct competition with ADA membership initiatives. Since there is little chance the AGD board will rescind its anti-ADA membership vote, future ADA recruitment strategies must address this challenge.

If present programming is any indication, the ADA's Division of Membership is capable of addressing any AGD advances. Independent of recent academy actions, the division has been actively involved in a wide array of recruitment initiatives directed at the emerging dentist. Its Field Service program, which includes the highly visible Transition Program, has been a major success.

To reach all dental students, the division offers the Student Communications program. This direct-mail plan, designed to raise awareness of ADA, sends welcome cards to first-year students, student appointment books to sophomores and juniors, and a congratulatory card to all graduating seniors. Regardless of how favorable these indirect approaches appear to be, a personal one-on-one relationship between the ADA and dental students should be promoted.

Consider:

The academy is working on a program that asks AGD-member dental school alumni to promote AGD membership among faculty and students. Recruitment information also is being distributed to part- and full-time AGD dental faculty, enabling them to influence students.

These programs and messages, delivered through the "voices of the general practitioners,"

coupled with an extremely low post-graduate dues structure, gives AGD a major financial edge over present ADA new-dentist programs. In fact, an academy proposal that calls for no AGD dues for the first year after graduation is on the drawing board.

No AGD dues + no need for ADA dues = Why not join? It's free!

If the profession is to continue speaking with one voice, the ADA needs to establish a continued presence in each dental school. That presence could be strengthened through the identification of a full-time faculty member who shares a commitment to professional dentistry along with a dedication to teaching. This individual should be highly visible and command the respect of the students. Once selected, the faculty member should undergo an ADA training program as extensive as those provided to dentist consumer spokespersons. To ensure success, appropriate resources should be made available.

This is not a contest between David and Goliath. The AGD and the ADA are both giants in their respective domains. If the ADA wishes to go head-to-head with the AGD—to win the professional souls of dental students—its recruitment programs must start with the student's admission to dental school.

At stake is who speaks for dentistry. Right now, it's ours to lose. ∎

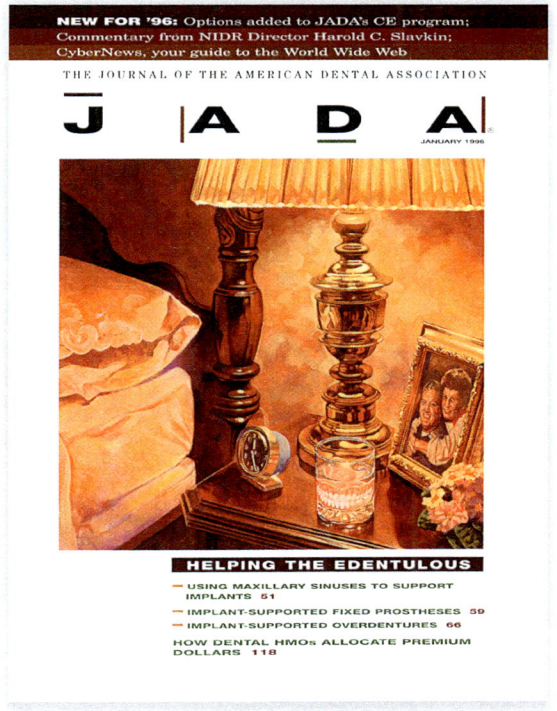

NEW FOR '96: Options added to JADA's CE program; Commentary from NIDR Director Harold C. Slavkin; CyberNews, your guide to the World Wide Web

THE JOURNAL OF THE AMERICAN DENTAL ASSOCIATION

# J |A D A|

JANUARY 1996

**HELPING THE EDENTULOUS**

— USING MAXILLARY SINUSES TO SUPPORT IMPLANTS 51
— IMPLANT-SUPPORTED FIXED PROSTHESES 59
— IMPLANT-SUPPORTED OVERDENTURES 66
HOW DENTAL HMOs ALLOCATE PREMIUM DOLLARS 118

# 1996

"Maintain your skills so that you never become outdated. Don't, regardless of the situation, attempt too much at the expense of yourself or your patients. And finally, if working ever ceases to be enjoyable, re-examine your criteria for success."

# Gold Hill revisited

*Originally published in JADA 1996 126: 12-14.*

"The man that will not read has no advantage over the man that cannot read."
— Mark Twain

Asking dentists if they read JADA is no different from asking patients if they brush their teeth. A negative response is unacceptable in either situation—especially if professional and societal expectations are to be met. Propriety might allow the respondent an answer such as, "Not as much as I should." But a definitive no? Absolutely not!

So back in the early 1990s, when word trickled down that JADA wasn't being read—that its contents weren't meeting the needs of practitioners—the ADA publishing subsidiary, suitably alarmed, investigated and, with a visionary willingness to rethink the past, acted.

Exactly 60 issues ago, and with the promise of improved relevance and readability, a totally revamped JADA was launched. Its dramatically changed format and content pleased some, offended others. As time went by, focused interviews with readers provided valuable feedback; some of the innovations were dropped or modified, while additional features were added. Editorial attention to reader suggestions continued until JADA constituents appeared satisfied that The Journal would work for them.

The editor's role is to ensure that reader needs are met. Doing so requires a continual search to attract contributions from the most knowledgeable clinician-researchers. Christensen, Mandel, Leinfelder—all frequent JADA columnists—exemplify that effort.

While the final determination of monthly JADA inclusions rests with the editorial staff, their decisions are heavily dependent on the peer review process. Each article published in JADA is reviewed by a minimum of three dental experts. More than 400 volunteers contribute to this process one or more times each year. It's their combined know-how that has provided JADA with its reputation as the profession's most widely read journal.

We don't expect that most readers will read JADA from cover to cover, because interests vary. That's why we place a prominently displayed abstract on the face page of each article—just browsing JADA's abstracts offers the dentist meaningful information. As to locating a particular article, JADA's table of contents is designed to be user-friendly, directing dentists to their interest areas without the need for skimming.

In our ever-changing professional world, JADA's continued relevance demands the timely inclusion of subjects that affect the majority of the profession. JADA's cover stories, usually two or three in number, are designed specifically to address that demand.

Balancing professional responsibility with editorial integrity, JADA operates independently from the parent organization. While it represents professional dentistry's interests, it does so in a manner that presents all aspects of an issue. The last five years have offered an unending series of complex issues: HIV, OSHA, health system reform, managed care, questions about amalgam, direct reimbursement and the Institute of Medicine study of dental education, to name just a few. Considerable space has been dedicated to these issues. It has been a time to respond to challenges, and we hope we have done so in an informative and objective manner.

Those involved with JADA's production, while taking pride in surveys that suggest increased readership, will not allow present success to hinder further proactivity. With five years passing since JADA's major overhaul, a re-evaluation of The Journal's readability and relevance has merit.

To accomplish this review in the most objective manner requires discarding the superficial do-you-read-JADA? readership surveys. This time, we

> **Exactly 60 issues ago, and with the promise of improved relevance and readability, a totally revamped JADA was launched.**

want to involve our readers in evaluating The Journal in depth, from cover to cover. Each JADA inclusion should be dissected and analyzed for readability and relevance.

An analysis of this magnitude could be costly and time-consuming. To have validity, it would require a large number of dental volunteers. Furthermore, the dental participants would have to make at least a year-long commitment, providing monthly reports.

Our readers are up to the challenge.

A single call for dental volunteers through the ADA News and JADA brought an overwhelming response from generalists and specialists alike. In fact, so many responded that within just two weeks, the enrollment had to be closed.

Starting this month and continuing for the next two years, these dentists will examine each article, each news item, even the advertisements for readability and relevance. To our knowledge, no professional journal has ever been subjected to such intense scrutiny.

Still, the editor and JADA staff will not wait months or years to change The Journal if early as-

sessments indicate the need for change. Indeed, even before the JADA review begins, you should know that substantial alterations in our continuing education program have been made. In addition, proceeding on reader feedback, we are not waiting for the review process to conclude to introduce a new section in JADA dedicated to clinical tips. This new section, called Clinical Directions and designed to help practitioners practice more efficiently and effectively, will debut later this year.

In January 1991, our editorial focused on the newly revised Journal. As an illustration, the column showed a road sign in Gold Hill, Colo. That picture is repeated here. Its not-so-subtle message—don't accept the bottom line without examining its components—is as appropriate today as it was then. It calls on all our readers to review their Journal and to let us know if we're on track.

In that regard, a personal request from your editor: With 150,000 issues of JADA circulating each month, only a small number of our readers share their thoughts with us on JADA's features. We need to hear the voice of the profession. Let's start with you. After all, this is your Journal! ∎

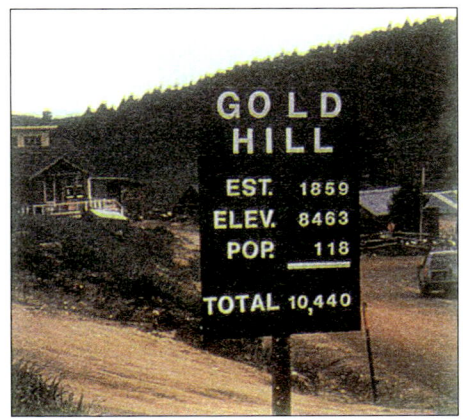

# Meaning is perception

*Originally published in JADA 1996 126: 154-156.*

As a frequent flyer who, until recently, was secure in the belief that the risks of flying were minimal, I found a report in a leading travel magazine very disturbing. The article suggested that breathing the air in an airplane cabin can lead to serious disease. Tuber-culosis, it seems, was spread from a crew member with active TB to fellow crew members and, so the author inferred, perhaps to some flyers on the plane.

I am now a concerned frequent flyer. Every unshielded passenger cough and sneeze makes me run for cover. I now "see" infectious droplets everywhere and can almost "feel" a sore throat coming on. Scientific research, the airlines maintain, indicates that the concentration of microorganisms in cabin air is less than that in many city locations. That finding does little to reduce my apprehension. I'm not going to stop flying, but I want evidence that the air surrounding me in my airplane is free of pathogenic organisms.

A similar scenario involving dental patients might be occurring in certain areas of the United States. Local media exposés of unsafe, "disease-causing" water coming from some dental unit water lines, or DUWLs, may be alarming some patients. As in the airline example, the information probably won't stop patients from making dental visits, but they would feel much better if they knew the water in the office wasn't contaminated. Until that assurance is offered, their dental visits will not be as comfortable.

To address this issue, the ADA, through its Council on Scientific Affairs, has just issued a policy statement calling on all interested parties to work toward developing dental equipment by the year 2000 that can deliver water that meets present standards used in hemodialysis units. While I applaud this recommendation, I believe the time line should and can be shortened.

> **If dentistry doesn't want to lose the positive public image it has created regarding the safety of dental visits, it can't wait five years for pure water.**

Let me explain.

The dental profession has been successful in assuring the public that a dental visit is safe. To lessen or eliminate the spread of infection to patients, barrier techniques are mandated for each office. Dentists sterilize everything. The office operatory equipment is scrubbed and wrapped. Den-tal team members are appropriately gloved, masked and gowned. All dental patients should be impressed with the precautions taken to ensure a sterile environment.

How then can dentists rationalize utilizing water, not even of potable standards, during the delivery of dental services? While no scientifically documented cases of serious illness in patients or dentists can be traced directly to DUWL contamination, there have been anecdotal reports of aerosolized infection in dentists.

Recent calls for research to refute or substantiate these claims seem reasonable, especially in light of documented waterborne disease outbreaks in hospitals. Cases of legionella infection have been linked to hospital water taps and shower heads. Of dental interest are a hospital case report that describes infection spread by gargling contaminated water before sputum collection, and a report of Pseudomonas infection after tap water was used to dilute antiseptic solution.

If dentistry doesn't want to lose the positive public image it has created regarding the safety of dental visits, it can't wait five years for pure water. I realize that the ADA has been proactive in dealing with this subject and has held several meetings with dental manufacturers and researchers to find solutions for this problem. However, much more needs to be accomplished.

I suggest as a first step that the ADA's Division of Scientific Affairs, in conjunction with the ADA Health Foundation, make a series of grants available to researchers interested in developing mechanisms to reduce or eliminate biofilms in dental equipment. This action would be timely since dentistry's research leader, the National Institute of Dental Research, has not demonstrated a major interest in this subject.

Ultimate resolution of the "bad" water issue will necessitate a two-pronged research effort. The highest priority should go to the development of technologies that will reduce or eliminate the effects of biofilm in DUWLs and concurrently address the issue of back flow. This latter subject is equally important, because failure to eliminate patient-to-patient contamination could compromise any new system. Second, research to ascertain whether there are any deleterious health effects from contaminated DUWLs also needs to be conducted.

Coupled with the research effort should be a continuing campaign to publicize any new technologic advances that might be readily incorporated into the practitioner's armamentarium. It appears that a device that employs chemical disinfection coupled with filtration may soon be available. At present, there are systems that feature autoclavable DUWLs.

While the initial purchase cost may be high, this type of unit may prove to be cost effective when measured over time. Meanwhile, you can reduce the CFU (colony-forming units) count in your DUWLs by following the advice offered by the Council of Scientific Affairs and printed in this month's Journal (see the cover story on page 181).

People too often assume that water that looks pure and doesn't taste or smell bad is OK. Dental patients are no exception. Any deviation from that perception could weaken the confidence the American people have in dentists and dentistry. The search to reduce present waterline contamination deserves the profession's highest priority. The year 2000 may be too late. ∎

# Dental licensure revisited

*Originally published in JADA 1996 126: 292-294.*

Critics of dental licensure exams have become more vocal since more than 1,000 of 1995's new dental graduates failed their initial licensing test. In questioning the validity of an exam routinely failed by a third or more of its applicants, these critics are making increasing demands for a total overhaul of the present licensing system.

For young dental professionals scrambling to balance recent practice commitments with the immediate need to retake the next test, their emotions parallel those of exam critics: "Validity? There is none." And as evidence they often point to the unexpected exam failure of one of their class's top clinicians.

Many of these young professionals are bitter, believing they deserve better after spending four arduous and costly years in training. Blame rarely falls on the educational institutions. More often, the licensing bodies or the American Dental Association are held accountable. As the results of board failures trickle down to next year's senior class, new apprehensions grow. Will anyone intercede? Can't anyone develop a more reasonable exam?

No one can argue that this year's low passing rate is just a blip—not after last year's results, which included candidate failures ranging from 50 percent to more than 80 percent at various testing sites. And present concerns are not limited to exam construction alone.

Also warranting attention is the need for a timely and appropriate appeals process, remediation opportunities for those who fail and an exploration of the ethical issue attendant to using live patients. What's more, while entry-level licensure may be the stimulus for change, no solution can be crafted that ignores licensure policies for currently licensed dentists seeking to relocate. Except for remediation, the testing issues are the same.

> **With two-thirds of the exam failures linked to clinical procedures, about 4,500 patients receive treatment that is judged substandard.**

It would be misleading to infer that nothing is being done to remedy dental licensure exam problems. The ADA and the American Association of Dental Examiners have agreed on guidelines for a common national clinical exam, and a committee of those two groups has noted progress by licensing agencies to employ these guidelines in their clinical exams.

The concept of a common clinical exam was recently put to the test. The Northeast Regional Board and the Central Regional Testing Service joined forces in the spring of 1995 to offer CORE, a single clinical licensure examination acceptable to both regional testing services.

Unfortunately, procedural differences, not the CORE exam itself, have temporarily shut down that initiative. But the word is that other regional boards are also talking "common exam." With 78 percent of all dental students graduating from schools within regional board states, an agreement that would create a common "clinical" exam would be a giant step in ending the mobility problem for future dental graduates.

Even with such an accord, the issue of the live patient still remains a major stumbling block to eventual acceptance of a common licensure exam. Simply stated: Is it ethical to use human subjects for the purpose of discovering incompetence? Dentistry stands alone among other health professions in its determination to continue the use of live patients.

And it uses quite a few. About 6,000 dentists are tested each year, and each will use between three and four human subjects during the exam. With two-thirds of the exam failures linked to clinical procedures, about 4,500 patients receive treatment that is judged substandard.

Since these individuals are patients of the examinee, not the school, responsibility for their future care is often ill-defined. Critics of the live exam contend that such patients are treated with no regard for a treatment plan, that the focus of examiners and candidates is rarely on the patient's welfare.

There is a division between educators and examiners on this issue. Most dental schools respond affirmatively to the question, "In your experience with clinical licensure examinations, do you believe that the use of human subjects raises frequent or significant ethical concerns related to the appropriate sequencing and/or timely provision of treatment?"

Only one of the 13 testing bodies answered yes to this question.

A recent experiment—a pregraduate exam—administered by the Southern Regional Testing Agency at the University of Tennessee gave greater protection to the patient and addressed the question of student remediation. Still, the ethical issue of using live patients remained. Dental testing boards stand firmly committed to the policy that they will discontinue the use of human subjects only when comparable methods of testing are available.

When will that be?

Sixteen months ago, an editorial entitled "Time for a Dental Board Checkup" appeared in this space. It addressed that year's high failure rate on dental boards by dissecting the components of the exam process and then offered potential solutions. One of those proposals called for the development of a Part III National Board Exam composed of interactive clinical simulations that would eliminate the use of live patients.

That suggestion could be on the verge of becoming reality. Today, 11 dental organizations representing education, testing and dental practice are actively developing a multiuse interactive simulation exam. Functioning as a nonprofit corporation under the name Dental Interactive Simulation Corporation, the group has made significant time and financial contributions to further this process. Considering the importance of entry licensure, additional assistance for the DISC operation may be needed to meet an accelerated timeline for a completed exam draft.

Once completed, all entry licensure candidates should be required to take the simulation exam to provide normative data. The results of both clinical and simulation exams could then be correlated with each other, as well as with the academic performance of the dental student. It can be hoped that, with continuous refinement, a "patient-free" exam might be ready to accompany the profession into the next century.

The term "multiuse interactive exam" is no misnomer. Properly validated, the Part III exam could be used to satisfy mobility licensure issues for the already licensed dentist—and even could serve as a nonpunitive mechanism for practitioners to assess their own continued competency.

The clock is ticking. The 21st century is not far off. ∎

# Diagnostic oddities of the strangest form

*Originally published in JADA 1996 126: 418-420.*

*"An investigation of the patient's background disclosed that she had been treated by 20 dental practitioners during a 4-year period, 12 of whom had treated her within a 10-week period, each unaware of the other."*[1]

Sometimes even the finest diagnosticians can be duped. Maybe it's happened to you. Then again, you probably wouldn't have known that one of your patients had succeeded in manipulating you into treating a fictitious disorder. Chances are they've already left your practice—to be treated elsewhere for the same condition. It may seem hard to believe that anyone would feign illness and submit to treatment. But it happens.

It's called Munchausen's syndrome, after an 18th-century German soldier known for fabricating fabulous stories. Most clinical descriptions of this intriguing oddity are found in the medical literature, although examples of patients feigning dental diseases also have been documented.

True cases of dental Munchausen's may be rare. A much larger percentage of the population, however, uses feigned illness to satisfy personal needs (drug habits, for example), a practice that complicates differential diagnosis. Somewhere between these two groups lies a collection of patients, many elderly, who manufacture dental diseases for personal attention.

Learning how to differentiate among these patients can curb potential problems for the dentist.

True Munchausen's subjects are pathological liars who, for reasons not clearly understood, want to be sick. They appear to seek nothing in particular, although some clinicians suggest they adopt the sick role in a quest for sympathy.

> **It's called Munchausen's syndrome, after an 18th-century German soldier known for fabricating fabulous stories. Most clinical descriptions of this intriguing oddity are found in the medical literature, although examples of patients feigning dental diseases also have been documented.**

Some Munchausen's subjects are self-abusive or abusive to the health care worker. They feign the physical signs and symptoms of a disease with the intent of becoming part of a treatment process. That treatment often can involve unnecessary and even life-threatening surgical procedures.

An especially bizarre twist on this phenomenon is known as Munchausen's syndrome-by-proxy—one person creates or fabricates the symptoms of illness in another. A mother, for instance, may report factitious symptoms of disease in her child. The literature includes cases of care givers for the elderly creating symptoms in their charges.

The British Dental Journal last year reviewed two cases of dental Munchausen's syndrome.[2]

The first case concerned a 31-year-old male who presented with pain in the left maxilla. To date, he is known to have subjected himself to two extractions and has 15 endodontically treated teeth. All treatments failed to relieve his reported pain. To the author's knowledge, the patient still is making the rounds of dental offices, looking for unsuspecting dentists to treat his "affliction."

In the second case, a 35-year-old female complained of pain in the submandibular gland. The gland was removed by an oral surgeon, but the surgical biopsy showed a normal salivary gland. The pain then reoccurred as a right glossopharyngeal neuralgia, which also was treated surgically. The pain then moved to the other side of the tongue, prompting further diagnostic involvement, including sialometry, sialography and scintiscanning. Still no resolution.

Piquing my interest in this topic was a true case of Munchausen's syndrome described to me by an oral pathologist. The subject, an elderly woman, apparently made numerous visits to dentists throughout a large Midwestern state. On each visit, she presented with oral ulcerations of unknown origin on her buccal mucosa. The biopsy report on the lesions consistently read, "tissue necrosis of unknown etiology."

The woman was referred finally to a dental school's oral pathologist who examined her and found no lesions. In the course of the examination, he briefly left the room only to find on his return that the lesions had appeared. He noticed, too, that a cigarette apparently had been lit and then put out, leading him to suspect that the burns were self-induced. Confronted with this observation, the woman fled the office, proclaiming that all dental practitioners were stupid.

Dentists may never encounter a classic case of Munchausen's syndrome, but patients whose symptoms mimic Munchausen's may contact hundreds of dentists over a period of years. These people, categorized under the psychological rubric of "malingering," can be differentiated from "pure" Munchausen's subjects by noting whether their motivation has some external objective—for example, a desire for drugs—other than just being ill.

Consider the patient whose dental pain from an extraction never seems to subside, and who calls continuously for refills of controlled substances. Is it really a dry socket, or is the patient constantly manipulating the tissues to retard the healing process?

What about the elderly patient who complains regularly of a "sore area" under his or her denture, which never seems to disappear regardless of treatment. The biopsy report repeatedly describes "tissue necrosis of unknown origin." Is this a form of attention seeking, or does the patient have a justifiable complaint?

And what of the patient who has 15 dentures made over a five-year period? Or the patient who complains perpetually of burning mouth?

Drug seekers, attention seekers or those with true Munchausen's syndrome—all can present diagnostic challenges to the unsuspecting dentist. Be on the alert for these oddities. Include them in your differential diagnosis. They may prove to be uncommonly common. ▪

1. Fusco MA, Freedman PD, Black SM, Lumerman H. Munchausen's syndrome: report of case. JADA 1986;112:210-2.
2. Scully C, Eveson JW, Porter SR. Munchausen's syndrome: oral presentations. Br Dent J 1995;178:65-7.

# You and your life's work

*Originally published in JADA 1996 126: 548-550.*

"In order that people may be happy in their work, these three things are needed. They must be fit for it. They must not do too much of it. And they must have a sense of success in it."
—John Ruskin

Dentistry's appeal to the independent-minded as a profession that allows its members to "be their own boss" continues to draw talented students despite its lengthy and costly training process. This successful recruitment of the best and brightest, which continues to include a high percentage of daughters and sons of dentists, is a reflection of how positive dentists feel about their work.

"I don't know any profession in the world that is better than dentistry. You're your own boss, you set your own hours, you can go anywhere in the world and practice. ... Your working conditions are ideal. Okay, they're physically hard, but there is nothing wrong with that."[1]

At a time when poll after poll indicates widespread dissatisfaction with work environments, a recent ADA survey of practitioners indicated that 88 percent of dentists were satisfied with their choice of profession. As a further endorsement, more than 50 percent indicated that dentists should "encourage young people to go to dental school."[2]

Quite a remarkable expression of satisfaction from a professional group that has seen major constraints placed on its independence.

No one can say that dentistry is an easy day's work.

"You don't make money unless you have your hand in somebody's mouth. It's not like any other business where you can get income by being away. Anytime you're not working on a patient, you're losing money. Your overhead continues."[1]

> Maintain your skills so that you never become outdated. Don't attempt too much at the expense of yourself or your patients. And if working ever ceases to be enjoyable, re-examine your criteria for success.

If you're an average dentist, you work full time (84 percent), practice solo (73 percent), own your practice and spend 48 weeks yearly practicing dentistry. You work an average of 34 hours a week, during which time you treat an average of 83 patients. That's more than 3,900 dental visits a year.[3]

How many times have you heard patients or friends say, "I wouldn't be a dentist no matter how much I was paid—and besides, don't dentists have the highest suicide rate anyway?" And how have you responded?

"Dentistry is very precise. No matter what you do, sometimes things don't go right. ... One of the big diseases dentists have is stress. The patients are in a tense position too."[1]

To the tens of thousands of U.S. dentists trained to be perfectionists in an imperfect world, the Ruskin quote has real meaning. Maintain your skills so that you never become outdated. Don't, regardless of the situation, attempt too much at the expense of yourself or your patients. And finally, if working ever ceases to be enjoyable, re-examine your criteria for success.

In the main lobby of the San Antonio Hilton Hotel, there is a wall plaque entitled "My Philosophy," written by the hotel's architect, H.B. Zachary. It's about work—and life. Its unique contents are both poignant and inspiring, and I often reread my copy. While coping with today's world of work, perhaps you, too, will find its contents a worthy stimulant for your thoughts. (We reproduce it here with the kind permission of H.B. Zachary Jr.)

"I do not choose to be a common man. It is my right to be uncommon if I can. I seek opportunity—not security. I will refuse to be a kept citizen, to be humbled and dulled by having my state and nation look after me. I want to dream and to build, to fail and to succeed—never to be numbered among those weak and timid souls who have known neither victory nor defeat. I know that happiness can come only from the inside through hard constructive work and sincere positive thinking. I know that the so-called pleasures of the moment should not be confused with a state of happiness. I know that I can get a measure of inner satisfaction from any job if I intelligently plan and courageously execute it. I know that, if I put forth every iota of strength that I possess—physical, mental, spiritual—toward the accomplishment of a worthwhile task ere I fall exhausted by the wayside, the Un-

seen Hand will reach out and pull me through. Yes, I want to live dangerously, plan my procedures on the basis of calculated risks, to resolve the problems of everyday living into a measure of inner peace. I know if I know how to do all this, I will know how to live and, if I know how to live, I will know how to die." ■

1. Terkel S. Working. New York: Ballantine Books; 1972.
2. American Dental Association. 1992 survey of dental practice. Chicago: American Dental Association; 1993.
3. American Dental Association. 1995 survey of dental practice. Chicago: American Dental Association; 1996.

# Join the electronic revolution now!

*Originally published in JADA 1996 126: 716-718.*

Interested in receiving quality continuing education without leaving your office or home—and at a fraction of normal cost? If the answer is yes, the first step is to join the more than 30 million people already communicating through the Internet. Don't worry about it becoming a high-cost adventure. Most dental office computers will need little or no modification, perhaps no more than a high-speed modem. And except for a small monthly cost to access the Internet, joining the electronic revolution requires only curiosity, coupled with the willingness to spend time surfing the Net.

You will not be alone.

The ADA, recognizing the infinite potential of electronic communication, has responded to this informational revolution by creating ADA ONLINE. Now, at your convenience, you and fellow dentists can access the latest in dental information by addressing "http://www.ada.org".

Considering that some dentists equate turning on a computer with changing a tire at 65 miles an hour, some will be reluctant motorists on the information superhighway. To them, and to those already using the Internet, let me propose an electronic opportunity that could elevate dentistry's most popular form of postdoctoral education to even higher levels of achievement.

Almost every dentist is, or has been, a member of a dental study club. While not unique to the dental profession, study clubs have become virtual institutions in dentistry, meeting a critical need for peer interaction and clinical updating.

Participating dentists travel like religious pilgrims to regularly scheduled meeting places, regardless of the weather or the loss of practice income. Their goal: to exchange experiences on clinical situations and to listen to the advice of visiting dental experts paid by the collective dues of the study club members.

What could be better?

Perhaps this scenario: The dentist, in the comfort of his or her office or home, turns on the computer, accesses the Internet and enters the address of his electronic study club, or ESC. Connected to all other members of the ESC, the dentist begins an electronic conversation with his or her new associate in Denmark. Plans to meet at an international meeting are completed.

The dentist then responds, again electronically, to a question posed by several ESC members on the setting time for a dental material. It appears that those ESC members having difficulty with the material live in arid climates where the low humidity may be the problem.

The ESC dentist then downloads software that enables him or her to use an audio/video CE program developed by an international expert on implants. The dental expert remains online to answer ESC members' questions.

After the live interaction at the ESC meeting, the dentist uses the study club's dental materials purchasing form to place an order. Group purchasing agreements with other ESCs have resulted in major savings for all.

Electronic study club members are asked to vote on a proposal to add a new clinical dimension to their organization. A leading dental manufacturer has offered to supply new dental products to club members for in-office testing. By entering their clinical observations on an electronic chart, the manufacturer and the clinical ESC members will gain first-hand information about new products. For ESC participation, the manufacturer also has promised to contribute to the club's speaker clinician budget.

These are but a few of the opportunities for those who join the electronic revolution and form the "new dental study club." Without geographic

> **The ADA, recognizing the infinite potential of electronic communication, has responded to this informational revolution by creating ADA ONLINE.**

limitations, participation is limited only by manageable numbers.

Today's greatest challenge is how to start an ESC. Most dentists don't have the knowledge to design and program the electronic space for a dental bulletin board. Help is needed and must come from those dedicated to promoting advanced education for dentists.

So look to the dental schools, the ADA and its constituent and component societies. Look also to existing dental study clubs and even dental manufacturers as groups that might assist in making your entry to the world of electronic dental education enjoyable and meaningful. ∎

# Kicking the habit

*Originally published in JADA 1996 126: 844-846.*

It's time to give tobacco another kick, and this time it's dentistry's turn. Just recently, the American Medical Association—with a great deal of public fanfare—called on all individual and institutional investors to divest their holdings in stocks or mutual funds that have interests in producing or selling tobacco.

This was not a frivolous act on the AMA's part. Neither was it a publicity stunt. Rather, it underscored the medical group's crusade to curb the morbidity and mortality directly linked to tobacco use, and for good reason. Tobacco causes cancer. It significantly increases the risk of cardiovascular incidents, and it severely reduces lung function. Almost 500,000 deaths each year can be traced to tobacco use, and that's probably an underestimate.

Aside from the pain and suffering of those with tobacco-related diseases, the economic costs are equally staggering: at least $100 billion annually and climbing.

If you believe that as a non-smoker you are immune from the effects of tobacco smoke, think again. Tobacco smoke is everyone's problem. The results of a national study that tested for serum cotinine (a major metabolite of nicotine) found that 92 percent of the U.S. population aged 4 years and older had measurable levels. More than 37,000 Americans each year will die of heart attacks fueled by passive exposure to tobacco smoke. Thousands more are at heightened risk of cancer or impaired lung function.

For these reasons, I believe the American Dental Association should follow the lead of its medical counterpart and call on its members and their associates to divest tobacco holdings from their investment accounts. Few dentists would deny their professional obligation to protect and promote the health of the American public. Joining the AMA in its recent call for tobacco divestiture falls within this scope.

Not that organized dentistry has been derelict in its personal campaign against tobacco. The ADA has adopted several policies taking a strong stance against tobacco use. The ADA, for example, "supports legislation and/or regulation that acknowledges nicotine as an addictive drug and that authorizes the FDA to regulate tobacco products as nicotine delivery devices and/or drugs." The Association further "urges that such legislation be promptly enacted so that the use of nicotine is restricted."

In a recent Survey of Current Issues in Dentistry, just 6 percent of dentists reported that they were current or occasional smokers, contrasting sharply with the 25 percent of the adult population who smoke. Among dentists, 23 percent were former smokers, and more than half said they routinely advised patients to quit. More than 90 percent of dentists said staff and patients were barred from using tobacco anywhere in the dental office.

Surely these statistics send a strong message that dentistry doesn't support tobacco. Why, then, the call for divestiture?

Because anti-tobacco campaigns aren't enough—especially when it comes to children. Consider these facts:

■ 44 million Americans have quit smoking, but 46 million still smoke;

■ the number of "heavy" smokers has not declined and remains at about 25 percent of all smokers;

■ 3 million U.S. adolescents smoke, another 1 million chew and the numbers are rising;

■ research conducted by the University of Michigan Institute for Social Research found that among eighth and 10th grade students, the percentage of those who had smoked in the previous 30 days has

> **The American Dental Association should follow the lead of its medical counterpart and call on us members and their associates to divest tobacco holdings from their investment accounts.**

risen 33 percent since 1991;

■ the average age of first-time smokers is 14 years. About 3,000 teens begin smoking each day, and 1 billion packs of cigarettes are sold each year to youngsters under 18.

Will eliminating tobacco stocks from your portfolio help reverse this disturbing trend? Probably not directly. Wall Street watchers inform me that such actions would be mainly symbolic. They say that most investors don't look beyond the performance numbers of their holdings. And even if they did, they would find it difficult to cull out tobacco companies, since so many of them are part of massive conglomerates with individual holdings that can only be found by studying lengthy prospectuses or annual reports.

But the AMA is trying to help investors divest. The April 24, 1996, issue of JAMA carried statistics on 15 of the largest mutual funds and examined their tobacco holdings. Unfortunately, nine of the 15 have tobacco stocks among their top 10 holdings.

Still, there are mutual funds that don't invest in tobacco: of the roughly 7,000 mutual funds, just 20 percent have tobacco holdings, though you may have to search for them. According to Morningstar, the company that tracks the performance of mutual funds, only 0.16 percent of the money in diversified stock funds goes to socially conscious funds.

What can the ADA do if it wishes to follow the AMA's lead? Perhaps the simplest and most effective response would be for an individual member or a constituent or component society to present a resolution to the 1996 House of Delegates calling on ADA members to divest themselves of tobacco holdings. This action would provide those with strong beliefs on this issue a meaningful forum for discussion and debate.

Regardless of that outcome, the ravages of tobacco require that health professionals seek responsible solutions to this devastating but preventable health problem. Would a symbolic call for divestiture make a difference? It depends on your unit of measure. According to mine, the answer is an unequivocal yes. ■

# Do we need another dental school?

*Originally published in JADA 1996 126: 1146-1148.*

Dentistry's educational landscape may soon change. After a decade of class-size reduction, marked by the closure of six private dental schools, a reversal is in the offing. Florida-based Nova Southeastern University has announced its intentions to open a new private dental school.

Rationalizing that unmet dental needs, plus a high demand for careers in dentistry by south Florida residents, can be addressed only by creating a new dental school, Nova Southeastern University plans to enroll a class of 75 dental students by fall 1997.

Moving quickly to meet this ambitious timeline, Nova Southeastern has asked the Commission on Dental Accreditation to review the school's initial educational plans. If the outcome of that review is favorable, the commission could grant the new school "Accreditation Eligible Status" and the right to begin interviewing applicants for the first school year.

This new educational venture has left many dental educators and practitioners puzzled. Why, at a time when most academic health centers are battling to maintain the fiscal integrity of their existing programs, is a new dental school being considered?

Even the medical schools in a number of university health science centers are struggling today, their revenues proving insufficient to sustain high quality. And the dental deans at these centers are worried that a "trickledown" effect, as the medical schools try to solve their fiscal problems, could adversely affect their dental programs.

Hardly seems the time to start a new dental school. Especially one that will depend on private funding.

Nova Southeastern must realize that underwriting a dental education program will be an expensive process—probably the costliest of all university ventures. Few would view a private dental school as a profit center.

There was a time—about 100 years ago—when expanding commercial opportunities created by the growing enforcement of dental practice acts led many dental entrepreneurs to start their own schools. From 1881 to 1900 the number of dental schools, almost all of them proprietary, rose from 14 to 57. But for-profit dental education didn't fare well. By 1929, the last proprietary school in the United States had disappeared.

Today, even with large financial contributions from carefully developed endowment funds and salary offsets from research grants and generous gifts from alumni, the burden of financing dental education rests mainly on student and institutional commitments. And most of that load is shouldered by the students.

Consider:

■ Income and expenditure records from existing private dental schools indicate that only 64 percent of a private dental school's yearly cost to educate a single student is covered by tuition or clinic income. At $45,000 per student year—a figure that closely approximates the true cost of private education—the unmet yearly cost per enrollee would be at least $16,000.

■ With annual tuition at some private schools already reaching $30,000, passing all or even some of that additional cost on to students in the form of higher tuition would be disastrous. At that price, access to a dental education soon would be limited to the wealthy or those willing to accept debts as high as $200,000 for the four-year program.

Nova Southeastern says it will help by anteing up about $45 million to build the physical plant, but what about the rest of the money? With a full

> This new educational venture has left many dental educators and practitioners puzzled. Why, at a time when most academic health centers are battling to maintain the fiscal integrity of their existing programs, is a new dental school being considered?

complement of 300 students, initial yearly expenditures could exceed revenues by $5 million.

While I'm still unsure of the rationale for and financial stability of this new school, I'm most concerned about the process of its creation. If we are to have a new dental school—the first of the 21st century—shouldn't it reflect what will be, not what is?

These and other questions need to be answered.

Will the dental school of the future have to own and manage its own clinics? Should the 21st century's new dental school share faculty with existing dental schools through the electronic media? For teaching preclinical sciences, virtual reality and other computer-driven simulations already are affecting basic dental education. How should these innovations be addressed, as the brick and mortar of the new school pile up?

Interviews with leaders in dental education and organized dentistry show that they had little opportunity for input on the Nova Southeastern initiative. The excitement and involvement that should accompany an undertaking of this magnitude appear to be lacking.

In the early 1960s, Dean Alvin Morris and the faculty of the new University of Kentucky dental school challenged the entire dental community to share in developing its innovations. Dentistry continues to reap rewards from those interactions.

A visionary message from that original faculty in Kentucky might be of value today.

*Dear Nova Southeastern University:*

*Dentistry doesn't need just another dental school. Existing schools could easily expand to address specific manpower requirements. If south Florida has unmet needs, why not let its present dental school fill that void?*

*If, on the other hand, you [Nova Southeastern] have an educational plan that supersedes the parochial goal of being just one of the gang—a real willingness to take chances, to go where others haven't been, to truly lead—if this is indeed your vision, let other dental educators and practitioners join with you in realizing that goal. All of dentistry would benefit.* ∎

# A breath of fresh air

*Originally published in JADA 1996 126: 1282-1285.*

Twenty-first century technology neatly packaged with attention-getting ads is providing a growing number of entrepreneurs with big profits. Promoting new cures for one of society's oldest and most troublesome social maladies, these super salespeople are coaxing people to "come out of the closet" to solve a problem of such a personal nature that those affected often will not discuss it even with family and friends.

The culprit is halitosis, malodor or just plain bad breath. Whatever the name, it is a prevalent affliction, affecting 25 million to 85 million Americans, depending on who supplies the data.

Ninety-two percent of dentists surveyed at the ADA's 1995 annual session reported that they had patients with chronic bad breath. Almost half reported seeing six or more patients weekly with unpleasant breath. Based on that statistic, those dentists would encounter roughly 500,000 halitosis patients a week.

Over-the-counter "cures" (mints, chewing gum, sprays and mouthrinses) for those seeking temporary solutions for their breath problem have created a $1 billion industry. Mouthrinses blending flavoring agents, alcohol and essential oils give the desired clean taste—but only temporarily, never longer than a few hours.

Four years ago Consumer Reports tested 15 mouthrinses, using "garlic pizza" breath as a standard. All worked for at least 10 minutes. After an hour some were still effective, but at the end of two hours little residual effect remained.

Considering America's preoccupation with pleasing social appearances, a permanent treatment for halitosis could ignite a multimillion dollar enterprise. No wonder many who seek new and profitable business opportunities are anxious to enter the bad breath market.

> **Considering America's preoccupation with pleasing social appearances, a permanent treatment for halitosis could ignite a multimillion dollar enterprise.**

Some aren't waiting. Franchises to treat bad breath are springing up throughout the country. Advertisements for these clinics promise cure rates of 98 percent or higher. And for those who are geographically unable to visit a clinic, home treatment programs are available.

The Internet also has become a venue for participants. People with a breath problem can now "talk" with halitosis experts without having to identify themselves. Treatment is readily available—just have your credit card handy and choose from the following:

- "Plagued by Dragon Mouth? Here's Good News."
- "For pennies a day ... starter kit is $29.95 plus shipping and handling. Money-back guarantee. You have nothing to do but lose your bad breath."
- "You can be reassured you have finally contacted a group of doctors that take your problem seriously."
- "Try the Bad Breath Self-Examination."

The news media also are promoting fresh breath. The Chicago Reader's "News of the Weird" section recently featured a Reuters news service report that profiled a New York City dental hygienist who charges $125 for a breath makeover.

USA Today, NBC's "Today Show" and ABC's "20/20" all have aired recent segments featuring bad breath treatments. Their conclusions were similar: bad breath can be controlled or eliminated with appropriate treatment.

The following dialogue, excerpted from the "20/20" bad breath segment, is typical of the presentations:

Bad breath sufferer to her fiancee: "Look at my tongue! I don't have a white coating on it anymore! Smell my breath!"

Interviewer: "Could you tell the difference in her breath?"

Fiancee: "Yeah."

Bad breath sufferer: "It was like a miracle. ..."

You can imagine the impact of that exchange on 20 million viewers, at least 2 million of whom suffer from bad breath. No wonder bad breath is becoming big business.

How does all this media exposure affect the everyday practice of dentistry? Is there an increased demand for malodor treatments? Dentists I've spoken with say no, the demand has not changed appreciably. Most dentists view the breath centers with skepticism and don't see themselves devoting extra time to treating this problem. "It's just a normal part of our diagnosis and treatment activities—no reason to change" is a typical view.

Dental schools show the same indifference. With few exceptions, dental schools don't emphasize the treatment of bad breath. Their curriculums give only minimal information about malodor and its treatment.

This attitude may represent an opportunity wasted.

In today's competitive marketplace, dental consumers are looking for the most service at the most reasonable price.

Dentists willing to give high visibility to in-office treatment of halitosis might find high interest among many of their current patients. Treating bad breath also could become a practice builder—attracting patients who, while initially seeking help for their problem breath, could eventually become a member of your dental family.

The ADA's survey showed that patients themselves initiated discussions of their halitosis with their oral health care providers. This is surprising in light of the potential embarrassment. Among those patients unaware of or unwilling to disclose their problem, a hygienist broached the subject 31 percent of the time, while a dentist brought it up 27 percent of the time.

From a treatment perspective, bad breath is similar to other body odors. It's generated by bacteria—usually under anaerobic conditions. Get rid of the bacteria and you'll probably "cure" the malodor. With at least 85 percent of bad breath originating in the oral cavity, it should respond readily and successfully to treatment.

The scope of treatment for bad breath falls within the normal limits of routine dental services. CDT-2 codes covering the oral hygiene, nutrition, periodontal and caries treatments most often used to eliminate malodor should ensure dentists compensation for halitosis treatment.

There is nothing unique in the treatment approach advocated by fresh breath entrepreneurs. Isn't it time to push their hype aside by giving this potential practice builder its appropriate place in your treatment armamentarium? ∎

# Facing up to phobia

*Originally published in JADA 1996 126: 1450-1452.*

The evidence continues to grow that universal precautions and barrier techniques have reduced to nearly zero the risk of transmitting the HIV bloodborne pathogen from patient to dentist. Those who question this statement need only examine the outcomes of health worker exposures to the AIDS virus. According to the Centers for Disease Control and Prevention, the risk of seroconversion in health care workers exposed to HIV-infected blood through the percutaneous route (needlesticks or cuts) is 0.3 percent. For those exposed by contact with mucocutaneous tissues, the risk is 0.09 percent. The risk is even less for skin contacts.

What's more, of the 49 health care workers who have seroconverted to HIV after occupational exposure, none was a dentist.

While its statistics may not be all-inclusive, the CDC surveillance system covers sufficient numbers within the dental universe to allow it to testify in a court of law that "treating HIV positive patients ... in a dental office does not pose a direct threat to the health and safety of others." That includes dentists and members of their dental office teams.

Risks for patients visiting a dental office also are negligible; only in the mystifying Acer case has HIV transmission from an infected dentist to a patient been recorded. The mode of transmission in that case still has not been established.

Acting on CDC treatment recommendations and scientific information, the ADA has declared the dental office safe for all participants. The strength of that commitment can be noted in the ADA's Principles of Ethics and Code of Professional Conduct, which includes the following: "A dentist should not refuse to treat a patient whose condition is within the dentist's current realm of competency solely because the patient is HIV infected."

While earlier surveys indicated a reluctance by some dentists to treat HIV-infected patients, recent assessments indicate that most dentists are adhering to the tenets of the ADA's ethical code.

Compliance, however, has not been universal, and more than one dentist has found that a reluctance to treat can subject him or her to court actions and substantial fines.

Since HIV infection has been labeled a disability under the Americans with Disabilities Act, legal encounters have centered on federal courts. To date, no legal argument has prevailed that questioned the classification of HIV infection as a disability. And no argument has prevailed that implied that HIV-infected patients pose a direct threat to the health and safety of others.

Attempts to discredit the effectiveness of universal precautions and barrier techniques have gained little credence. Inevitably, such arguments collapse under the huge body of evidence that dental procedures are safe, that the risk is infinitesimal.

I concur with the CDC and ADA positions. The science supporting universal precautions and barrier techniques is irrefutable. However, I would like to advance a proposition for those dentists experiencing excessive mental stress when called on to treat the HIV-infected patient.

Please note that I limit my proposal to dentists who are sincerely fearful of the consequences of treating the AIDS patient, even though they are aware the risk is small. Excluded are dentists who would deny care due to certain prejudices.

On several occasions, dentists have confided to me that their fears of infectivity make it difficult—even impossible—to carry out an effective treat-

> Fear has not been an acceptable legal defense for failing to treat the HIV-positive patient. But anxiety and uncontrollable fear are legitimate psychiatric disorders. Fear has not been an acceptable legal defense for failing to treat the HIV-positive patient. But anxiety and uncontrollable fear are legitimate psychiatric disorders.

ment plan. Forcing them to treat could cause damage to both patient and dentist. As one who finds it difficult to stand on a six-foot ladder without dizziness, I am sympathetic.

How many dentists fall into this category? I don't know. There may be only those few who have spoken or written to me. Or there could be hundreds more too fearful to speak out.

I would predict that most of these dentists, knowing the career-damaging consequences of their fears, would willingly offer treatment if they could control their anxieties.

For dentists in this phobic state, chances are that many are mid-career. They entered the profession with no thought that they would ever be in a situation—no matter how small the risk—where they might contract a fatal disease. For such dentists, the profession should offer programs to help them deal with their fears.

Fear has not been an acceptable legal defense for failing to treat the HIV-positive patient. But anxiety and uncontrollable fear are legitimate psychiatric disorders. Unwarranted, illogical fear of a situation can, on the one hand, manifest itself in simple curtailment of normal function. On the other hand, it can produce extreme panic leading to illness or bodily injury.

This editorial does not suggest that dentists who refuse to treat AIDS patients be allowed to use fear as a legal argument. What it does recommend is that the two, 20 or 200 dentists who legitimately are not in total control of their professional skills, hamstrung by their fears of HIV, be treated as phobic.

Such treatment is available and often successful; 90 percent of phobias respond to therapy. Programs using accepted therapies—desensitization, behavior modification, visualization—can assist needy dentists, not punish them.

Just as peer boards have been established to support the HIV-infected dentists, so should professional boards be created to assist those dentists who have nothing to fear but fear itself. ■

# 'To dream the impossible dream ...'

*Originally published in JADA 1996 126: 1568-1571.*

"To fight the unbeatable foe ... to reach the unreachable star."[1] Spirits uplifted, inspired, few theatergoers leave a production of "Man of La Mancha" without secretly desiring to emulate the knight-errant Don Quixote's quest to "right the unrightable wrong."

Few actually do. But now and then ...

Consider the example of an ophthalmologist from Salem, Ore., who this month has given the voters of his state the chance to ban capitation as a means of paying for medical care.

Talk about tilting at windmills.

Many doctors would view this proposed legislation as far exceeding Don Quixote's wildest dreams. Imagine trying to outlaw a payment mechanism presently used to pay the health care bills for more than 60 million Americans.

The bill's preamble—"because patients have the right to be protected from unscrupulous practices which reward health care providers for withholding standard patient care"—gives insight into this doctor's rationale for an action that most would consider unthinkable. Obviously, he feels that market forces have failed and that only his legislation can stop fragmentation of the patient-doctor relationship.

His action has not been easy or cheap. Without major organizational assistance and at his own expense (an estimated $67,000), he obtained the necessary 76,216 signatures required to get the issue on the ballot.[2]

Support for the measure from the Oregon medical establishment has been limited. Opponents of the ophthalmologist's initiative include the powerful Oregon Medical Association and HMO insurers—now partners in their attempt to defeat the measure.

They appear to have the upper hand. A poll of physicians indicated that two-thirds would vote against the initiative. But in a state where 44 per-

**All participants must agree that the primary standard for judgment must be the placement of patient welfare ahead of any other consideration.**

cent of the population obtains care through HMOs—the highest in the country and twice the national average—who would expect the physicians to vote against their bread and butter?

Powerful foes do not appear to deter or alter this warrior's quest to "right the unrightable wrong." Capitation, he has been quoted as saying, is a "plundering of the heart and soul of the profession."

With that type of conviction, one or two windmills just might topple.

After all, he isn't alone in his admonishment against capitation. As higher and higher profits appear in the earning statements of national HMOs, critics wonder if profit is perhaps achieved by rationing needed care—that patient health is being compromised to enhance the stockholders' bottom line.

Both scientific and anecdotal reports are fueling the flames of this argument. At this year's American Heart Association annual meeting, a research report indicated that in a study of Medicare claims, victims of heart attack treated by cardiologists had a 15 percent lower risk of dying than those treated only by a general practitioner.

Recent national media reports have sensationalized instances of patients' being denied needed care. Time magazine's in-depth coverage of "The Soul of an HMO" lends de facto support to the Oregonian initiative by questioning "whether patients, especially those with severe illnesses, can still trust their doctors."

Defenders of HMOs argue otherwise. They refute the denial-of-care arguments and point out that if health care costs are managed, more people have access to affordable health care coverage. The quality issue, they contend, would become moot if an objective scorecard were available.

Regardless of its outcome, the Oregon initiative already has served to enhance discussion on one of medicine's burning issues. Dentists should take note: it applies to all health providers if passed.

While commending the Oregon ophthalmologist's dedication, I can't share his view that the only way to counter capitation is to legislate it out of existence. HMO supporters, using similar arguments, could introduce legislation to ban fee-for-service as a payment method, citing examples of payment excesses as their rationale.

Instead, the marketplace should remain the arena for ultimate decision making. Let all payment methods be judged against each other. Examine and compare cost, quality and provider remuneration. But before the assessment begins, all participants must agree that the primary standard for judgment must be the placement of patient welfare ahead of any other consideration.

A comment in a recent editorial in the New England Journal of Medicine concisely summarizes this position: "Patients are vulnerable and dependent and need to know that their physicians are not only at their side but on their side."[3]

Dentists should agree. The ADA Principle of Ethics and Code of Professional Conduct states unequivocally that "dentists may choose to enter into contracts governing the provision of care to a group of patients; however, contract obligations do not excuse dentists from their ethical duties to put the patients' welfare first."

To ensure a fair evaluation, the competing payment systems must be on an even playing field. Many health care workers complain that this hasn't been so. However, recent legislation may be leveling the field. For example, many practitioners are heralding the recently revised antitrust guidelines, which will allow physicians and dentists greater freedom to form fee-for-service networks.

Health care providers are also hoping for the passage of H.R. 2400, The Family Health Care Fairness Act. Introduced by dentist-turned-legislator Charles Norwood (R-Ga.), the act "sets a ground floor, a minimum set of standards that all health care plans must follow."

While normally not an advocate of greater government controls, Norwood appears committed to provide legislative protection for patients who are subject to managed care abuses.

As federal activity continues, professional attention is directed to the Oregon initiative. Regardless of the vote's outcome, capitation will continue to be a major payment method for health services. The ultimate judgment will be made not by voters in one state, but as an eventual summation of a variety of different assessments.

The real victor in Oregon—even if the vote is not in his favor—will be the ophthalmologist, whose unflagging persistence and conviction gave the voters a choice.

Who would have ever thought that possible?

Perhaps only Spanish philosopher Miguel de Unamuno y Jugo, whose inspirational message "Only he who attempts the absurd is capable of achieving the impossible" provided the foundation for the musical creation of "Man of La Mancha." ∎

1. Wasserman D (book), Leigh M, Darion J (score). Man of La Mancha. 1965.
2. Page L. Ophthalmologist asks Oregon voters to outlaw capitation. Am Med News 1996; Aug 26:3,20.
3. Kassirer JP. Managed care and the morality of the marketplace. N Engl J Med 1995;333(1):50-2.

# Would you do it again?

*Originally published in JADA 1996 126: 1696-1698.*

For the price of a postage stamp, thousands of JADA subscribers use our Question of the Month to register their views on dentistry's issues. Their thoughts are tabulated and published in The Journal. Unlike most polls that boast accuracy within a standard deviation of a few percentage points, the JADA survey makes no claim to represent the perspectives of anyone beyond the dentists who respond.

Given this limitation, my concern about the response to July's question may merit little consideration. That month we asked readers, "If you had to do it again, would you become a dentist?" Forty-four percent of respondents said they would not.

No doubt every profession has unhappy members who, given the opportunity, wouldn't do it again—or at least say they wouldn't do it again in some anonymous poll.

The intensity of clinical practice, however, may cause more postgraduate dissatisfaction in dentistry than in other fields. Ours is a profession that demands perfection from its members. Dentists are known to be highly self-critical—even though their patients value their services and give them high marks for competence and caring.

So maybe dentists, by professional nature, will find fault regardless of reality. If so, this might explain the high number of dentists who answered "no" when asked if they would "do it again."

Although this may be a legitimate explanation, certain write-in responses to July's question warrant consideration. Citing economic hardships, heavy-handed outside regulation, high stress and loss of autonomy, these respondents reveal serious underlying concerns for themselves and their profession.

Younger dentists, for example, wrote that student loans are adversely affecting their enjoyment of professional life. "Though I love what I do," wrote one young dentist, "my student loan debt is so overwhelming, I cannot properly provide for my family the way I thought dentistry could."

Older dentists focused more on the office environment. Noted one, "It is a highly work-intensive or labor-intensive profession fraught with much politics regarding the work environment ... no other profession is held to the high standard that dentistry is." Wrote another, "OSHA overregulation, PPO, HMO, managed care—dentistry is now seen as an industry instead of a profession."

With no relief in sight from the cost of dental education and little chance of fewer outside intrusions, today's practitioner can expect stress levels to continue rising.

Some who answered the July question showed concern for those who have not yet entered the profession. Said one, "Someone should get the message to incoming students—they have no idea." Asked another, "Why didn't someone tell me what dentistry is really like?"

In response to these concerns, let me offer a suggestion.

> **Dentists are obliged to inform their patients of all positive and negative aspects of proposed dental treatments. They should do the same for students considering a dental career.**

Dentists are obliged to inform their patients of all positive and negative aspects of proposed dental treatments. They should do the same for students considering a dental career. Students deserve complete information about the practice of dentistry—even if it dissuades them from pursuing a dental career.

Such information should include a detailed analysis of the cost of dental education, a review of current dental practice issues and a description of the physical hazards practitioners face. And this information should be provided to those who directly influence career choices.

Dental school admissions counselors may argue that they already are informing students about potential career problems. I hope they are. But they're not the first to counsel young people on career choice, and they're not the primary audience for this initiative. By the time students enter a dental school's admissions offices, most already have opted for a career in dentistry.

It's the predental advisers—faculty members in colleges and universities—who serve (usually gratis) as first-stop advisers for those considering careers in the health professions. And it is these advisers, usually biology or chemistry teachers, who should be targeted. Few possess the in-depth knowledge of dentistry needed to assist students in making informed career choices.

What is needed is a joint initiative of the ADA and the American Association of Dental Schools to develop an informational packet for these predental advisers. This information also could be pack-aged as a video or CD-ROM for easier access.

While this packet may prove sufficient, I would further suggest that dental schools, in cooperation with local ADA representatives, hold on-campus seminars for these advisers. During my tenure as dean at Colorado, such meetings were well attended and helped foster good relations with one of dentistry's most important recruitment partners—the faculty member.

In the clinical setting, no one expects informed consent to assuage all patient concerns. Nor would educational informed consent necessarily prevent all future dentists from becoming disillusioned with their profession. But such a program would constitute a professional best-effort to assist in a decision that has lifelong implications. ∎

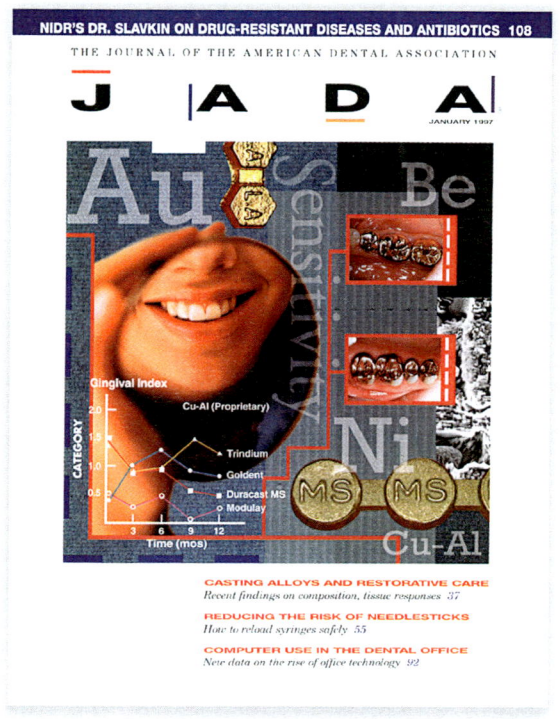

# 1997

"In response to one Consumer Reports query, more than 80 percent said their dental works was 'very good' to 'excellent.' Ninety-six percent said they had confidence in their dentist's technical competence."

1997

# Privacy at risk. Whose? Yours!

*Originally published in JADA 1997 128: 8-10..*

**Y**our internist says you have high blood pressure. That information becomes part of your permanent record. A police officer gives you a speeding citation. Another entry. Academic achievements, credit ratings, armed service records, IRS returns, a refund to a dental patient. It's all on your ever-expanding personal ledger.

Such records present few problems if they remain under your control. Unfortunately, the massive storage capacities of computers have made it virtually impossible for the average citizen to keep track of who knows what about his or her past. Unable to determine or control who might access or use such personal records, many Americans are seriously concerned about invasions of privacy.

Consider the ramifications of being told you have high blood pressure. Life and disability insurers are interested in that information. They may want to extract higher premiums from you on future insurance applications. Even if the condition is being controlled successfully, you must respond in the affirmative to their question, "Have you ever been treated for hypertension?" And once you have answered yes, your response is shared with the entire insurance industry.

Such things happen in other industries as well. What you consider private becomes another routine entry in a growing dossier on you. Those troubled by this continual infringement on privacy seek protections that would give them access to their personal records but restrict public access. Their one major success—the Open Records Act—allows them to see what's inside their file. But the act doesn't prohibit others from seeing as well and from using the information.

This may change soon, spurred by grave concerns about those involved in genetic testing. It appears that genetic discoveries with the potential to predict diseases—some untreatable and eventually fatal—have caused the medical, legal and ethical communities to look for ways to protect those whose genetic makeup has been revealed.

The recent discovery of breast-cancer–related mutations in the BRCA1 and BRCA2 genes illustrates the need for immediate action. Women with these genetic mutations have a lifetime risk of breast cancer that approaches 85 percent.

The most beneficial outcome of genetic testing would be preventive treatment for those with a genetic predisposition to breast cancer. But oncologists can't offer definitive treatments. It isn't even clear from the literature that "preventive mastectomies" are effective.

Knowing your genetic makeup in this case could be a problem. What you know can hurt you. A negative test, for example, might be falsely interpreted as a lifetime guarantee against breast cancer. It isn't. A positive test, without the promise of successful treatment, would lead to further concern and heightened emotional distress. For those who test positive, still more harm could come if the results are communicated to their employers, their health insurers or even to their family members.

Once insurers get the test results, higher premiums or denied coverage could be expected. Employers, wishing to minimize their financial risk, could compound the problem by choosing not to hire—or to dismiss—workers with positive test results.

Family complications are another possibility. Who, for example, speaks for the 8-year-old girl whose BRCA1-positive mother wants her daughter tested for the mutant gene? The mother's rationale: if the test is positive, removing the child's breast buds could prolong her life.

Does a parent have the right to invade a child's privacy before the child has the knowledge and ex-

> **As a health professional, chances are that you will be drawn eventually into a confrontation that pits genetic testing against personal privacy.**

perience to make her own judgments? Does a child have the right of privacy, even if exercising that right may harm her in the future? There are no easy answers.

As a health professional, chances are that you will be drawn eventually into a confrontation that pits genetic testing against personal privacy. Would you, for example, hire a receptionist who has reported to you that she has the BRCA1 mutation? If your answer is yes, you risk increased health and disability insurance premiums for your entire office. Failing to hire, on the other hand, might make you the target of a lawsuit for discriminating on the basis of an applicant's predisposition to a disease.

At least 12 states have been sufficiently concerned about the right to genetic privacy to pass laws declaring that "genetic information is the unique property of the individual ... and that the intent of the statute is to prevent information derived from genetic testing from being used to deny access to health care insurance, group disability or long-term care insurance."[1]

National legislation, similar in design, was introduced last spring. It failed to receive Senate attention before the session ended but is likely to be reintroduced during the next term.

Genetic discoveries continue at an accelerated pace. Within a few years, science will have mapped and sequenced the entire complement of human genes. And in the not-too-distant future, you may be asked whether you want to know about your DNA.

At a recent conference on genetic testing, a group of ethicists, health care providers and lawyers were asked to respond to this statement: "I would want to know about my DNA, but it should not become part of a central repository." Their answers: 27 yes, eight no.

There is a genetic test that can identify a very rare form of Alzheimer's disease, a form that accounts for about 1 percent of all existing cases. If your family has a history of Alzheimer's, would you want to be administered this test? And if you tested positive, would you want anyone besides yourself to know the results?

Whose privacy is at risk? Yours is. ■

1. Colorado Senate Bill 94-058, Concerning Limitations on Genetic Testing; signed June 2, 1994, Gov. Roy Romer.

# Patients first and always

*Originally published in JADA 1997 128: 138-140.*

Pressured by third-party insurers, health plans and HMO trade groups, the American Medical Association is moving ahead with a major accreditation program for physicians. If you thought, as I did, that all U.S. practicing physicians already were accredited through licensure and clinical boards—and you question the motive for such a program (and the impact it might have on dentistry)—further clarification is in order.

With "If we don't do it, they will" as their rationale, the AMA will seek information on the clinical operations and management systems of a physician's office as well as the basics of his or her academic training. Plans are to "enhance" the accreditation packet with measures of the physician's clinical performance and patient care results.

Some specialty physicians believe this initiative will undermine the importance of board certification. Despite their objections, however, the concept seems to be gaining acceptance. At least 10 state medical societies are interested in partnering with the AMA on this accrediting venture.

Can you imagine the response from dental practitioners if the ADA were to propose a similar program? How many dentists would favor a new regulatory program that might restrict their ability to practice—especially if it was designed to please a third party? Using the rationale that "we have to do it before it's done to us" is like handcuffing yourself to prevent someone else from doing it. Either way, you've lost control.

Unless things have changed without our noticing, the true test of a profession's effectiveness is measured by the public's well-being—not the size of the insurer's bottom line. The ADA Principles of Ethics and Code of Professional Conduct clearly states that the dentist's "primary professional responsibility shall be service to the public." I don't

> **How many dentists would favor a new regulatory program that might restrict their ability to practice—especially if it was designed to please a third party?**

see any movement within dentistry to alter that charge.

What is needed, however, is objective feedback from the public to monitor the dental profession's performance in fulfilling its professional role. Three independent studies in the last two years have addressed this issue.

A 1994 study commissioned by the ADA found that most Americans gave dentistry a rating of either "good" or "excellent." Sixteen percent gave it a grade of "fair," while only 2 percent checked the "poor" column. Scores were even higher when quality of care was assessed. Fifty-five percent said they received "excellent" care, 31 percent said the treatment they received was "good" and just 1 percent were unhappy with their care.

Those responses speak well for the dental profession. Third parties that aid in financing dental care should be satisfied that their contributions are well-spent.

Still, some of dentistry's detractors still might say, "It's an ADA study—what would you expect?"

Public opinion expressed through a similarly designed investigation conducted by an "unbiased" university-based research group should allay any criticism. As in the first study, the results were largely positive. Responding to a question designed to elicit the degree of public trust in dentistry, 35 percent said they held "a great deal" of trust in the profession, 50 percent "a moderate amount" and only 2 percent "none."

Questions measuring public respect for dentistry resulted in even higher scores. Ninety percent of respondents answered either "a great deal" or "a moderate amount" to the question, "How much respect would you say you have for the dental profession?"

A study published in the December 1996 issue of *Consumer Reports* provided dentistry with what I consider its best and most accurate evaluation.

Fifty-two thousand Consumer Reports subscribers participated in a survey on dental care. I think it would be fair to characterize these respondents as enlightened and responsible consumers—people who would be more thoughtful in their assessments of dentistry than the general population.

In response to one Consumer Reports query, more than 80 percent said their dental work was "very good" to "excellent." Ninety-six percent said they had confidence in their dentist's technical competence. In evaluating overall satisfaction, only one reader in 20 voiced any level of dissatisfaction.

There were some negatives, however. Ten percent of the readers complained that dentists rush through the dental visit. Much more alarming, 40 percent said their dentist never discussed the costs of restorative care in advance, and 50 percent reported that the dentist failed to lay out treatment choices beforehand.

These criticisms should not blur the outstanding report card that dentistry has received from the public. There is no current need for accreditation of dental practitioners. Let the insurers, the HMOs, the trade groups—let everyone—examine how well dentistry is perceived by the public.

On the other hand, professional complacency cannot be tolerated. Issues of patient communication, case presentation and sensitivity to the cost of care need to be addressed. Doing so may prevent a future call for the accreditation of dental practitioners. ∎

# A dental rip-off

*Originally published in JADA 1997 128: 264-268.*

The February issue of Reader's Digest implies that dishonest dentists are ripping off the American public. Actually, the magazine does more than imply. On newsstands, it carries a second front cover with the eye-catching headline, "Exclusive Investigation: How Dentists Rip Us Off."

Inside, the cover exposé is accompanied by the too-familiar graphic depiction of a dentist menacingly hovering over a patient with the dreaded drill in hand. Add to that picture an accumulation of noncomplimentary adjectives about dentists—describing, for instance, the dentist's "nutcracker" handshake—and you have all the ingredients for a full-fledged bashing of the dental profession.

Judging by the public response logged on the Reader's Digest Web home page, the dental exposé more than fulfilled the magazine's desire to generate controversy and boost sales. One Digest reader commented, "Dentists cannot be trusted! I do not let anyone mess with my teeth. I remove my own tartar ... anyone who sees a dentist should have their head examined, not their teeth! They are ALL crooks!!" Another wrote, "I was hoping that I would be living in one of the cities that had one of the good dentists listed. Unfortunately, I live in a city where the author did not have a good experience." Responses by dentists, while strongly admonishing the magazine for inflammatory reporting, often degenerated into windy rhetoric as they tried to refute the article's charges.

From the dental perspective, there is indeed a rip-off going on. But it's dentists, not the public, who are the victims. By the author's skillful manipulation of words, variations in dental practice patterns have been incorrectly presented as evidence of dental dishonesty.

Had the Reader's Digest presentation suggested that dental treatment plans can be quite variable and encouraged the public to seek additional opinions, I wouldn't have taken offense. It's the dishonesty theme that I find unacceptable. Questions about a profession's veracity and insinuations of collusion to rip off the public cannot be left unanswered.

Let's start with what we know about our profession. While it is definitely science-based, no one would say that we have all the answers. Indeed, basic information regarding disease processes and outcomes is still incomplete. To my knowledge, no one can say with surety whether it will take an untreated, incipient carious lesion six months or six years to reach the dental pulp. Nor do we have data that can predict the longevity of a cast full crown. Empirical evidence still remains a dentist's major source of information.

Don't anticipate definitive information about risk, progression of disease and outcomes of treatment in the near future. Dental research still channels most of its resources into the development of new and better dental materials. Until a significant portion of these resources is diverted to investigate outcomes of dental treatment, dentistry will remain vulnerable to further public scrutiny.

The following excerpt from a recent review of variation in dental practice offers the best description of the present state of the art. The authors write that "a substantial proportion of the variation may stem from differences in dentists' beliefs about dental diseases and their treatment—such as diagnostic criteria, knowledge of risk factors, rates of incidence, prevalence and progression—and the outcomes of alternative treatments." The authors conclude that "information which a lay observer might assume to be the very bedrock of the dental profession all too often resembles quicksand."[1]

Much of this "quicksand" is located in one of the fastest-growing areas in dentistry: aesthetics. In-

> **From the dental perspective, there is indeed a rip-off going on. But it's dentists, not the public, who are the victims.**

creasing numbers of patients are demanding more than restoration of function. Enhancing a patient's overall appearance by altering the configuration of the mouth can have aesthetic as well as psychological benefits.

Regardless of the sincerity of the dentist in presenting the treatment plan, the perception of what is aesthetically pleasing rests in the eyes of the beholder. Under these circumstances, inconsistencies in dental treatment plans with aesthetic components will occur. They should be viewed as an honest effort to benefit patients—not an attempt at a rip-off.

To Reader's Digest and the author of "How Honest Are Dentists?": Please take note of the following true scenario.

DENTIST: "Larry, this isn't a beauty-vs.-the-beast discussion. Your wife is already very attractive. But help me to convince her that closing that diastema between [teeth] No. 8 and No. 9 will render her forever beautiful. Just look at this before-and-after computer projection."

These are the words of our family dentist, who sincerely believes that closing a small space between my wife's maxillary central incisors would enhance her appearance.

Although our dentist is highly skilled and literate in the art of aesthetic dentistry, his yearly prescription for cosmetic improvement continues to fall on deaf ears. The patient, convinced that her diastema is an integral part of a personal signature, continually rejects his plan. Undaunted, convinced that he can make a difference, he will present his aesthetic blueprint again and again.

An attempted rip-off? Absolutely not! A dishonest practitioner taking advantage of a patient? Hardly. Just an ethical dentist presenting what he sincerely believes would enhance the oral appearance of his patient. ∎

1. Bader JD, Shugars DA. Variations in dentists' clinical decisions. J Public Health Dent 1995;55(3):181-8.

# We are the world

*Originally published in JADA 1997 128: 392-396.*

Few question the primacy of American dentistry. After all, aren't we the world? This superior attitude, which admittedly ignores the many contributions of countries with well-developed dental standards, can be justified by considering the evidence.

U.S. dentistry is supported by the most extensive network of state-of-the-art technology and research expertise in the world. Hundreds of dental researchers are employed full time seeking new knowledge. Professional oversight ensures that dental education meets uniform standards of excellence. Short-term, high-quality continuing education programs are accessible and affordable.

These factors, coupled with the research, education and professional communities' historical commitment to improve the nation's oral health, provide the basis for the supremacy claim.

Some dental leaders would contend that being "the dental world" is not without added responsibility and that we have social and moral obligations to share our expertise with all who desire it. Realistically, considering the intensely competitive nature of present-day dental practice, I doubt if many U.S. practitioners have the time or inclination to become involved outside of their present scope.

Nonetheless, there are dentists who, at the appropriate time, will participate in information exchange programs. The following suggestions are directed at those willing to share their dental knowledge with interested dentists from other countries. These proposed strategies should be relatively easy to introduce.

The frequent traveler knows that hearing the personalized perspectives about a foreign country from one of its residents often results in a more enjoyable and memorable experience, much better than the conventional tourist itinerary. Unfortunately, while many prefer to cultivate a foreign contact, finding one can prove difficult if not impossible.

New York City has recognized the importance of making visitors feel at home and has solicited 500 volunteers willing to spend 3 or more hours with a foreign guest.

Japan features a person-to-person system that matches tourists with families located throughout the country. The fortunate traveler involved in this type of program gets a firsthand view of country life and insights into politics, economics, religion and family life that no ordinary tourist could experience.

> **Until you actually engage in a dentist-to-dentist interaction, you cannot fully appreciate the importance of sharing your expertise with those who do not have our resource base.**

Building on this successful theme, why not create an international dentist-to-dentist program? Dental societies worldwide could collect the names of local dentists willing to give a few hours of their time to meet with a dental visitor. The next step would be to find a mechanism that would provide for a rapid interchange when a request is received.

Perhaps the ADA could act as the clearinghouse for collecting and distributing names of foreign and U.S. dentist-to-dentist volunteers. Coordinating a program of this type should not be expensive and might provide the ADA with the impetus to increase its international presence.

For dentists unwilling to wait for the development of such a program, I would suggest using the classified section of JADA. I remember an ad placed in The Journal by a French dentist who was seeking a U.S. experience for his 16-year-old daughter. The dentist promised, in return, a similar opportunity for the children of his daughter's host. He received an overwhelming response to that ad.

Dentists choosing the classified route should be able to establish contacts in almost any country in the world. With almost 4,000 foreign dentists presently receiving JADA, either as a benefit of affiliated membership or through a paid subscription, finding dental contacts should not be a problem.

Other dentist-to-dentist opportunities might be arranged during the ADA annual session. Depending on the meeting site and joint sponsorship by the FDI World Dental Federation, anywhere from 1,000 to more than 3,000 attendees come from foreign countries.

ADA members desiring other exchange opportunities can participate in hands-on service and education programs. Call or write the ADA for its second edition of "International Dental Volunteer Organizations: A Guide to Service and a Directory of Programs," available through the ADA Department of International Health (Ext. 2726 at headquarters). This comprehensive guide provides invaluable advice for the dentist considering any type of volunteer work. It contains detailed information on how to get started, types of equipment needed, how to fund projects and a comprehensive list of established organizations seeking dental volunteers.

While these programs require a hands-on commitment, other, less time-consuming opportunities await those wishing to share their knowledge with foreign dentists. Consider using your computer and the Internet to establish a dental bulletin board or an international study club. For that first adventure, try using the Internet to find an electronic dental "pen pal."

Until you actually engage in a dentist-to-dentist interaction, you cannot fully appreciate the importance of sharing your expertise with those who do not have our resource base.

I am presently communicating with a dentist in Bhutan, a small kingdom sandwiched between India and Tibet. As one of only six dentists serving a country of about 1 million people, he has no access to any formal continuing education programs outside his country. He must rely on books, journals and perhaps audio or video cassettes. These items are costly—a year's subscription to JADA represents an entire month's salary.

In our communications, the Bhutanese dentist has written, "I look forward to receiving anything on dentistry that will assist in improving the quality of dentistry in Bhutan so that I can serve my King, people and the country in better ways."

With that kind of request, how can we refuse involvement?

After all, when it comes to dentistry, "we are the world." ■

# Putting choice back into the health care equation

*Originally published in JADA 1997 128: 536-540.*

**U**ntil a few years ago, the ability to exercise unrestricted choice of one's health care provider was generally taken for granted. Not so any more. Responding to escalating health care costs, employers and government officials have instituted a variety of health programs that now affect long-standing provider-patient relationships.

One of the most visible changes has been interference in the patient's ability to freely choose health care providers. By requiring high deductibles and copayments from program enrollees who go "out of the system" for care, insurers hope to contain costs by minimizing choice.

Their strategy is working. As the price of choice goes up, increasing numbers of patients are fiscally unable to continue their health care relationships with nonpreferred practitioners.

To blame only insurers for restricting free choice of provider would be incorrect. Some network providers, who not long ago thrived through free-choice mechanisms, have become major proponents of limiting choice options. Caught in the national feeding frenzy to protect and build patient markets, they, too, are advocating financial penalties for those seeking care out of their network.

I can attest to this from personal experience.

Until recently, my employer, the University of Colorado Health Sciences Center, has supported a health plan allowing free choice of health providers with no penalty. No longer.

Claiming a need to ensure enough patients for educational purposes as well as to promote its practice plan, the Health Sciences Center instituted a plan (Gold) that provides maximum bene-

> **By requiring high deductibles and copayments from program enrollees who go "out of the system" for care, insurers hope to contain costs by minimizing choice.**

fits to those who use the university's physician network. To placate those who still wish free choice of provider, a second plan (Silver), requiring high deductibles and coinsurance, was offered at a price 21/2 times the monthly premium for the university plan.

Because our family wished to continue its relationship with our previous health providers, we selected the Silver plan. It cost more, but so what? We didn't want to change providers. Apparently, too many university employees felt the same way. This year the Silver plan was modified.

Employees in the university network plan received a monthly premium increase of 6 percent. Those of us in the "free-choice plan" saw our premiums zoom by 48 percent.

The squeeze play worked. Enrollment in the Silver plan fell 50 percent. Now the university benefits office is talking about getting rid of the Silver plan altogether. They say that point-of-service opportunities in the university Gold plan will handle those who still want choice. They neglect to emphasize that any requests for out-of-network payment will be reimbursed at just 60 percent of cost. Recently, we learned that their next move is to develop an HMO Gold plan with no provision for out-of-network services.

No choice at all?

In the United States, most pre-Medicare health benefits are tied to employment. Few people, including me, are in a position to change jobs because of unhappiness with the health plans offered. Fortunately, there is a program already in place that can restore choice—and much more.

This potential savior is the medical saving account, or MSA, which was modeled after the highly successful tax-exempt retirement account. The concept did not become a viable option until this year, when the federal government gave the green light to a four-year limited test. Up to 750,000 self-employed workers or employees of small companies with two to 50 employees will be allowed to participate.

Even with limited fanfare and publicity, the Jan. 1, 1997, introduction of the MSA test has received a thumbs-up from both consumers and employers. The enrollment cap for the pilot test is expected to be reached by year-end.

This is how the MSA works:

During the four-year trial period, MSA participants need to be enrolled in a high-deductible health plan. Deductibles for individuals must be at least $1,500, and not more than $2,500. For families, the deductible must be at least $3,000, not exceeding $4,500.

Depending on the worker's status, MSA contributions will be made either by the employer or by the self-employed worker. Decisions on medical services used rest with enrollees. If questioned, they must deal directly with the Internal Revenue Service.

Economists from MIT, Stanford and Harvard used past health-program data to estimate that, with MSAs in place, 90 percent of employees would have at least $25,000 at retirement; 50 percent would have $50,000 or more; and just 20 percent would have less than half their contribution.

How will MSAs affect dental services? One of the concept's designers and major proponents, Ger-

ald Musgrave, believes that the spinoff from "transforming money and power from large bureaucratic institutions to individuals and encouraging vigorous competition in the market for health services" will be exceedingly positive for dentistry.[1]

Specifically:

- Individuals could maintain separate dental coverage even though they had an MSA.
- Dental services are a valid expense under an MSA but presently would not count toward the deductible.
- Those who end up with major positive balances in their MSAs at retirement could use them to purchase benefits, such as long-term care policies, or to continue insurance plans that offer subsidies for dental care.
- Since dental services can be purchased through the tax-free dollars in the MSA, the average worker can effectively reduce the price of dental services by up to 50 percent.
- Economists predict that the demand for dental services by MSA holders will increase as soon as they note excess dollars in their MSA accounts.

All in all, a major plus for dentistry.

To further the expansion of the MSA program, dentists must become fully conversant with the concept. They need to endorse it vocally, even participate if possible. But most important, they should support congressional efforts to extend MSA benefits to all who wish to join.

Let's help put choice back in the health care equation! ∎

1. Goodman CJ, Musgrave GL. Patient power. 2nd ed. Washington, D.C.: Cato Institute; 1994:134.

# What do dentists do when they don't do dentistry?

*Originally published in JADA 1997 128: 682-686.*

It would be the rare dentist who, in moments of frustration, did not consider changing careers—letting his or her mind drift to some less stressful and more rewarding occupation.

Few do more than dream, but some do change. I know of a dentist who decided, after practicing for 16 years, to leave the profession to "move snow and dirt" in Aspen, Colo. He is now baking bagels in Oregon. Was it dissatisfaction with dentistry that motivated his career change? No, he says. "Where is it written that you can have only one career?" he asks.

Dentists usually leave the profession because of disability or retirement. Those exiting to another career are in the minority, but they attract the most professional attention. After all, it's hard not to be intrigued by those who defy social convention and seek more than a single career during their lifetime.

Who are these mavericks and what do they do after dentistry?

An in-depth study of former dentists who volunteered to tell why they left dentistry is under way at the University of Minnesota. Among the 32 former dentists studied, the list of new career tracks is long and varied. The roster includes ministers, a writer, a wildlife expert, an actor, a cartoonist, a financial planner, a photographer, a psychotherapist, a filmmaker and a househusband.

Many study subjects admitted to lifelong dreams of the occupations they now follow. Others said the stimulus for change had been talents or interests that developed during their lives as practitioners. Almost all were happy with their decision to leave dentistry.

Yet most dentists don't leave.

Could the reasons include the high cost of leaving? The large capital investment in the office? The need to pay off educational debts? The stigma of leaving a high-visibility health profession? The inability to receive equivalent economic return in alternative professions? The difficulty of pursuing a new career that requires retraining or new credentialing? Or the fact that dentistry offers little opportunity to transfer clinical skills to other professions, except possibly medicine? Any or all of these reasons could keep dentists from making career shifts.

Then there are the retirees, the largest group that has left dentistry.

In 1995, there were 182,306 living dentists, of whom 153,346 were considered professionally active. That leaves 28,960 who had retired or were no longer in active practice. This already sizable group will be joined by thousands of new retirees over the next 15 years.

Also in 1995, 23.4 percent of professionally active dentists were 55 years of age or older. The numbers of dentists over 55 will rise to 33 percent of the profession by 2005, and to almost 40 percent by 2010—all resulting from the bulge created by the dental graduates of the 1970s moving through the system.

How well these dentists plan for retirement will determine their future options. Having sufficient financial resources to live a comfortable retirement is a high priority for most Americans, and dentists are no exception.

Assuming financial stability and good health, what will these dentists do when they don't do dentistry?

Some retiring dentists will leave their professional involvement behind completely and concen-

> **Retired dentists will want—will need—to remain active in their profession in some capacity. The question is: does the profession have a place for them?**

trate on travel, golf or other hobbies. Some will open a small business. For others, the total separation from a profession they have devoted their lives to will leave a void. These dentists will want—will need—to remain active in their profession in some capacity. The question is: does the profession have a place for them?

Unfortunately, this growing resource of experience and knowledge has not been factored into future professional planning. Yes, those who have been members for 30 years get a nice certificate of life membership and pay no further dues. But what else? If they want JADA or the ADA News, these are out-of-pocket expenses.

Why isn't the profession courting this group? Its members could represent a major asset to the ADA Health Foundation, both as solicitors and donors. Many retired members still have political clout, keeping in touch with former patients who hold elective office and other influential positions.

The interest is there for life members. They represent 13 percent of the ADA's grassroots army. Some are in their 80s and even their 90s. Old? Sure, but so are some of our legislators.

One of the great frustrations of retired dentists is the difficulty they encounter when trying to volunteer their services to treat the underserved. A dentist writes, "When I wanted to volunteer my expertise, I couldn't without taking another state board. Apparently, ample credentials and a highly successful, documented track record count for very little."

Perhaps it's time for the ADA to push for a National Service Corps of Retired Dentists. Because of licensing restrictions, such a group's activities may have to be confined initially to federal sites, but the ADA could take an active role in helping constituent and component societies to establish local sites for volunteers among retirees. With President Clinton's national emphasis on volunteerism, ADA support for such action would demonstrate dentistry's continuing commitment to the underserved.

Today, only the fledgling American Society of Retired Dentists—with 300 members—is available to help meet the needs of thousands of dental retirees. With a massive increase in numbers already on the horizon, professional dentistry must take note and serve this group. These dentists have a great deal to offer and want continued professional involvement.

Not long ago, I had the privilege of interviewing a 97-year-old dentist whose words are a testament to the vitality and spirit of our retired dentists. "I'm not getting old, just older," she said. ■

# An oversupply in the offing?

*Originally published in JADA 1997 128: 802-804.*

Critics of excessive or frivolous federal spending must be having a field day with the announcement that the federal Health Care Financing Administration will pay selected New York hospitals $400 million to reduce the number of physicians they train.

To reap the benefits of this unusual offer, 41 New York hospitals have agreed to cut their residency slots by 20 percent or more over a 6-year period. HCFA believes this fiscal incentive will slow the "oversupply" of physicians.

If there are hospitals in other states looking for a share of the HCFA money, don't bother to apply—only New York hospitals are eligible. Furthermore, HCFA has said nothing about extending the program to address real or imagined imbalances in other health care fields.

For many JADA readers, this HCFA announcement must bring back memories. In the 1970s, the federal government predicted that the United States soon would face a shortage of dentists and physicians. To offset this approaching shortage, the government offered dental and medical schools large sums of money to boost class size.

The predicted shortage never came, of course, and the result was was an oversupply of dentists that took a couple of decades to level out. Wait long enough and the pendulum makes a complete swing.

When market forces acted to correct dentistry's personnel imbalance, entering dental class sizes fell from 6,301 in 1978 to less than 4,000 in 1989, and there has been little fluctuation in class size since that time. However, because of dentistry's recent economic successes, class sizes soon may begin to rise again.

Consider the following:
- Between 1990 and 1994, the average income of a general practitioner rose 17.2 percent in real dollars (adjusted for inflation).
- The pretax net hourly rate for dentists now exceeds the hourly earnings of medical generalists, internists and pediatricians.

These income figures have not gone unnoticed. An economic measurement called "rate of return" often is used to predict the demand for more candidates to enter an occupation or profession. The formula accounts for the cost of education and years of income lost during the educational period. It then projects future economic return, amortizing educational expense against anticipated future income.

Even allowing for the high cost of a dental education, future dentists have a high rate of return (according to this formula) resulting in rising numbers of qualified dental school applicants—and growing pressure on dental deans to increase class size.

Reflecting dentistry's favorable rate of return, the number of applications to U.S. dental schools rose by 2,590—a 51 percent increase—between 1991 and 1995. In that same period, first-year places in dental school increased by just 120 seats. That translates into 22 applicants for each new position.

Increased interest in dentistry as a career option comes at a time when most dental schools are cutting budgets. If this trend continues, however, how long will it be before class sizes begin to climb?

The rate-of-return formula has its limitations. For one, it usually estimates future incomes using present conditions, which may not be valid. Public demand for dental services may be high today. But what will the future bring? Who can assure prospective dentists that they will have 30 years of prosperity?

For those involved in predicting the demand for dentists, the article "Trends in Dental Care Among Insured Americans: 1980-1995," which appeared in

> **While public demand for today's dental services may be excellent, what about the future? Who can assure prospective dentists that they will have 30 years of prosperity?**

the February issue of JADA, should be required reading. The data for this report are limited to an insured population. But if the authors' assumptions prove correct, a major decline in demand for restorative procedures is on the horizon.

The study showed that for those 35 years old and younger, the need for "extractions, endodontics and crowns all declined appreciably." This is the first report of its magnitude to be published; it would be unfair, therefore, to draw any definitive conclusions from it. Nevertheless, this study could have a profound influence on the demand for future dentists.

The dental gurus who predict such things are interpreting these results with caution—and properly so. Many other factors must be studied as well.

Still to be addressed are the dental care utilization and health patterns of those without dental insurance. This population segment, which constitutes the majority, must be an integral component of any personnel planning.

Also requiring study is the impact of implants and cosmetic dentistry, the fastest growing areas in dental care; the aging of America and the fact that more people are keeping their teeth in later life; and the fact that the profession itself is aging, with more than 40 percent of dentists expected to be past their most productive years by 2010.

Earlier attempts to predict the demand for dental personnel have been, at best, an inexact science, a process fraught with difficulty. Dental policy planners would agree that the large number of uncontrolled variables in dentistry makes a truly perfect prediction virtually unattainable. Still, an ongoing assessment of need is critical to those in practice and to those who wish to consider careers in dentistry.

The newly established ADA Health Policy Resources Center will be addressing the future demand for dentists, a clear indication of this issue's importance to dentistry. ∎

# Do it or lose it

*Originally published in JADA 1997 128: 1058-1060.*

Like the aftershocks of an earthquake, the February Reader's Digest's special report titled "How Honest Are Dentists?" continues to provoke discussion. Some of the discourse has focused on my editorial defense of dentists' honesty in the treatment planning process. While respecting the comments of those voicing opposing views, I remain firmly convinced that the science necessary to bring objectivity to dental treatment planning is virtually nonexistent and that until sufficient data become available, dentistry will be vulnerable to outside attacks.

However, unlike the arguments I used to rationalize the idiosyncrasies of dental treatment planning, I offer no rebuttal to Mr. Ecenbarger's criticism that "only 21 [of 50 dentists surveyed] conducted the ADA-recommended oral cancer screening." His comments reflected what previous research from a National Health Interview Survey already had documented: just 15 percent of U.S. citizens aged 40 years and older recollect ever having had an oral cancer examination. That percentage does not come close to the screening recommendations of the American Cancer Society, which call for an annual exam for those over 40 years of age.

For a disease that is dentistry's to prevent and treat, we have demonstrated a singular lack of progress in controlling the occurrence of oral and pharyngeal cancer, especially when compared with the major inroads that have been made in cancers of the prostate, breast and colon.

Consider this abysmal record. Each year, 30,000 U.S. citizens are diagnosed with oral cancer—a number that has shown no meaningful decrease in the last three decades. From the oral cancer morbidity pool, about 8,000 deaths are recorded each year; that is more than one oral cancer death per hour.

While the oral cancer death rate exceeds that

registered for either cervical cancer or malignant melanoma, it does not get anywhere close to the national attention directed toward early detection of the latter two.

It should. It must!

The oral cancer 5-year overall survival rate of 56 percent is strongly skewed by the low 19 percent survival rate in advanced cases. If cancer is detected early, the survival rate for those with localized lesions reaches 80 percent. Discounting the potential life-saving aspects of early diagnosis, detecting oral cancer in its early stages will alleviate the disfigurement and diminished quality of life associated with late-stage carcinomas.

Interestingly, while the dental profession vigorously pursues programs designed to educate patients about the need for good oral health and regular dental visits, major professional campaigns focused primarily on the oral cancer detection issue have been virtually nonexistent.

> **If significant numbers of dental practitioners do not fulfill their responsibility in oral cancer detection, the medical specialties will move quickly to become the oral cancer experts.**

If the deliberations of a committee consisting of experts in dentistry and related health professions come to fruition, needed changes may follow. Last August, a national conference that included representatives of organized dentistry, government, industry and the nonprofit public and private sector set goals intended to reduce oral cancer morbidity and mortality. The group called for implementation of a national campaign to prevent and control cancer of the oral facial region and pharynx.

No expensive new initiatives are needed to increase the percentage of dentists who perform routine oral cancer exams. Every practitioner has had extensive training in the visualization and interpretation of oral lesions. All that is necessary is for dentists to uniformly apply that skill to each of their patients.

No age group should be excluded from examination. Adults with histories of heavy smoking and alcohol use are at high risk of developing oral malignancies. Anaplastic lesions have been noted in teenagers who chew tobacco. With 8- and 9-year-old children experimenting with different forms of tobacco, they too must be examined for lesions that could become problematic at some future time.

To advance the goal that 100 percent of all dental patients be given a yearly cancer exam as an integral part of their complete oral exam, let me propose that the American College of Dentists and its colleagues in the International College of Dentists sponsor multisite continuing education programs designed to reinforce practitioner skills in the detection of oral cancer. While these programs might involve some costs, this type of activity would be in keeping with the public service mandates contained in the charters of these honorary societies.

Research to develop more sensitive measures of oral disease also needs support. Think of the impact the Pap test has had on cervical cancer detection. The prostate-specific antigen test, a recent development, has accomplished the same for early prostate cancer detection. The pending FDA application to use toluidine blue O as an adjunct in detecting oral malignancy may provide an early step in this direction.

For those involved in developing codes on dental procedures and nomenclature, there is a need to expand the code descriptor for oral exams to include a specific reference to oral cancer detection.

Additionally, dental policymakers should give more than lip service to public education that stresses the importance of yearly oral cancer exams. Their messages should alert the public that early detection can save lives and that dentists are the health professionals most competent to perform the exam.

In a time when health care competition is the new order, in which new territories are being staked out by the medical specialties and subspecialties, the issue of who performs what procedure(s) has taken on new importance. If significant numbers of dental practitioners do not fulfill their responsibility in oral cancer detection, the medical specialties will move quickly to become the oral cancer experts.

Dentists have all the skill and training necessary to prevent, diagnose and manage oral cancer. To abrogate that responsibility would be unconscionable. The message could not be clearer: "Do it or lose it!" ∎

# A kinder, gentler approach

*Originally published in JADA 1997 128: 1195-1196.*

"Look to your right, look to your left, look at yourself," says the dean. "One of the three of you won't make it to graduation."

A few decades ago, depending on the dental school, thousands of dental freshmen heard such words as they embarked on their journey to a dental career. Intimidation, fear and humiliation were the time-honored teaching techniques of the day.

Dentists who remember their student years as educational pain are not good targets for dental school fund-raising campaigns. With a few notable exceptions, dental deans soliciting major contributions from these older graduates usually fall short of expectations. "They didn't care about me then," these graduates observe. "Now they want my money? No way!"

But dental education has changed dramatically over the years. No longer is denigration of the student an acceptable component of dental teaching. Today, the dental school's philosophy is: "How can we help you?" For the struggling student, tutors often are made available at no charge.

Many of our colleagues consider this mollycoddling. "If I went through it, so should they," these dentists insist. They would be appalled to find that many of the hands-on, basic laboratory techniques we suffered through have been replaced by simulation exercises capable of giving objective feedback without public humiliation.

These changes do not mean that getting a dental education today is stress-free. Hardly. Dental school is still an enormous challenge, but that's mainly because of the growing body of knowledge that must be assimilated in a short period—not because of personal intimidation.

Recent graduates are more likely to view their dental schools as places where they can seek advice and continue their education. Even with limited resources, they support their schools with donations. And the schools respond in kind, seeking ways to enhance the careers of their graduates.

One educational institution, the dental school at the Univer-sity of Minnesota, has taken this concept a giant step further. Three years ago it launched a venture with a monumental goal: to warranty its educational program. Describing the program as a "Guarantee of Quality," Minnesota pledges to each of its graduates that graduation does not conclude the school's responsibility to the student.

The University of Minnesota dental school, while believing it offers one of the nation's best undergraduate dental programs, understands that under certain circumstances the new graduate will need the continued assistance of faculty.

A prime example is what happens if a new graduate fails the state board examination. Before the Quality Program was introduced, graduates had no mechanism to remediate and prepare for the next exam. Often, months would pass before the second exam was given. During this period, failed graduates had no way to hone their skills beyond self-study and heavenly guidance.

Minnesota then said, "Let's give educational opportunities to all our new graduates, not just to those whose board performance required remediation." For the last 4 years, all new graduates have been given the opportunity to build their knowledge base in general dentistry by

- free attendance and unlimited access for 18 months to all the dental school's didactic and clinical continuing education courses;
- unlimited clinical opportunities for a period of up to 1 year in the school's Comprehensive General

> **No longer is denigration of the student an acceptable component of dental teaching. Today, the dental school's philosophy is: "How can we help you?"**

Dentistry Clinic. (No tuition is charged regardless of the amount of additional instruction received.)

The new dean of the Minnesota dental school, Dr. Michael Till, is pleased with the program. Dr. Till says the Quality Program shows new graduates that "their school will not abandon them in time of need." He notes, too, that "since most new grads don't have the tuition money for continuing education, the program assures that financial circumstances will not be a barrier to receiving the continuing education they need during their transition to practice."

Recent Minnesota dental graduates appreciate the program. "The rigors of dental school often can leave a student frustrated once he or she graduates," says one. "This program helps to ease its burden and also helps us to realize that the school is truly behind its new graduates and its profession." Says another, "I just want you to know it has saved me $1,800 in CE. I could not have paid for it otherwise."

As an added bonus, former students can use the school's Dental Placement Service at no charge for 18 months—a critical period for those seeking either an associateship or practice location.

Since the program's inception 4 years ago, the dental school has recorded 233 uses of either CE programs or involvement in the Comprehensive Clinic.

Some dental educators have voiced concerns that graduates not accepted into formal General Practice Residency programs might create their own de facto residency by adding another year to their training at no additional tuition cost. Dr. Till is not concerned. "If they think they need more training, that's what this program is about," he says.

To my knowledge, the Guarantee of Quality program is unique among educational programs in the health sciences. Minnesota should be commended for its pioneering efforts. Other schools should be aware, however, that a program of this type can have considerable fiscal impact. While economies of scale exist for CE lecture courses, the cost for faculty and auxiliaries in hands-on clinical programs can be quite high.

This new approach linking students to the dental school after graduation should benefit both graduates and the school. New graduates are made life-long learners at no personal expense—and one thing they learn is that their dental school still cares.

Minnesota will not go unrewarded. The good feelings generated during the students' years in dental school will translate into support for the schools.

Providing a dental education, even with today's high tuitions, is an expensive proposition. State and federal support of both private and public dental schools is waning. The schools must cultivate other revenue sources—including their own graduates. ∎

# Much ado about nothing

*Originally published in JADA 1997 128: 1347-1348.*

Antifluoridationists must be having a field day with actor Mel Gibson's comments about fluoride in the recent blockbuster movie, "Conspiracy Theory." His character thinks the government uses fluoride more to control people than to prevent tooth decay. Nothing new in that paranoid view. I doubt that it will stimulate any increased interest in the antifluoridation movement.

But a new regulatory action by the U.S. Food and Drug Administration on labeling of fluoride toothpastes could give those who question the safety of fluoride new life. A glance at a tube of fluoride toothpaste produced since April 7 tells why.

The new federal decree requires that the following warning appear on all tubes of fluoride-containing toothpastes: "If you accidentally swallow more than used for brushing, seek professional help or contact a poison control center immediately."

The FDA poison warning will now accompany the ADA Seal of Acceptance on the labeling of fluoride toothpastes. The present ADA directive ("Do not swallow. Use only a pea-sized amount for children under six. To prevent swallowing, children under six years of age should be supervised in the use of toothpaste.") appeared to have withstood the test of time. Its wording is concise and easy to follow. Yet, for a variety of reasons, those instructions—at least in the government's view—were insufficient to protect the American public.

The new labeling has received a great deal of publicity, both here and abroad. People who have seen the labels or the media descriptions are wondering whether they were prompted by some new information that counters long-held views on the safety of fluoride toothpastes.

What makes this warning even more difficult to accept is that some substances known to cause real harm to children—spit tobacco, for example—are readily available. Many do not carry meaningful warnings on their package. The labels on some chewing tobaccos warn that "this product may cause gum disease and tooth loss," or the product "is not a safe alternative to cigarettes." Such statements hardly have the same impact as "contact a poison control center immediately."

The ADA has taken the position that the FDA warning overstates "any demonstrated or potential danger posed by fluoride toothpastes." The Association cites a long list of actions demonstrating that the ADA has been proactive in this area for decades.

For example, realizing that excess ingestion could be a problem, the ADA for more than 30 years has required that no more than 260 milligrams of fluoride be added to any tube of fluoride toothpaste. Promoting the use of "pea-sized" amounts of toothpaste, coupled with parental supervision for those under age six, also has been a long-standing recommendation from the ADA.

The Association has always monitored any adverse reactions to fluoride toothpastes through surveys of incident reports in emergency rooms and through contacts with regional and national poison centers.

The results of this surveillance leave no room for disagreement: incidents involving fluoride toothpastes do not lead to major adverse outcomes. It appears that other toothpaste ingredients—the humectants and surfactants they contain—will induce vomiting long before any toxic effects of fluoride can take place.

This unnecessary labeling requirement is part of a larger FDA initiative to address potential hazards connected with over-the-counter drug products. It is not an isolated action aimed solely at fluoride-containing toothpastes. In fact, if it had not been for the persuasive arguments developed

> **This new warning label probably will result in an untoward number of costly and worrisome visits to emergency rooms.**

by a coalition of dental manufacturers and the ADA, the required warning probably would have been much stronger.

The FDA action qualifies as just another bureaucratic happening. Their rulings make no allowance for products to be treated differently, even when they do not pose similar risks.

Unfortunately, this new warning label probably will result in an untoward number of costly and worrisome visits to emergency rooms by parents unable to discern how much toothpaste their child actually ingested.

Is this another case of good intentions causing more harm than good? I would say so. The FDA has an excellent track record; I applaud the agency's efforts on safety. But here is a case where policy needs to be reexamined. Unfortunately, changing government regulations has not been an easy task. Other solutions need to be considered.

The U.S. Public Health Services' National Fluoridation plan encourages manufacturers to develop a toothpaste that can be delivered in a dose-limiting container. If people can be convinced that two or three doses are not better than one, this type of container might provide a viable solution to the dosage issue.

Those who suggest that the best solution would be the development of a lower-dose fluoride toothpaste for preschoolers must understand that such a venture would be costly, with no guarantee of marketplace success. Since there is no evidence that a lower-dose fluoride dentifrice would have the same caries-reducing effect, expensive clinical investigations would have to precede any FDA clearances.

The antithesis to this much ado about nothing situation recently appeared in media reports warning that children in families that consume bottled water may not be getting enough fluoride. Some dentists are recommending fluoride supplements for these children.

A thought: perhaps the FDA should require a warning label on bottled water. The warning would advise parents that if their children do not drink fluoridated tap water, then the children should ingest a little fluoride toothpaste each day. A facetious comment? Of course. But then, I find the FDA's rationale for its new labeling on fluoride-containing toothpastes just as ludicrous. ∎

# The great American sell-a-thon

*Originally published in JADA 1997 128: 1488-1492.*

The American Dental Association calls upon dentists to follow high ethical standards which have the benefit of the patient as their primary goal."[1]

What's in a name? Money and lots of it if you're Pepsi, U.S. West, Coors and other influential members of corporate America. For years, they have promoted their own brand of philanthropy, blending promises of significant financial support with conditions for exclusive rights to advance their products. Apparently, the quid pro quo of these philanthropic deals has been sufficiently lucrative to stifle any criticism.

But when the most influential health organization in the country—the American Medical Association—revealed its exclusive product endorsement deal with the Sunbeam Corp., questions about the ethical nature of the contract drew national attention.

Critics of the AMA action focused their attention on the exclusivity of the proposal, the failure to require testing to back up its endorsement, contract clauses allegedly supporting larger payments if the products were successful in the marketplace and loss of professional credibility as an impartial source of health information.

The rationale for the agreement—that the revenues received by the AMA would be used only to enhance its public service, medical education and scientific research agendas—doesn't seem to have prevailed.

AMA president-elect, Nancy W. Dickey, was quoted in the Sept. 1 issue of *American Medical News* as saying, "The motivation of the Sunbeam agreement was appropriate to find a nondues revenue source to allow the AMA to advance its agenda in the interest of patients and physicians. But if that motivation creates problems from ethical and other perspectives, we have to rethink the deal."

In response to widespread negative publicity, a restructuring or elimination of many of the questionable aspects of the Sunbeam/AMA agreement was under way at this writing.

During the early explosion of criticism over the agreement, media attention also was directed at other health care organizations—including the American Cancer Society, the American Heart Association and the ADA—all known to have endorsed commercial products.

Criticism of all but the ADA program was noted. Dental professionals were heartened by reports, which indicated that dentistry, while supporting an endorsement (acceptance) program, only charged fees to help cover costs. One national publication praising the ADA's Seal program noted that the ADA may have devised the model commercial arrangement for a health care organization.

I'm sure the intensity of the public outcry caught the AMA off-guard; after all, the practice of selling endorsements by medical groups goes back years. And if you view today's medical care as a major commercial industry that emphasizes stockholders and profit statements, a financial arrangement such as this should have come as no surprise.

Medicine hardly stands alone in wooing industry to increase discretionary dollars. The public appears to be equally or even more susceptible. With a perception of too-high and too-many taxes, the door has been opened to industry to exact major concessions for its philanthropic dollars. Some of these partnerships are so commercial that the propriety of public-supported institutions that enter into them becomes questionable.

Examples of these sell-a-thons abound. In a Denver suburb, a large school district has cut a deal with Pepsi and U.S. West to build a $5 million-plus football stadium. These two companies have agreed

> **With a perception of too-high and too-many taxes, the door has been opened to industry to exact major concessions for its philanthropic dollars.**

to put up 80 percent of the cash for this enterprise. In return, Pepsi will be allowed to sell its products exclusively in the district's 140 schools and to advertise its wares in district stadiums, fields and gymnasiums.

With access to the school district's 88,000 students, Pepsi's actions can hardly be considered philanthropic. For its contribution, U.S. West will imprint its name on the new stadium, become the district's preferred phone carrier and, as an added incentive, sell its credit card with the district emblem.

Except for a few negative letters in the local paper, taxpayers in the school district seem pleased. Industry has relieved them of one more tax burden. The propriety of allowing product exclusives in a public-supported enterprise has not been questioned.

Nor has the more basic issue of whether advertising of any form should be allowed in public education institutions. With the solid support for this arrangement as a precedent, opportunities for new commercial deals will be limitless, as companies look for exclusive rights to build product identification and loyalty in the developing minds of schoolchildren.

The actions of the AMA and this Colorado school district have undermined the credibility of these institutions; if the price is right, what isn't for sale? Can you maintain public trust with that philosophy? We know the ADA needs additional nondues revenue to advance its agenda for patients and dentists. To date it has toed the ethical line—perhaps at the expense of not fully achieving that goal.

In a time when selling one's name for gain is the rule rather than the exception, let's run the risk of becoming an anachronism and hold on to our ethical principles. Perhaps we will be viewed as stupid not to join in the search for gold. But then, what's new about that? After all, what health profession has so totally committed itself to its own dissolution than dentistry with its unwavering support of fluoridation?

If that's stupid, so be it! ∎

1. American Dental Association. ADA Principles of Ethics and Code of Professional Conduct. Chicago: American Dental Association; 1997:2.

# The Pledge Allegiance Generation

*Originally published in JADA 1997 128: 1616-1620.*

Creating descriptives for generational subcultures of the American population has been a successful activity for journalists. Who among us has not heard terms like "the Pepsi Generation," "the baby boomers," "the Me Generation," "the Beat Generation" or "Generation X"?

In developing this month's editorial, I've exercised my editorial prerogative to coin a term describing my own generation. Let me introduce to you the "Pledge Allegiance Generation."

This generation dutifully, and without question, opened each school day with a pledge to the American flag. There was no discussion as to why we recited this pledge or why America needed or deserved our loyalty. The pledge was just part of being an American.

This willingness to make unqualified commitments to the country translated years later to professional membership in the American Dental Association. Here, too, there was no question as to the benefits of joining. Our dental class joined because that's what professionals did.

Today, with a membership rate exceeding 80 percent, our Pledge Allegiance age group contains the highest percentage of dentists who are members of the American Dental Association.

Our commitment to professional affiliation, as exhibited in this membership percentage, is in jeopardy. Of the dentists who have graduated within the last 12 years, more than 13,000—about one-third of those graduates—have not joined the ADA. Discovering how to entice them into membership has become one of organized dentistry's major challenges.

Unfortunately, this has not been an easy process. The needs and attitudes of young dentists

> Take young nonmember dentists to lunch; take them to dental meetings. Convince them that membership in the ADA is crucial for their professional growth as well as for the public's well-being.

have changed. Reliance on past recruitment initiatives has not been totally successful. To paraphrase President Kennedy's famous speech, it appears that it's no longer what you can do for your profession but rather what your profession can do for you that pushes the membership button.

The ADA has responded to this new reality and now offers an extensive line of personal- and practice-oriented financial services. As an ADA member, you can get a mortgage, obtain all types of insurance, join a variety of retirement programs, receive special financial credits and conduct your banking. Recent graduates who are ADA members may be interested in programs that offer educational loan consolidations as well as financing toward setting up dental practices.

All of these are important offerings, but they should not be the primary reason for joining a professional dental organization. A question raised by a freshman dental student creates an opportunity to present a rationale for this view.

Each fall I present the ADA's Principles of Ethics and Code of Professional Conduct to the incoming freshman class of the dental school where I teach. The concepts in the document, I explain to the students, delineate dentistry's commitments to society and to fellow health professionals.

A student asks, "If a dentist is not a member of the ADA, is he or she bound by the tenets of the document?" My response is guarded. Theoretically the answer is no, but I qualify my response by sharing with the class the following excerpt from the ADA's mission statement:

"The mission of the ADA presents a significant opportunity to improve the public's health and the well-being of the entire profession. For this mission to be achieved, however, strong and stable membership and financial support will be needed. Thus, all dentists should be members of the ADA, since its mission benefits all dentists and since universal membership will provide a strong voice for dentistry … ."

In that regard, consider two recent actions by the ADA that reinforce my argument for universal membership without qualification. The first is the recent ADA Board of Trustees' approval of a supplemental financial request to send member dentists a document concerning what to do after percutaneous exposure to HIV-infected blood. This information is essential to all dental workers, as new information has demonstrated that an 80 percent reduction in seroconversion can be achieved if treatment is instituted within two hours of exposure.

The ADA believes all dental workers should have complete access to this information. Nonmembers will be informed that they can receive this document for only printing and mailing costs—an action in keeping with the ADA philosophy that we must safeguard all dental workers regardless of membership status.

The other example concerns patients' rights.

The continuing effort to serve patients' needs with quality care is of the highest priority to the profession. Concerned that organizational systems that herald their ability to contain health care costs may be accomplishing their goals at the public's expense, the ADA is supporting a bill before Congress that would ensure the public's right to quality care.

Introduced by Rep. Charlie Norwood, himself a dentist, the Patient Access to Responsible Care Act, or PARCA (H.R.1415/S.644), is attracting significant bipartisan support. At the ADA meeting in Washington, D.C., hundreds of dentists gathered on the steps of Congress to voice their support for this bill.

And when the ADA speaks, Congress listens—because it knows that the ADA's membership represents the profession of dentistry.

Both examples demonstrate how a profession can promote the welfare of its members and the public it serves. However, continued public and professional efforts will succeed only if professional dentistry is able to maintain its reputation as the voice of dentistry.

To ensure that future, a special effort to recruit the 20,000 non-ADA members who were graduated less than 10 years ago needs to be begun. This initiative must go beyond what the ADA presently offers. It must take on a personal dimension that conveys the sincerity of the member dentist.

I'm calling on all ADA-member dentists who identify with the attributes of the Pledge Allegiance Generation to share their commitment with these young nonmembers. Take them to lunch; take them to dental meetings. Convince them that membership in the ADA is crucial for their professional growth as well as for the public's well-being.

And maybe, just maybe, a few will view you as the professional mentor they have always sought and will take your advice. ∎

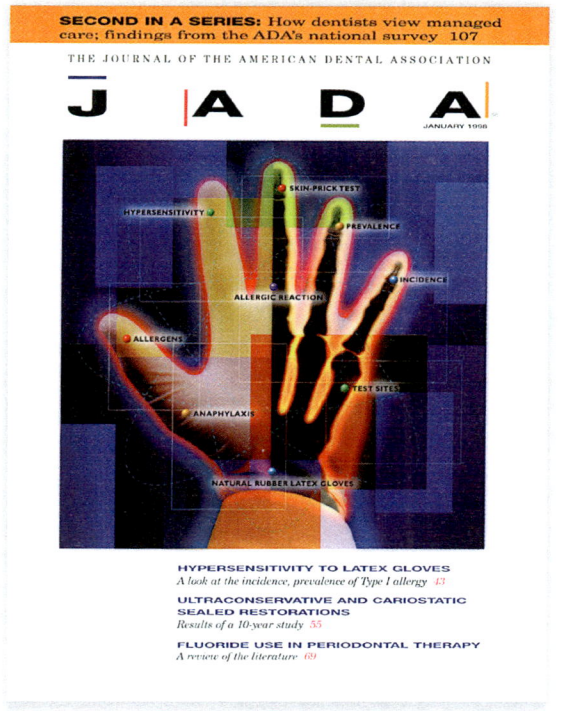

# 1998

"The key to the future health and well-being of dentists will depend on organized dentistry's ability to ensure that the environment for the practice of dentistry continues to offer high levels of professional satisfaction. Therein lies the great challenge."

# Focal infection: back with a bang!

*Originally published in JADA 1998 129: 8-9.*

Latter-day Ponce de Leóns searching for their personal fountains of youth have introduced a new culture of health behaviors. In their quest to extend longevity or enhance quality of life, they follow each new medical news release by yet another visit to a health and nutrition outlet or to the family physician.

And why not? In one week's time, the lay press reported that cognitive performance and social functioning improvements could be had by an over-the-counter purchase of an extract of gingko biloba. Readers were probably doubling their intake of vitamin E after they heard the announcement that it had properties that prevented colon cancer. Women were heartened by the news that exposure to sunlight could reduce their risk of breast cancer because it enhanced vitamin D production. As too much sun causes skin cancer, why not load up on vitamin supplements with lots of "D" ?

What about the announcement that DNA can stimulate the production of new blood vessels? HMO gatekeepers are going to have a difficult time convincing their enrollees with severe cardiovascular disease that gene therapy is not covered under their health plans.

Dentistry has been virtually excluded from these "life-extending" press announcements. The media, rather than promoting quality-of-life enhancements that can be achieved from a dental visit, have focused on dirty waterlines or the potential dangers of dental materials.

Well, dentistry's time to shine may have arrived. Research has identified periodontal disease as a major risk factor for cardiovascular disease, or CVD, and stroke. It even may be a risk factor for the production of low-birthweight babies. While the subject has received some press coverage, a major public response has yet to surface.

But it will! It's only a matter of time until one of the major TV networks does a showcase piece on

**It's only a matter of time until one of the major TV networks does a showcase piece on how a trip to your dentist could be a lifesaver.**

how a trip to your dentist could be a lifesaver. After all, periodontal disease can be cured! With more than a million people dying each year of CVD, the prospect of prolonging life through a few trips to the dentist should motivate millions of Americans to queue up for their periodontal treatments.

Insurers of dental care will have to redefine their benefit packages. Dentists, especially general practitioners, will have to expand their capacity to treat periodontal disease. When the news hits, expect the dental hygienists to intensify their efforts to become private entrepreneurs so that they can cash in on the action.

Pressure to create low-cost periodontal treatment programs for those unable to afford dental care will come from candidates seeking political office. If someone's longevity can be significantly extended, shouldn't access to periodontal treatment be a right extended to all Americans?

Expect to see repeats of the 1960s and 1970s, when new dental schools were opened and existing dental schools received government subsidies to expand class size.

Enough of these delusionary thoughts? What scientist, remembering how the focal theory of infection was discarded years ago, would care to suggest that periodontal infection could be a major risk factor for CVD, stroke or other life-threatening diseases?

The answer to that rhetorical question is that the focal theory of infection is back—at least for periodontal disease—and it is world-class researchers with financial support from the National Institutes of Health, or NIH, who are providing the evidence.

While none of these researchers is ready to incriminate periodontal disease as the cause of a variety of systemic diseases, the evidence they have collected continues to support this hypothesis. This is what's known:

■ Subjects with high levels of substances related to inflammation were at increased risk of experiencing heart attack.

■ The theory is that periodontal inflammation works to increase plaque buildup in the arteries, thus increasing the risk of heart disease. Suggested mechanisms have periodontal disease serving as a reservoir of lipopolysaccharides, which could be the source of potentially harmful lipid mediators and cytokines—both of which have been implicated as possible contributors to CVD.

■ Aspirin's effectiveness in reducing the risk of myocardial infarction demonstrates that anti-inflammatory agents may provide some assistance in preventing CVD.

■ Related research[1] linking periodontal inflammation and preterm low birthweight strongly suggests that eliminating periodontal disease would be a significant public health achievement. The authors of this research estimate that more than 18 percent of preterm low birthweight may be attributed to periodontal infection. If their prediction is accurate, reduction in periodontal disease could save millions of dollars.

■ The NIH is definitely interested. Current research is evaluating whether an intervention of periodontal therapy lessens the risk of preterm low birthweight. Support for this type of intervention can be found in the literature. Research reports indicate that when bacterial vaginosis is treated with an antibiotic, there is a 50 percent reduction in vaginosis-related preterm birth and preterm rupture of membranes.

As the hypothesized mechanisms of causation are similar, a positive research outcome in the birthweight area would boost investigations to test the effect of periodontal intervention on CVD. Interventions to reduce the incidence of stroke also will be added to that agenda if a recent report from Europe—that strokes are 2.5 times more common in people who have poor oral health—proves to be correct.

There will be those who question how a localized infective process, such as periodontal disease, could present such a major systemic threat. I ask them to consider the following comment from one of the pioneer researchers in this area1: "[As] the surface area of the periodontium may cover as much area as the entire ventral surface of the arm … logically … if the entire forearm were inflamed with gross suppuration and radiographic evidence of osteomyelitis, one would not be surprised if there were systemic sequelae."

Eighteenth-century anatomist William Hunter,[2] who chastised the dental profession for "allowing chronic abscesses and other forms of chronic suppuration to continue in the mouth," would surely agree. He firmly believed that "septic infection is without exception … the most important and prevalent cause of and complication of many medical diseases." He concluded, "Its ill-effect extends to all systems of the body."

Practitioners, get ready. Sharpen your curettes; hone your periodontal skills. In a society bent on prolonging life, once the word is out, the rush will begin. ■

1. Offenbacher S, Katz V, Fertik G, et al. Periodontal infection as a possible risk factor for preterm low birth weight. J Periodontol 1996;67(10): 1103-13.
2. Hunter W. Role of sepsis and antisepsis in medicine. Lancet 1911; Jan. 14.

# A gentle touch is not enough

*Originally published in JADA 1998 129: 136-137.*

The ad in the yellow pages boasted, "Smiles—By Women Dentists With A Gentle Touch." The inference: female dentists—at least those who placed the ad—believe that a gentle touch is a desired component in the delivery of quality dental care. Apparently unwilling to concede that a gentle touch can be offered solely by women, male dentists were responsible for two additional ads promoting the gentle-touch theme.

In a profession shadowed by past negative images, it appears that the "touch" may have value as an indicator of high-quality dental care. Do you have the right touch? Can dental patients tell whose touch is gentle and whose is rough? Would you be willing to be compensated on the basis of how employers, insurance companies and patients rated your touch?

Nonsensical drivel? Perhaps. But not if you consider what is going on in the health care marketplace. Purchasers and users of care are demanding quality assessments of provider services—report cards—to make their health plan choices. To address the need for assessment, various groups are using the components of structure, process and outcome to develop their quality yardstick.

Health care professionals also are interested in measuring quality. They are concerned that with increasing pressure to deliver services at reduced cost, quality could be compromised. If that proves to be the case, they want the consumer to know who's to blame.

If a direct relationship between cost and quality of care existed, the issue of quality measurement could be quickly resolved. All that would be required would be to determine the cutoff point at which reductions in cost result in less-than-acceptable quality of care.

> **For the dental profession, the assessment of quality still remains a professional judgment call usually based on the technical excellence required to produce the treatment.**

Unfortunately, the concept of quality does not lend itself to simple measures. The variables that affect quality of health are numerous and often obscure. Anyone attempting to measure quality of health care must be aware that this is a highly complex venture not amenable to "shake and bake" solutions.

In dentistry, a health profession still relatively free from managed care pressures, patients' assessments of quality of care are based on dentists' reputations, cost of service and word of mouth. For the profession, the assessment of quality still remains a professional judgment call usually based on the technical excellence required to produce the treatment.

This empirical, rather than scientific, approach to assessment is not unexpected. Demands for technical perfection during dental training translate into a practitioner philosophy recognizing only excellence—an excellence that equates with permanence. It is a rare dental school which teaches that a restoration properly placed and cared for should not last a lifetime.

The dental literature demonstrates otherwise. Clinical studies indicate that more than 50 percent of the average dentist's chairside time is spent in rerestoration and retreatment procedures. Are these treatment failures signs of poor quality? Without further definition and objective assessment of treatment outcomes, quality in dentistry remains vested in the eyes of the beholder.

Our profession and society demand more.

The 1997 ADA House of Delegates responded to this challenge by supporting a resolution calling on the ADA to develop objective indicators for oral health care. The dental care indicators would be based on the ADA's dental practice parameters, scientific data and professional consensus. A commendable resolution, but not an easy task.

Process and outcome measures are the two criteria most often used to characterize quality. The former evaluates the procedures that are considered prerequisites for good outcomes—number of people receiving radiographs, frequency of recalls, infection control, oral cancer exams, smoking prevention, perhaps even "touch." While this is the least expensive way to measure quality, relating these process factors to disease outcomes is a difficult task.

Patient-reported satisfaction from questionnaires also can provide information about quality. Responses to such questions as "How much were you helped by the care you received?", "What is your overall satisfaction with the quality of care and services provided you?" and "How willing are you to recommend us to your family and friends?", while not treatment outcome measures, can affect decisions by consumers of health services.

Measuring clinical outcomes of care is the most desirable measure of quality. However, doing so is labor-intensive and costly and, in the case of chronic diseases, requires inordinate amounts of time for observation of the effects of treatment. Nevertheless, treatment outcome information has become the measure most often sought by employers and patients.

Unfortunately, dentistry has little documented evidence of successful treatment outcomes. This became quite evident in last year's Reader's Digest debacle, in which dentists stood accused of greed in providing a variety of treatment plans to address the dental needs of the same patient. Without documented outcomes of dental treatment, the profession remains vulnerable to criticism.

The American Academy of Periodontology is addressing that issue. Each year, a group of experts collates and analyzes treatment information in one or more subject areas. The results are shared with members through the publication of position papers.

This initiative needs to be expanded to include all areas of dental treatment, and the ADA is the most logical choice to underwrite this effort. Providing ADA constituents with evidence-based treatment outcome information would be a membership benefit appreciated and used by all.

Don't look for any immediate action in this area. There appears to be little grassroots interest beyond the present initiative of developing process indicators to measure quality. Documenting outcomes of treatment hasn't waved the immediacy flag necessary to open the ADA's pocketbook—but it will. Dentistry's ability to function in the competitive world of the new millennium depends on it. ∎

# And then there were none

*Originally published in JADA 1998 129: 274-275.*

Dental educators and practitioners were stunned by the announcement that Chicago's Northwestern University, or NU, planned to discontinue its dental education program. For more than 106 years, the dental school that G.V. Black nurtured has been an integral component of NU's prestigious educational offerings.

No longer! NU's dental school appears targeted for extinction by a university seeking to rearrange its portfolio of schools and programs. It doesn't have a "cachet" any more, said the NU spokesperson who responded to questions about why the school is being closed. "Cachet," in this usage, is defined as a feature or quality conferring prestige.

How do you measure prestige? NU's dental school has been blessed with a quality applicant pool. Last year's entering class had a grade point average of 3.4 and the fifth highest academic and second highest perceptual ability Dental Aptitude Test scores among all U.S. freshman dental students.

With this strong applicant pool, the NU dental school accepted a smaller percentage of total applicants (10 percent) than did all of the university's professional schools except the medical school. NU's Kellogg School of Business—often top-ranked nationally—accepted from 14 percent to 37 percent of its applicants, depending on the specific program.

No, it wasn't cachet. It's really a matter of money—and lots of it. Do you think NU or any other university would close a program if it were profitable? "It doesn't have the cachet" really means, "We don't want to subsidize the dental school any longer. Let's grab the cash and run. After all, haven't six other private universities closed their dental schools in the last decade?"

In contrast, medicine, which has almost twice as many schools—and a reported large surplus of physicians—has had no school closures in the comparable period. The difference? On average, medical schools generate more than 70 percent of their operating revenues independent of state or university contributions. Dentistry's educational programs are the opposite. They depend heavily on tuition and state contributions, garnering 65 percent of their operating revenues from those sources.

In addition to the large differences in self-generated revenues between dental and medical schools, it costs considerably more to educate a dental student than a medical student. The differential is directly related to training costs in the clinical years. Medicine sends its students to hospitals for their third and fourth years of training—at no cost.

Dentistry provides its own clinical facilities for its students. That's costly. About a third of a dental school's budget is consumed by its clinical operation. This increases the cost of training dental students by tens of thousands of dollars over the cost of training their medical counterparts.

> **Six dental schools have already closed, and there have been a number of initiatives to close others. The underlying rationale is always the high cost.**

This high cost is no secret. As noted earlier, six dental schools have already closed, and there have been a number of initiatives to close others. The underlying rationale is always the high cost.

As evidence, consider this quote from a state legislator who introduced a bill to close a state-funded dental school: "The dental school might be a good school. That's not the point. The point is that the institution is soaking up funds that could be used elsewhere to provide education to a far greater number of students."

Those most vulnerable to the high cost of dental education have been the dental students. The debts of graduating students continue to rise. Graduates of private dental schools are now reporting an average debt of $113,128. Graduates of state-related schools report an average debt of $93,583, while graduates of state-supported schools have an average debt of $66,669.

The real jolt comes when the new graduates start paying off their debts, plus interest. During those early practice years, some graduates report difficulty meeting basic personal expenses. The pressure to pay off debts affects practice decisions for these young dentists.

The highly ambitious plan set forth by ADA Past President Arthur Dugoni to create a $1 billion education endowment from professional contributions could provide some debt relief, buying down the interest on student loans.

Using its potential $60 million annual yield for loan payment reductions of 3.5 percent, each new graduate would save $20,000 over the life of a 10-year $100,000 loan. While helpful, this effort would not appreciably alter a student's monthly debt payment (reducing it from $1,161 to $989).

As well-meaning as the Dugoni plan is, I view it as a Band-Aid approach. To ensure the long-term stability of dentistry's educational base, major changes will have to be made that permeate the entire fabric of the educational process. And change must begin now! Unless costs are controlled, more schools will close, and the entire educational system eventually will be compromised.

I have a proposal. It calls for an unprecedented professional and financial commitment to address the cost of dental education. It asks for trust and sacrifice from all dentists—and it requires a substantial out-of-pocket contribution.

The first step in the plan would be to assemble dentistry's most creative thinkers and charge them with the responsibility to develop methods and programs that could significantly reduce the cost of dental education. To convert their recommendations into action, special project grants, using contributed funds, would enable qualified individuals and organizations to field-test the recommendations.

I am convinced that when the necessary resources are applied, a significantly altered but high-quality dental education program will emerge. The difficulty will not be to find solutions but to assemble the dental support necessary to launch this venture.

Most dentists have little concern about the closing of a dental school, unless it's their alma mater. Some may even be pleased about a closing—believing that we have too many dentists. One or two may speak out in support of the schools, but their voices eventually fall silent, muted by the lack of peer support. It's so much easier to conduct business as usual.

But if no one speaks this time, or the next time, or the next, soon there will be no opportunity to speak—for there will be no schools left to speak for.

A few years ago, there were three dental schools in Chicago. Soon there will likely be only one. ∎

# 'I think I can … I thought I could'

*Originally published in JADA 1998 129: 402-403.*

Remember that classic childhood story of the Little Blue Engine that, against immeasurable odds, successfully chugged up and over a mountain to bring toys to deserving children? Of course. Who could ever forget "The Little Engine That Could"?

"I think I can," and then "I thought I could," the Little Blue Engine cried out, imparting an inspirational message for all ages: what initially appears to be impossible may, with superlative effort, be achieved.

Dentistry and the American public are witnessing a replay of the Little Blue Engine's ride to success. Following that story line, it appears that a few years ago a group of distraught townspeople gathered together to discuss how to stop the continued erosion of their relationships with their health care providers.

They were especially concerned that administrators of their health plans were denying or delaying needed care, often refusing to allow referrals and then claiming they were not accountable when deleterious outcomes resulted.

The concerned citizens debated what to do. "Our rights as patients are being violated, and we have no one to protect us," they said. "We need a spokesperson. We need action. We need legislation. But who will represent our interests? Who is willing to speak for us? Who can move us out of this quagmire?"

Turning to the biggest engine—the insurance companies—they asked, "Will you help us?"

"Why should I?" the insurance companies replied. "Helping you will adversely affect our bottom line." And the insurance companies chugged off.

The townspeople then turned to the next biggest engine—the largest association of American physicians—and asked for help.

"No!" it replied. "That agenda is way too complex to support, especially the antidiscrimination clause. Besides, I'm a very important engine indeed. I won't pull the likes of you." The physicians' group huffed and puffed, and it chugged off.

"Who can we turn to now?" cried the people. "We need help!"

Then they saw the American Dental Association engine coming down the track. "Could it help us?" they wondered. "No, it's not big enough to carry our message because it represents just over 4 percent of the $1 trillion U.S. health care expenditure."

But they asked anyway. And to their surprise, the ADA engine said, "I think I can." And so, led by one of their own, Rep. Charlie Norwood of Georgia, the ADA three years ago became one of the primary supporters of the Patient Access to Responsible Care Act (PARCA, HR1415).

Carefully constructed to address the concerns of a growing number of patients, PARCA proposes to re-establish the patients' right to choose health providers within a plan. It also offers the option of joining a point-of-service plan outside the network. Additionally, patients would be assured of prompt care, access to care within reasonable distances from their home and emergency care without prior authorization from their health plan.

PARCA would ensure that patients would not be denied specialty care and would eliminate the use of gag rules prohibiting health care workers from providing patients with information on appropriate treatment options not covered by the plan.

Quality of care also would be emphasized under the proposed legislation. Through periodic assessments of the health plan's review and administrative operations, PARCA is designed to protect patients from health plans that place bottom-line profit ahead of quality and access to care.

The accountability components of PARCA call for

> **PARCA supporters want those making medical decisions to be held responsible for their actions— even if they are not physicians.**

sweeping changes over present-day practices that restrict many patients from pursuing legal action for negligence against health plans. This option currently is denied to 125 million workers enrolled in employer self-insured health plans.

This inability to hold employer self-insured plans liable for negligence springs from the Employer Retirement Income Security Act, or ERISA. Initially designed to protect employee pensions, it unfortunately contains language allowing self-insured health plans to bypass state accountability laws.

PARCA has attracted the support of 221 bipartisan members of the U.S. House of Representative and scores of national health organizations. Adding to PARCA's momentum has been the highly visible letter-writing and personal visits with legislators by ADA grassroots members.

This support has not gone unnoticed by the bill's opponents. Powerful politicians in the House of Representatives have begun a vocal bombardment against the bill. Insurers and employers also are lining up to defeat the bill, claiming that its provisions could drive up the cost of insurance by 23 percent to 39 percent.

The naysayers argue that if this bill became law, it would cause "thousands" of employers to stop offering insurance. They also maintain that the higher cost of premiums will force millions of lower-income workers to drop their insurance.

PARCA supporters say these cost estimates are exaggerated. They point to a recent study by a national actuarial firm estimating premium increases only in the 0.7-to-2.6 percent range. They also cite the recent experience with PARCA-like legislation in Texas where premiums climbed just 1 percent—nowhere near the 28 percent increase forecasted by those against patient protection.

What may derail PARCA is not the threat of increased premiums but its liability provisions. The insurance companies are obviously concerned because PARCA will hold them liable. Employers also are fearful, even though Rep. Norwood has added a provision that would protect them from malpractice suits.

The battle lines have been drawn. PARCA supporters want those making medical decisions to be held responsible for their actions—even if they are not physicians. Opposing them are the heavily financed insurance and business lobbies, who are stepping up their efforts to defeat PARCA.

It's conceivable that PARCA might not survive in its present form—only time will tell. But even if it doesn't, it has placed the issue of patients' rights on the nation's front burner. Eventually some form of legislation will pass—that's a given. Additional legislative actions will follow and will continue until patient rights are fully acknowledged and protected.

The American Dental Association—its Washington office and its grassroots supporters—should take pride in bringing this issue to national prominence. Others, far better positioned, were unwilling to do so. The ADA's efforts truly represent the wisdom professed in "The Little Engine That Could."

"I think I can ... I thought I could." ▪

# Proceed with caution

*Originally published in JADA 1998 129: 530-531.*

Last fall, Washington politicians passed what some see as the most important legislative health initiative of the decade. The legislators pledged to spend $40 billion over the next 10 years to promote child health. If dentistry chooses to participate, it could mean millions, even billions, of new federal and state dollars to fund dental services for the underserved.

The initiative—the Child Health Insurance Program, or CHIP—recognizes the efforts of parents who work but lack the income to afford health insurance coverage for their families. The congressional intent is to extend health coverage for as many as 11.3 million children who presently fall above the level set for Medicaid participation.

Unlike Medicaid guidelines that require a state/federal dollar-for-dollar match, the CHIP program will be funded mainly with federal funds. States that wish to participate must ante up a lesser contribution of new state dollars. Before receiving any CHIP funds, the states also must submit their coverage and benefits plans to the feds for approval.

CHIP programs do not have to contain a dental component. In fact, dentistry can be included only if state officials and dental leaders offer an acceptable plan of dental coverage and benefits for CHIP enrollees.

The omission of mandated dental coverage for CHIP enrollees is bad news, say some dental leaders. They note that low income is the single best predictor of high caries experience in children. Dental benefits, some leaders say, should have been one of CHIP's highest priorities.

CHIP critics also contend that not requiring dental benefits as part of the initiative gives the states a financial excuse to abrogate their responsibility to improve the dental health of these low-income, but above-poverty-line, children.

These views are not universal in the dental profession. Some see the omission of mandated dental benefits in CHIP as an opportunity—a chance to develop programs that will offer these children the benefits of dental insurance while avoiding the administrative quagmire of red tape and underfunded benefits. They point to the present Medicaid dental program as an example of what such a program shouldn't be.

Where do grassroots dentists stand on CHIP? In a nonscientific sample of 50 Colorado dentists, I found that not one of them recognized the CHIP acronym. Ensuing discussions showed that most of these dentists would reject participation in another Medicaid-type program. Dentists don't want another "black eye," they said. Because CHIP programs can be construed in a number of ways—the easiest being a simple extension of Medicaid—it's understandable why, for many dentists, their first impression of CHIP may not be positive.

Dentists should know that there are alternatives to CHIP-endorsed Medicaid extensions. States can develop their own programs, and many anticipate doing just that. Chances are that state officials won't include dental coverage in these new programs unless they are approached by a representative member of the state's dental community.

Herein lies an opportunity for dentistry. In a number of states considering CHIP programs other than Medicaid clones, dentists from the community have submitted dental coverage programs that provide comprehensive services for the children plus dentist compensation at prevailing market rates. With input from local dentists, two states already have included well-funded, comprehensive dental programs in their CHIP plans. Others hope to

> **If dentistry chooses to participate in the Child Health Insurance Program, it could mean millions, even billions, of new federal and state dollars to pay for dental services to the underserved.**

follow suit.

Dentistry's CHIP experience has not been positive in all cases. At least one state has not included a dental plan because the amount of CHIP funds offered to dentistry was not sufficient to fund a quality program. This decision to exclude dental services is commendable but not without risk.

Being branded with a self-serving label is always a possibility when dentistry says it can't deliver comprehensive services without adequate compensation. So what's new? Let's not let the threat of future labeling stop dentistry from voicing its priorities. After all, if dentistry doesn't promote opportunities for improved dental health in needy children, who will?

Moreover, dentistry's absence in CHIP health planning activities could open the door to "alternative" primary dental providers. I am sure there would be more than a few nondentists who wouldn't mind being named a CHIP provider—

even if their duties were initially limited to preventive services.

Participation in CHIP also might positively influence other government programs that involve dentistry. For example, the process of negotiating acceptable dental fee schedules in CHIP programs also might stimulate increases in dental Medicaid payment levels. All but two states are reporting surpluses this year. If there ever was a time to properly fund dental programs, this is it.

With valid arguments pro and con about dental participation in CHIP, this is definitely a "proceed with caution" situation. Dentistry should be at the table in each state contemplating a CHIP program. But dentistry's participation should not be equated with capitulation. Only when the profession is assured that the resources will be there to provide the necessary services should it agree to participate.

No more black eyes! ∎

# Research interpreters wanted: apply within

*Originally published in JADA 1998 129: 668-669.*

Too bad the National Institute of Dental Research, or NIDR, isn't listed on the New York Stock Exchange. If it were, it would be every stockbroker's top pick for its return on investment. In its 50-year history, $3.2 billion has been invested in dental research and development. In return, NIDR generates "revenues" estimated at $4 billion a year in reduced health care costs—and the yields continue to compound with each new research discovery.

Not too shabby by any standard.

This year marks NIDR's golden anniversary. Its future challenge—to match or exceed its earlier contributions—could be a formidable task. Indeed, if all NIDR had achieved over the last half century were its fluoride discoveries, that alone would have been sufficient to justify its existence.

But there has been so much more. For the dentist and patient, NIDR's development of the high-speed handpiece truly revolutionized restorative dentistry. Many of us still remember preparing a tooth for a crown with burs revolving at 1,500 to 2,000 rpm. Not a pleasant experience for either patient or dentist.

Add to this achievement a few more of NIDR's contributions—sealants, digital radiography, an array of new restorative materials, and new techniques to manage periodontal disease, xerostomia and pain—and you quickly grasp how important dentistry's own research institute has been to the profession and the public.

So what can we expect for NIDR's 50th anniversary celebration? The fanfare will probably include a Washington-based research symposium. There will be dinners with congratulatory speeches by National Institutes of Health bigwigs, perhaps a few members of Congress, representatives of organized dentistry, dental educators and NIDR's industrial partners. What's missing from this picture? Grassroots dentists.

For all its national glow, NIDR's image remains somewhat tarnished by the lack of a strong national advocacy for NIDR as well as groundswell support from those who benefit most from its work: dentists and patients. Dental research, it seems, has always suffered from the perception that it "lacks relevancy to hands-on dental practice." And if dentists fail to see the value of dental research, how can they or the public be expected to beat the drum for NIDR?

To gain the support of the grassroots dentist, NIDR must establish that research and relevancy are synonymous for both dental practitioner and scientist. NIDR understands this, and to its credit has made the issue of "science transfer" a top priority for many years.

For example, since 1977 NIH has convened 108 consensus conferences designed to evaluate safety and efficacy issues related to major health concerns. NIDR has been directly involved in six of these conferences and has cosponsored three others. Topics included dental implants, removal of third molars, dental sealants and pain management. NIDR also sponsors Technology Assessment Conferences related to biomedical technology. The most recent (1996) featured the management of temporomandibular disorders.

What's more, NIDR has worked to help scientists break out of their ivory towers. Researchers often see peer-reviewed publication of their findings as the end point of their work, but NIDR has been actively engaged in pushing them one step further: sponsoring yearly symposiums where world-renowned scientists speak directly to practitioners about their research and its clinical applications. Unfortunately, only a comparatively few

> **NIDR generates "revenues" estimated at $4 billion per year in reduced health care costs—and the yields continue to compound with each new research discovery.**

dentists are able to take productive time away from their offices to attend.

Past efforts not withstanding, the responsibility of how to transfer science effectively from researcher to practitioner does not rest totally on the shoulders of NIDR. Other groups are actively engaged in transfer initiatives. For example, the ADA last year offered those attending its national meeting the opportunity to question experts on "the critical issues in dental practice today." Those present took home vital information.

In the specialty area, the American Academy of Periodontology is seeking ways to provide dental practitioners with the results of their analysis of what works in periodontal therapy. Others attempting to bridge the research transfer gap include the hundreds of clinicians who share their interpretations of research findings as part of their continuing education offerings and the industrial "reps" who often interact one-on-one with dentists.

What is missing in this researcher-to-dentist-to-patient equation is coordination. While well-intended, the present shotgun approach is grossly inefficient and gives no guarantee that new information will reach those who need to be informed.

To tackle this issue, a coalition of researchers, educators, representatives of industry and organized dentistry and grassroots dentists needs to be formed. This group would designate the science-transfer topic areas most relevant to clinicians, arrange for translation of research into language understandable to practitioners and then ensure that the information gets to practitioners in the most effective way.

Dentistry need not reinvent the wheel to accomplish these objectives. For starters, consider a research-and-relevancy model for dentistry based on the highly successful agriculture extension system offered by most land-grant colleges and universities. These networks reach into every hamlet with the newest information, translated for public use. As many of you know from personal experience, it's a great dissemination system. Why not a similar one for dentistry?

NIDR is heavily involved in science that will dramatically change the scope and nature of dental practice. Advances soon will be forthcoming in gene-mediated diagnostics and therapeutics. The science necessary for replacing body parts such as teeth, bone and salivary glands is on the horizon. Dentistry must have a mechanism in place to ensure that its constituents receive this new information in a timely and understandable format.

The future of America's oral health depends on it! ∎

# No sex, please

*Originally published in JADA 1998 129: 815-816.*

A young woman steps from her bath wearing nothing but soapsuds and a smile. A young man clad only in a towel greets her. He, too, is smiling.

This may sound like something from late-night cable TV, but it isn't. The scene is from a highly provocative ad for 1-800-Dentist. Exactly what message the advertiser is trying to convey escapes us. What we do know is that this particular ad—or ads like it—will never appear in an ADA publication. Elsewhere, yes, but not in JADA or ADA News.

Some may call us old-fashioned, unhip, not with it. We don't care. Our business is transferring clinically relevant information to our readers, not promoting human sexuality. We'll leave that to Dr. Ruth.

How well is JADA doing in meeting ADA members' clinical information needs? Not too badly, if we can believe what we read and hear in the letters, calls from readers, the comments from focus groups and the results of periodic readership surveys.

Often this sort of feedback is considered biased because it's "in-house" or anecdotal. Now, however, we have an independent study of the entire dental publishing industry conducted annually by the Perq/HCI Corp. Its 1998 results are exceptionally good news for those responsible for producing JADA.

We have been told that JADA's readership scores, though always strong, have improved dramatically within the past year. The Perq/HCI Corp. survey showed that JADA is the best-read journal in dentistry.

Indeed, among all dental publications (including tabloids), JADA ranks second, just one percentage point behind the industry-leading ADA News. We were especially pleased to note that for dentists who have been in practice 15 years or less, we are

tops. Since these dentists represent dentistry's future, this news is particularly encouraging.

But this is no time to pat ourselves on the back. Status quo only means that soon we may be looking up at the leader, not down from our perch. We need to construct a JADA that is even more useful to its readership.

Our readers tell us to make The Journal more relevant, improve the timeliness of its content and expand its coverage. They want more information on practice management, esthetic dentistry, new restorative materials and biotechnology. We are encouraged to extend our coverage of both pharmacology and the relationship between medicine and dentistry. Foremost, readers have urged us to seek new pathways that would accelerate the flow of information in all subject areas.

Our initial response to these suggestions was to expand JADA's Editorial Board, adding three outstanding dental practitioners who have general practice and esthetic dentistry backgrounds. Our new appointees—Drs. Cherilyn Sheets, Daniel Castagna and Michael Rainwater—already are providing invaluable advice on the future composition of JADA.

Next, we established a panel of five associate editors and specifically charged them to harvest the most current offerings in their areas of expertise—and to bring that information to JADA.

On practice management, we have asked Dr. Leslie Seldin, a seasoned practitioner with experience as past chairman of the ADA Council on Insurance, to direct this critical area. Dr. Karl Leinfelder, already a frequent contributor to JADA and past JADA Editorial Board member, was chosen to act as JADA's liaison to the community of scientists in dental materials and biotechnology. Dr. Paul Moore, a University of Pittsburgh researcher and author of dozens of articles on phar-

> **An independent study shows that JADA is the best-read journal in dentistry. But status quo only means that soon we may be looking up at the leader, not down from our perch.**

macology and dental care, will bring monthly contributions in this subject area to JADA.

We know our readers want more about esthetic dentistry. To address this need, we have successfully recruited author/lecturer Dr. Jacqueline Dzierzak to canvass her peers for potential contributions to JADA.

Finally, we couldn't go forward with our new initiatives without recognizing the importance of the growing number of interrelationships between medicine and dentistry. Dr. Michael Glick, a member of ADA's Council on Scientific Affairs and director of Programs for Medically Complex Patients at the University of Pennsylvania School of Dental Medicine, will be responsible for this endeavor.

This is truly an all-star lineup. During the course of this calendar year, each one will come on board with his or her contributions. Special graphic icons will mark their sections.

We know that most JADA readers will not read every article. To help them choose, we are developing a new abstract format to accompany every JADA research article. The abstract will be comprehensive in scope and give the reader a capsule of relevant information, including the article's clinical implications. Readers can then decide if they wish to read on for more detailed information.

Just as some readers will be satisfied with reading only the abstract, others will desire even more information than that contained in the article. Those of you who access ADA ONLINE on the World Wide Web know that JADA has a new monthly feature called "Ask the Author" that allows JADA readers to pose questions to the author or authors of a selected JADA article. What a great way to access some of dentistry's top experts.

What has always been the quiet issue of JADA, our December issue, should prove to be just the opposite. Working with the ADA's Dental Economic Advisory Group, JADA will be featuring an annual report on the state of the dental economy. Featured will be updates on current conditions in dentistry, such as changes in net income, total dental expenditures, fees, financing methods and managed care.

Other changes will follow. When surveys on the benefits of ADA membership are analyzed, receiving JADA always ranks near the top. We take this responsibility seriously. "Better" to us means getting pertinent information to our constituents in a clinically relevant form. This demands all our energies.

No sex, please. ■

# Who's in charge? You are

*Originally published in JADA 1998 129: 1070-1071.*

In the late 1960s and early '70s, many dentists were convinced that dentistry was facing an impending shortage of dental-office personnel. To address that "problem," dental leaders seriously considered expanding the clinical duties of dental auxiliaries.

At a national meeting called to address this issue, a prominent dentist arose and declared: "God made dentists to do dentistry—no one else!" While his words were cheered, clinical studies soon proved him wrong.

Dental auxiliaries can be trained to meet acceptable standards for selected dental procedures. Perhaps what this dentist should have said was that "dentists and no one else" should be responsible for the oversight, management and continuity of America's oral health care.

While this has been the prevailing philosophy of the dental profession and the goal of its educational training programs, there are nondentists who constantly challenge the exclusivity of this mandate. They wish to replace the dentist, arguing that they can provide the same dental services to more people and at lower cost.

Although the literature does not substantiate their claims, they have convinced some lawmakers to change their state dental practice acts. They are relentless in their apparent quest to fragment the delivery of dental services.

Organized dentistry's efforts to defeat these initiatives have proved to be both time-consuming and costly. Yet, a relaxing of professional vigilance could prove more harmful to the welfare of dental patients than any intrusion by third-party financial entities.

You be the judge.

If you are traveling in Vail or Winter Park, Colo., this fall and for whatever reason need your teeth whitened, radiographs taken or blood pressure checked, or if you wish to have an oral cancer screening, needle-free anesthesia, periodontal therapy or perhaps "decay-preventive sealants" placed on your children's teeth, you need look no farther than the U.S. West Yellow Pages.

Here you will find one of Colorado's "unsupervised" dental hygiene practitioners ready to assist you—no dentist needed. Oh, yes, insurance is accepted.

As many of you know, Colorado is one of five states that allow some form of unsupervised practice by dental hygienists. The state's hygienists earned that designation by convincing the legislators they could do more than dentists were presently doing for Colorado citizens. As hygienists in other states seek similar arrangements, their legislative arguments remain the same.

So what does the record show? Ask the Colorado Dental Association, which has had to deal with this legislation. Recently, after reviewing the Yellow Pages advertising of three unsupervised dental hygienists' offices, the CDA wrote to the Colorado Board of Dental Examiners seeking a judgment on whether this advertising "constitutes a violation of the Dental Practice Law," specifically as it applies to "advertising which is misleading, deceptive or false."

The CDA contends that the dental hygienists who place these advertisements "imply that they can provide services to the public which they cannot, as dental hygienists, provide without the authorization of a licensed dentist."

Although the board has yet to rule, the Dental Practice Act of the state of Colorado is explicit: "The responsibility for diagnosis, treatment planning or the prescription of therapeutic measures in the practice of dentistry shall remain with a licensed dentist and may not be assigned to any dental hygienist."

> **Dentists and no one else should be responsible for the oversight, management and continuity of America's oral health care.**

The concerted efforts of auxiliaries to carve out their own niche are not limited to dental hygiene. For example, if you think that denturism is on the wane, you're wrong. Those who monitor legislative activity affecting dentistry have seen an increase in denturist promotion in a number of states, and dental boards have had their hands full countering illegal activities in several states.

Some denturists have set up their offices on Indian tribal lands to escape state dental practice acts. Would-be denturists have received a boost for their professional goals by recent action in Washington state. Authorized by a voter initiative in 1994, Washington denturists now can construct both complete and partial dentures—no dentist needed.

The denturists' legislative arguments—that they can provide greater access and lower-cost prosthetic services—have been disproved. A report out of Canada last year showed no substantial cost differential between fees charged by dentists and fees charged by denturists.[1]

So what else is new?

As hygienists scramble to gain unsupervised status and add to the services they can perform, they're often vigorous in their opposition to those who might intrude on their territory.

For instance, for many years dental assistants in Kansas had performed coronal scaling. In 1995 the state hygienists' association asked the attorney general for a ruling on the legality of that service. It was declared improper.

There is little doubt that the American Dental Hygiene Association's leadership will continue to press for more autonomy. An editorial in the January 1998 issue of ADHA Access states, "The ADA delegates passed resolutions aimed at returning the 'dental family' to those halcyon days before dental hygienists came to realize that D.D.S. and God are not synonymous designations."

The editorial continues, "In time, even organized dentistry's deep, deep pockets will have nothing left but the jangle of loose coins and the unmistakable odor of tawdry crusades and misdirected resources."[2]

Where is the patient in this scurrilous denouncement? Never mentioned.

Those pursuing this course should remember that oral health care is not elective health care. It is an integral component of health care and must be viewed in that dimension. Just consider the emerging relationships between oral infection, low birth weight and cardiovascular disease. Show me the training that qualifies the nondentists to manage these conditions.

There are those who will say that this is a new world. That health care delivery has changed. That dentists are no longer able or interested in providing oversight of the patient's total oral health needs. That others can do it as well or better and cheaper with better access.

I say no! ∎

1. Abrams SH. Denturists: do they really provide more affordable care in Ontario? J Can Dent Assoc 1997;63(10):771-4.
2. Gervasi R. Legislative drama and marketplace realities [Editorial]. Access 1998;12(1):4.

# 'Public health malpractice, plain and simple'

*Originally published in JADA 1998 129: 1191-1192.*

I am a former cigarette smoker, one of 30,000 or more ADA members who reportedly have kicked the habit. During my smoking period, which spanned almost two decades, I had no idea that I was exposing anyone, including myself, to life-threatening toxic agents.

In l964, I watched as a group of America's top scientists appeared on national TV to describe the relationship between tobacco and morbidity and mortality. Their conclusions were definitive: tobacco use and cancer were inextricably linked. One of the committee members threw down his cigarettes and announced right there he would never smoke again. Others, including myself, followed his lead.

Gains in the ranks of those who were able to give up smoking came slowly. Reductions in the number of new smokers occurred at an even slower pace.

The committee's disclosure of a causal relationship between tobacco and a multitude of life-threatening diseases was vigorously resisted by tobacco interests. For years the tobacco industry used its enormous wealth and political influence to discredit research that demonstrated negative outcomes from tobacco use, which can be linked to nearly 500,000 deaths each year. Aside from the pain and suffering of those with tobacco-related diseases, the economic costs are equally staggering: at least $100 billion annually and climbing.

Recent legal actions holding the tobacco industry responsible for the deaths of cigarette smokers are altering this negative equation. The tobacco industry now indicates a willingness to take some responsibility for the deadly effects of its products.

Congress has responded with proposed federal legislation designed to settle all pending state and local lawsuits, impose tobacco advertising and marketing restrictions and set smoking reduction targets for America's youth. The bill was introduced by Sen. John McCain, an Arizona Republican.

One of the bill's major thrusts was to add a $1.10 tax on each pack of cigarettes. Market research had affirmed that this tax increase would significantly decrease the number of first-time smokers while concurrently reducing the quantity of cigarettes purchased by current smokers.

This was legislation that should have had total bipartisan support. However, a massive $40-million public education campaign by tobacco interests and the vociferous opposition by key members of the Senate scuttled any hope of bringing the legislation forward for a vote. The protobacco message: this was just another tax increase to fund big government.

The nation's health leaders were not pleased. After the Senate failed to move the McCain tobacco bill to the floor for a full vote, former U.S. surgeon general and tobacco opponent Dr. C. Everett Koop lashed out at the Senate leadership. "What they have done today," he said, "is public health malpractice, plain and simple. [By] ignoring the advice of every health professional in America, they have chosen only to listen to a handful of television ads and a lot of PAC committees."

The American Medical Association later reaffirmed its support for antitobacco legislation. Specifically, an AMA resolution favored directing substantial proceeds from settlements in tobacco lawsuits toward preventing children from smoking, helping smokers quit and protecting nonsmokers from environmental smoke.

At this juncture, where does organized dentistry stand?

As a strong advocate for federal, state and local activities that would "strengthen and expand their roles in tobacco-use education, prevention, research and cessation efforts," the ADA played a major role

> **Tobacco use can be linked to nearly 500,000 deaths each year, and the economic costs are equally staggering: at least $100 billion annually and climbing.**

in supporting the McCain bill.

The Association focused its efforts predominantly on chewing tobacco and its deleterious effects, especially on youth. Without this ADA involvement, smokeless tobacco—spit tobacco—would have been given short shrift when compared to the mandates and quota proposed for cigarettes.

Specifically, the ADA's Washington office successfully altered the McCain bill through an amendment that tightened how the incidence of underage tobacco use is measured. The suggested method using monthly—rather than daily—measures proved far more representative of how young people use various tobacco products. It will be critical to ensure that any future legislative bill contains this proviso.

National antitobacco legislation is not dead. There will be future legislative bills. Politicians facing re-election, take note: national polls taken after the defeat of the McCain bill still indicate that voters, by a two-to-one margin, will favor candidates who favor antitobacco legislation.

It's time to unleash dentistry's grassroots army. Every member of Congress must get a personal message: dentists do not support tobacco use in any form! As members of the health professions, dentists cannot allow a known killer to infect our children, or our adults.

Let us never forget what is now considered common knowledge. Smoking causes cancer and emphysema, complicates pregnancy and even enhances the development and severity of periodontal disease. Many of these warnings can be found printed on cigarette packs.

Organized dentistry must expand its advocacy role beyond spit tobacco, broadening its attack to include all forms of tobacco. It must actively promote the dental office as a place where smokers can receive professional help in smoking cessation.

Dentists report that lack of reimbursement mechanisms, the amount of time required, patient resistance and concerns about effectiveness are barriers to effective office cessation programs. An ADA priority to seek solutions to these issues could provide the incentive for more dentists to join in tobacco-use-cessation activities.

To continue to demonstrate the ADA's strong commitment, perhaps a component, constituent or even an individual member could introduce a resolution to the ADA House of Delegates reaffirming the Association's dedication to antitobacco legislation. Such action would proclaim dentistry's resolve to have a leadership role on this critical national health issue.

There was a period when we didn't know. But now we do. We also know that they knew—from the beginning. Isn't it time to stop the charade and put tobacco where it belongs? Failure to do so is "public health malpractice, plain and simple." ∎

# DMSOs: a reality check

*Originally published in JADA 1998 129: 1359-1360.*

Would you like to be associated with a large number of fine people under one roof who would pat you on the back when things have not gone right at home? Would you like to be connected with the most progressive dental organization in the world? Would you like to have your money in the business you were helping to build up, which would bring you large interest and in which you could still participate after your death? We would be pleased to explain further regarding our cooperative plan.

—Excerpt from letter soliciting Colorado dentists to join the Painless Parker Dental Clinic, Oct. 26, 1923

**M**odern-day Painless Parkers, sensing high-profit opportunities in dentistry, are sending messages like the one above to dental practitioners throughout the country.

And why not? With "sales" of close to $50 billion annually, dentistry's 100,000 or so individually owned and operated dental practices are ripe for consolidation by astute business interests.

Dentistry's Achilles' heel—a general lack of business acumen—has given these entrepreneurs the opportunity to penetrate the dental marketplace. Packaged as dental management service organizations, or DMSOs, they have already captured 2 percent of dental practices, and that number is growing.

DMSOs come in two sizes. The first provides an array of management services, such as billing and collections, patient scheduling, facilities and personnel management, group purchasing and a variety of other services designed to make the dentist more efficient. Dentists pick and choose which services they want. Ownership of the practice remains with the dentist.

The second type of DMSO is far more control-

> **With 'sales' of close to $50 billion annually, dentistry's 100,000 or so individually owned and operated dental practices are ripe for consolidation by astute business interests.**

ling. This DMSO actually acquires the hard assets of one or more dental practices. These offices are often absorbed into multilocation group practices and conform to standardized management procedures designed to enhance efficiencies and provide a more profitable bottom line.

A number of legal caveats exist for the DMSO arrangement. Of primary interest is the question of whether a nondental entity can actually own, control or manage a dental office. While a number of states appear to restrict this type of ownership, some are giving the issue more latitude—accepting nondental ownership as long as the dentist's control over treatment decisions is maintained.

Frankly, I am surprised at the growing number of dentists who seem interested in pursuing a relationship with this latter form of DMSO. Giving up control, even if it is only managerial control, doesn't fit with the personality type that normally chooses dentistry. Incoming dental students always rank "being one's own boss"—independence—as the major factor influencing their choice of a dental career. Is this motivation no longer valid?

The questions that should arise in practitioners when they first consider joining a DMSO are numerous. Would they be content to be employees, not owners? Would joining have an impact on their practice decisions? Would it affect patient relationships? Would the dentists lose control over certain aspects of practice in a way that they find personally unacceptable? Would this lack of control place them in potentially ethical conflicts, and—if the arrangement fails—leave them in financial jeopardy with long-term personal consequences?

Currently, the biggest audience for the DMSO concept appears to be dentists looking to sell their practices. With escalating student loan debt, and no debt relief in sight for recent dental graduates, young dentists are less able to purchase practices. Dentists seeking a buyer may find the DMSO's offer their only option.

The growth of the DMSO monoliths should trigger certain concerns within the profession. What impact will DMSOs have on dental practices if they gain control of a geographic area? The thought of dental Wal-Marts replacing dentists operating traditional practices is not pleasant.

With only a small percentage of dental practices actually in the DMSO fold, is there enough substance in the DMSO concept to put the profession on the alert? Surely, if you are an orthodontist, the success of the Orthodontic Centers of America, or OCA, has to be acknowledged.

Started in 1984, OCA currently has management or consulting arrangements with 238 orthodontists practicing in 413 centers in 41 states. With net revenues up 51 percent over last year—and net income per share up 53.9 percent—it's no wonder OCA shareholders are cheering.

Business analysts credit OCA with increasing public awareness of the need for, and value of, orthodontics. They predict that orthodontic DMSOs will end up with 20 to 35 percent of the orthodontic market in five years.

Success attracts imitators, and almost 20 DMSOs are either publicly traded or planning to go public. Most of these companies are in the general dentistry area, but speculators anticipate that OCA-type operations will soon surface in the periodontal and oral surgery specialty areas.

Is there a DMSO in your future? Management services say that the top candidates are practitioners who will retire within the next five years. Sound counsel provided in the April issue of the ADA Legal Adviser cautions that anybody entering a DMSO who is 45 years of age or younger should think about having some kind of a safety valve—that is, if there is nonperformance over a couple of years—some kind of buy-out arrangement allowing a return to private practice.

Not all DMSOs succeed. First New England Dental Centers Inc. in Massachusetts filed for Chapter 11 bankruptcy in February. Reporting losses in the millions during its short existence, this DMSO left its dental "employees" with unpaid salaries plus substantial rent and equipment debts.

What goes up can come down. Dentists observing the increase in stock prices for some DMSOs should be aware that many of these companies are selling for far below their initial offering price. Accepting long-term "restricted stock" for what is to be the underpinnings of retirement income could be risky.

Don't look for the ADA to advocate or condemn the DMSO concept. Rather, if you are contemplating an association with a DMSO, look to the ADA for assistance in the decision-making process. Read all the informational materials. Use the ADA Contract Analysis Service.

While this is a matter with legal implications, it is mainly a practice management and personal issue. A decision of this magnitude should never be made until a thorough investigation of all its ramifications has been made.

Make it wisely! ■

# A few piercing thoughts

*Originally published in JADA 1998 129: 1519-1520.*

"Scraping the balls on the insides of the teeth produces quite a noticeable sound. You will frequently notice the wearers doing this as rapidly as possible to generate as much noise as possible. [If you are at party] it is a great way to break the ice."[1]

—A body-piercing studio's Web site[1]

Gripping the tongue with her forceps, the piercer begins the process of fastening a piece of jewelry through the tongue somewhat anterior to the frenum attachment. The 14-gauge needle used to open a passage for the jewelry will be passed completely through the midline of the tongue. The client's jewelry—a tongue barbell or ring—then will follow the needle.

Anesthesia? None. The explanatory pamphlet handed out to prospective clients states that most tongue piercings are "grit-your-teeth-and-bear-it" procedures.

To dentists, who dedicate themselves to making dental procedures painless, envisioning a 14-gauge needle making its way through the unanesthetized tongue must evoke a feeling of personal discomfort. Even more so considering that a 14-gauge needle has a diameter seven times greater than the needle routinely used for dental anesthesia.

Makes you wince just thinking about it.

Yet, a local piercer tells me that at her parlor they do at least 50 tongues a week, and the number continues to climb. "While everybody isn't doing it, people you would think wouldn't are," she says. Tongue piercing, she notes, continues to grow in popularity among the young and not-so-young alike.

Body art apparently is no longer confined to tattooing. The display of metallic jewelry in unconventional places—such as the lips, tongue, eyebrows and cheeks—is becoming commonplace. With a preponderance of these piercings taking place in or around the oral regions, it's a rare dental office that has not noted at least a few patients with one or more pieces of jewelry emerging from those regions.

Dentists are often the first to note any negative effects from the piercing process or from the jewelry itself. A study published in the California Dental Association Journal[2] indicates that these effects are numerous enough to alert the profession to the problems arising from oral piercings.

The article featured the responses of a convenience sample of 51 tongue-pierced people who filled out a questionnaire left at two piercing parlors in San Francisco. Two sought medical help for complications arising from the piercing. Thirteen people (26 percent) reported chipping damage to teeth. Four people reported gingival injury. Sixteen percent of the respondents reported increased salivary flow.

Lip piercing was much less damaging to oral structure. Of 24 people, three reported gingival injury and 13 percent reported increased salivary flow.

Aside from the teeth and gingival injuries, other reports indicate that piercing in the orofacial region has been associated with prolonged bleeding, permanent numbness, loss of taste and interference with speech, mastication and deglutition.

Concerns also have been expressed about compromised airways resulting from swelling or aspiration of jewelry. The National Institutes of Health has identified piercing as a possible vector for transmission of bloodborne hepatitis B, C, D and G. The possibility of HIV transmission has been noted.

Concerns about these side effects have caught the attention of professional dentistry. Last year, the Rhode Island Dental Society called on the ADA to develop a policy on this issue. The House of Delegates unanimously approved the request, and the

> **Most tongue piercings are 'grit-your-teeth-and-bear-it' procedures.**

House was expected to vote on a policy against piercing in San Francisco.

At this writing, the result of the House vote is unknown. If the policy is approved, dentists will have to be cautious in how they implement it. Too strong a stance against tongue piercing may alienate those who might benefit from dental counseling.

Those considering piercing might be reluctant to seek dental advice because of possible admonishments from practitioners. People who make the choice to undergo piercing might seem irrational and disagreeable, but to them it is a form of body art and self-expression no different from wearing earrings. Indeed, those over the age of 18 years legally have the right to do with their bodies what they wish—even if it is not in their best health interests.

These statements notwithstanding, dentists should be willing to counsel potential piercers about associated health risks. They should be aware that alternatives to piercing do exist.

For piercing wannabes willing to accept the "look" without actual tissue trauma, dentists can suggest magnetic jewelry. Apparently, the powerful magnets work quite well for lip, ear and nose jewelry. A major caveat: magnets used on the tongue could be swallowed.

Dentists failing to dissuade a patient from undergoing the piercing should inform him or her of the concepts of universal precautions. As a minimum, piercing clients should find out if their piercing parlor has an autoclave and offers them needles in sterile packages, and whether the piercer uses sterile gloves.

Unfortunately for those being pierced, most operations take place in parlors whose "practitioners" are unregulated, have no set training standards, and do not face OSHA or any other form of state or local regulation. The piercing practitioners I have interviewed all share a desire for regulations covering both training and health standards. They believe such rules would significantly reduce infection.

One piercer estimated that up to 50 percent of piercings are done by kids, on kids. Most are unsuccessful.

Considering the problems that commonly arise from oral and perioral piercings, dentists may find it difficult to support these piercing parlors in their desire for regulation. That would be unfortunate. Many piercing clients are young. They make decisions based more on emotion and peer pressure than on words of wisdom from more knowledgeable sources.

As with other fads, this one will pass. Until that time dentistry should support the regulation of the piercing industry. Remember, many of its clients are or could be your patients. ∎

1. Perforations Body Piercing Studio. Facial piercing. Available at: "http://www.perforations.com/educate/tongue.htm". Accessed: Aug. 18, 1998.
2. Boardman R, Smith RA. Dental implications of oral piercing. CDA J 1997;25:200-7.

# Healthier, wealthier and wiser

*Originally published in JADA 1998 129: 1660-1661.*

**M**ean, median or mode—no matter how you measure it, today's average dentist appears to be healthier, wealthier and wiser than his or her counterpart of 20 or 30 years ago.

While all dentists may not have prospered equally—few dentists are "average"—the last decade has been especially good for the majority. But will these gains continue? What does the future hold?

With the millennium rolling toward us, dental futurists soon will be filling the professional media and lecture halls with their predictions. Taking advantage of my editorial pulpit, I'll jump-start the process with some professional introspection that could prove advantageous as you enter the next decade of practice.

First, an observation on wealth as measured by yearly dental income. After years of flat or even decreasing take-home income, substantial increases recently have been noted. Since 1986, net real income for all dentists has increased 31 percent; for specialists, 40.9 percent. These percentages equal or exceed income growth in the other health professions. In fact, the average real income of general-practice dentists has surpassed that of physician family practitioners.

Young dentists have not been left out. Dental graduates with fewer than 10 years of experience are reporting average net incomes of $100,000. If they are specialists, add an additional $50,000.

These monetary gains have been achieved by dentists devoting a higher percentage of their office hours to treating patients—not by extending their hours. Annual office hours worked have remained constant.

Also, dentistry's $5 billion industry seems to be running against the trend toward "bigger is better." Economic advantages are not apparent in large, multidentist offices compared with one- and two-dentist offices.

It's always good news to hear that the economic status of your profession is on an upswing—even better if you are sharing in that prosperity.

Will the good times continue?

Dental care is a price-sensitive health service. With little anticipated growth in dental insurance, any downturn in the economy could have a negative impact. However, increases in esthetic dental procedures coupled with the treatment required by a now-dentate older population should help offset any economic slowdowns.

Wealthier? Yes. But healthier?

Despite continued exposure to various hazards, dentists appear to be thriving. In response to September JADA's Question of the Month, which asked about dentists' health and well-being, all but a few respondents checked "good" or "excellent." Many added personal comments that emphasized the importance of regular exercise and proper nutrition.

Stress was the one negative factor that received frequent mention. One dentist noted, "I feel like I'm going to have a medical meltdown."

The stress factor cannot be ignored. A past JADA Question of the Month (September 1996) asked dentists whether they would reconsider their careers if given the chance to "do it over again." Those who said they would reconsider cited stress as the major consideration.

The 1997 survey of current issues in dentistry underscores the immediate need to discover ways of containing or lessening stress. In that ADA survey, one-third of all dentists responded that the strategies they use for stress management were ineffective. About the same percentage answered "yes" to the question, "In the last two years, have you thought you might be experiencing burnout?"

The stress issue always leads to the inevitable question of whether dental stress leads to the high

> **The average real income of general practicing dentists has surpassed that of physician family practitioners.**

suicide rate publicly associated with the dental profession. The literature on this subject is equivocal. There are as many studies that say yes as there are that say no.

Of interest to ADA members is a study of more than 100,000 male dentists conducted between 1960 and 1965. The study examined suicide rates depending on whether the dentist was an ADA member. For ADA members, the rate was the same as that for the general population; for nonmember dentists, the rates were much higher than expected.

The ADA's annual Health Screening Program, or HSP, conducted at the annual session since 1964, provides additional evidence that dentists are in generally good health. For example, the HSP disclosure that dentists using precapsulated mercury exhibited lower urinary mercury levels than those using bulk amalgam resulted in policies that dramatically reduce urinary mercury. Levels of 15 micrograms per liter in the 1980s have fallen to the present low of 4 mg/L.

Also noteworthy has been the use of HSP data to recommend hepatitis B vaccination. Today's dentists have the highest rate of compliance of all health professionals.

Good news also from HSP findings is that antibodies to HIV among the 17,000 dentists screened through 1997 were virtually nonexistent. This has to be reassuring to dentists who conscientiously employ comprehensive infection control procedures.

So what about dentists' health and well-being in the future? Frankly, I'd expect little change from the present status. The potential for continued stress in a profession that demands perfection from its members is further compounded by the self-critical nature of dentists.

The salvation is that most dentists like what they are doing. When asked when they would retire, one-fourth of them said "never" because they enjoy practicing too much.

The key to the future health and well-being of dentists will depend on organized dentistry's ability to ensure that the environment for the practice of dentistry continues to offer high levels of professional satisfaction.

Therein lies the great challenge. How do we use our newfound wisdom to attain that goal?

Futurists agree that technology—especially information technology—will be the key to professional success. Dentistry is no exception. Its ability to provide continuous opportunity for professional satisfaction will depend on obtaining and assimilating information in a rapid and timely fashion.

The technology to provide this flow of critical information is available. But the construction and maintenance of this communication infrastructure will require the use of new and continuing resources. Some existing programs may have to be sacrificed. Doubters will flourish; the status quo is always easier.

Once in place, this infrastructure should give dentistry the ability to be continually proactive. This will require vision on the part of dentistry's leaders—a vision to recognize trends and predict their potential impact, to develop programs that address future outcomes, to anticipate, to lead.

A wiser profession will succeed. ∎

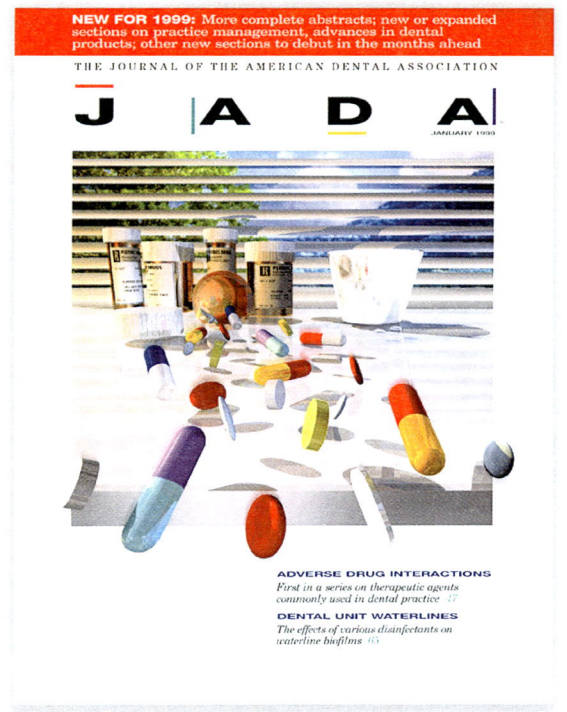

NEW FOR 1999: More complete abstracts; new or expanded sections on practice management, advances in dental products; other new sections to debut in the months ahead

THE JOURNAL OF THE AMERICAN DENTAL ASSOCIATION

**J |A |D A|**

JANUARY 1999

ADVERSE DRUG INTERACTIONS
*First in a series on therapeutic agents commonly used in dental practice*

DENTAL UNIT WATERLINES
*The effects of various disinfectants on waterline biofilms*

# 1999

"At a time when poll after poll indicates widespread dissatisfaction with work environments, a recent survey of practitioners indicated that 88 percent of dentists were satisfied with their choice of profession."

# Pew!

*Originally published in JADA 1999 132: 12-13*

Few "wet-gloved" dentists are aware of the recently released Pew Health Professions Commission report, "Strengthening Consumer Protection: Priorities for Health Care Workforce Regulation."[1] They should be. This report calls for all health professionals to pass periodic written exams and undergo in-office patient observation and record inspection by state regulators at least every seven years.

The commission minces no words, characterizing current state regulators as addressing only the deeds of the "egregiously incompetent." It maintains that "to become a viable element of consumer protection in health care, professional regulation must demonstrate that it unequivocally serves the public good—[presently] the ostensible goal of professional regulation—to establish standards that protect consumers from incompetent practitioners." Serving the public good, the report suggests, "is eclipsed by a tacit goal of protecting the profession's economic prerogatives."

Clearly, the commission members want immediate action. They believe that the states, which have the ultimate responsibility for consumer protection, aren't doing the job and that the assistance of the federal government is required.

The commission calls for "Congress [to] establish a national advisory board that will research, develop and publish national scopes of practice and continuing competency standards for state legislatures to implement."

ADA President S. Timothy Rose recently confronted the issue of monitoring continued dental competency head on. Citing the recent Pew Commission report, he stated, "We can ignore this issue and let some other group or agency develop a competency evaluation system for our profession, or we can be proactive and begin to define competency for new graduates and the currently practicing dentist."

> **Most dentists face only one competency assessment in their entire professional lives: their entry licensing exam. That, most dentists would argue, is the way it should be.**

Few issues in dental practice are so contentious. Most dentists face only one competency assessment in their entire professional lives: their entry licensing exam. That, most dentists would argue, is the way it should be, offering as evidence the extremely small percentage of dentists (1 to 3 percent) who actually face some form of punitive action for practice violations.

Those of the "don't-fix-it-if-it-ain't-broke" school cite other compelling evidence for their position. The December 1996 issue of Consumer Reports indicated that among the more than 52,000 survey respondents, more than 80 percent said their dental work was "very good" to "excellent."[2] Ninety-six percent said they had confidence in their dentists' technical competence. Only one reader in 20 voiced any level of dissatisfaction.

Proponents of periodic evaluation argue that patient complaints resulting in censure represent only the tip of the iceberg—that varying degrees of undiscovered incompetence are actually rampant, affecting the overall quality of dental care offered to the public. They cite to the Reader's Digest exposé ("Can You Trust Your Dentist?"[3]) as evidence that a significant number of dentists are less than honest.

The system for consumer protection presently relies on passive- accreditation mechanisms, licensing exams, character checks, continuing education and punitive interventions from peerreview hearings. In a few instances, civil or criminal actions are noted.

According to the Pew Commission report, the public is entitled to better—much better—protection.

Here's the issue for dentistry in relation to the Pew Commission recommendations: Is it possible to develop a program that satisfies the public need and concurrently provides objective feedback to dental practitioners regarding their state of practice knowledge?

Ideally, such a program would be constructed in a format that was neither intrusive, threatening nor punitive. If the accountability initiative were multidimensional and consisted of a portfolio of assessment instruments or techniques from which dentists could select, the answer to the question posed above would be "yes." Accountability is an area in which a great deal of energy and creativity already has been expended. Many instruments already exist. For example, the American Board of Dental Examiners has produced a list of nine such instruments, many of them already available.

Other possible contributions include the California Dental Association's Quality Improvement Through Lifelong Learning Program. It offers dentists the opportunity to measure their performance without being intrusive. The state of Utah's Continuing Quality Improvement Program, which the Utah Dental Association is delivering to its members, also deserves consideration.

Consider, as well, the concept of written recertification exams developed along the lines of those presently used by the Academy Board of Pediatric Dentistry and the American Board of Oral and Maxillofacial Surgery. Why not include the popular fellowship program of the Academy of General Dentistry? It surely has the potential to address the competency issue.

High-tech developments also hold promise. The first dental patient simulation on CD-ROM from the Dental Interactive Simulation Corp. should be available this spring. Sponsored by 12 major dental organizations, the CD simulations will allow practitioners to assess their medical and dental history skills, diagnostic capabilities and even clinical acumen in the privacy of their offices or homes.

The components are available. Putting together a working model acceptable to state regulatory agencies requires professional input and support. In dentistry, it's the ADA that is best positioned to develop these programs— not federal or state governments.

A go-ahead for Association involvement would require a reassessment of a resolution defeated by the 1997 House of Delegates. It's time to have that debate again. The oft-heard statement "If we don't do it, someone else will" takes on real meaning if that someone else is the U.S. Congress acting on behalf of its former leader, George Mitchell—who just happens to be the chairman of the Pew Commission.

If you believe outsiders can't force changes in dental practice that are opposed by dentists, think again. Read or ask about the MinnesotaCare Law. This legislation requires all dentists who provide dental care to people working for the state of Minnesota also to provide care to residents eligible for medical assistance.

If a dentist chooses not to participate, he or she is not allowed to provide care to any of the 150,000 employees and family members enrolled in state health care programs. Dentists are required to treat these medical assistance patients until their numbers reach 10 percent of the total patient population (until recently it was 20 percent). Minnesota dentists complain that current reimbursement under these programs does not even cover costs of providing these services.

Can you imagine a federal or state consumer initiative that sends its state employees only to dentists who have passed their continuing competency exam? I can.

All too many times I've heard, "Where was the ADA? Why didn't it anticipate this?" ADA President Rose thinks the Association should be out in front on this issue. I do too. ∎

1. Finocchio IJ, Dower CM, Blick NJ, Gragnola CM, Taskforce on Health Care Workforce Regulation. Strengthening consumer protection: Priorities for health care workforce regulation. San Francisco: Pew Health Professions Commission; 1998.
2. Keeping your teeth in shape. Consumer Reports 1996;61(12):43-8.
3. Eckenbarger W. Can you trust your dentist? Reader's Digest 1997; February:50-6.

# The great dental give-away

*Originally published in JADA 1999 130: 154-155*

Community fundraisers don't consider dentists big givers, something I learned when I co-chaired my university's charitable fundraising campaign.

When the dental school's donations failed to meet campus goals, professional fundraisers assured me that my experience with dental faculty reflected their experience with the charitable behaviors of dentists in private practice. Dentists in general, they said, have a reputation for clinging tightly to their purse strings. But on closer examination, this reputation may be unwarranted. Aside from the obvious—dentists may have chosen to donate to charities other than the community-wide combined campaign—a majority of dentists give continuously and substantially "at the office."

The 1997 ADA Survey of Current Issues in Dentistry offers some major revelations about the charitable care dentists provide needy patients. Almost two-thirds of respondents said their primary practice provided charitable dental care, with elderly and low-income nonelderly patients heading the list of the recipients.

These contributions were self-reported and possibly inflated. But even if they are discounted by as much as 50 percent, the volume is substantial. Consider the following: Dentists who indicated charitable involvement provided treatment to a yearly average of 42 patients at no fee, and another 103 patients at a discounted rate. In dollars, that's a yearly average of $8,912 of free dentistry, plus discounted fee savings of $31,145—about a $40,000 total charitable contribution per dentist.

Those wishing to design a publicly funded nationwide dental health program should take note. With no incentive for dentists to provide care at a reduced fee or without charge, national health planners would have to add about $4 billion to the costs of the program just to cover the present level of contributed dental service. That's almost 10 percent of the total yearly expenditure for all dental care.

These dollar amounts do not include dental services donated outside of the practitioner's office. The charitable survey indicates an average of nine hours of discounted care and four and one-half hours of free care donated each month by dentists treating patients in hospitals, community clinics or other public health settings.

Why do so many dentists donate their time and skills to the needy? The November JADA Question of the Month asked, "Do you donate your services?" Those who said they do emphasized the importance of charity. "Because ... it's the rule!" said one respondent. "I was taught to give back what I've been given." Others answered, "I enjoy it," or "I have been given a gift and should share it with those less fortunate."

Those not donating their services gave equally cogent responses. "Since dentistry is what I always do, I would rather volunteer in other endeavors," said one. "HMO discounted fees are about all the charity I can afford," said another.

It is impossible to name the hundreds of donated dental service enterprises that exist in every state. Traditionally, they represent a coalition between community resources and the dental profession. All are worthy, and most could expand their operation if more resources were available.

Let me describe a few of these groups that have caught my attention.

One program worth mentioning is the Dade County Dental Research Clinic. Don't be dissuaded by its name. While some research may be conducted under its aegis, its main thrust is a low-cost continuing education program for community dentists and an opportunity for the area's needy and disadvantaged to avail themselves of high-quality dental care.

**Almost two-thirds of dental practitioners reported their primary practice provided charitable dental care, with elderly and low-income nonelderly patients heading the list of the recipients.**

A good example of the value of this cooperative effort is the clinic's program in basic implantology. Dentists in the implant program pay a minimum fee of $45 a year and receive 22 full days of instruction spread over a two-year period. Initiated in 1981, this program has trained more than 200 local dentists who have placed more than 1,000 implants in the mouths of the area's dental needy.

The Smiles for Success, or SFS, program of the American Association of Women Dentists is one that I find especially appealing. Recognizing that a pleasing, healthy smile may be critical in obtaining a job, the SFS program offers free dental care to women in "transition from welfare to workfare."

There is no doubt that an attractive smile can enhance an applicant's chances of success in a job interview. In New York City, the SFS program partners with the AAWD's "Suited For Success" program, providing needy job seekers with clothing suitable for an interview. Combining appropriate business attire and a pleasant dental appearance makes the transition into the work world much easier.

Organized philanthropic programs aimed at providing dental services to needy children can be found in many U.S. cities, often operating on a shoestring, totally dependent on time contributed by local dentists and their staff. The materials and equipment used in these programs often come from the goodwill and largess of area dentists. But long-term commitments often are difficult to secure because of the soft funding base for these programs.

One program that has a firmer financial base for its operations, and may be a useful prototype for other such programs, is the Children's Dental Center in Inglewood, Calif. Now entering its fourth year, the center employs a multidisciplinary part-nering approach to achieve its objective of providing "the latest in dental care for children of working families who have no access to dental care."

A successful volunteer program that has attracted nationwide attention for many years is the Denver-based National Foundation of Dentistry for the Handicapped. Through its DDS (Donated Dental Services) program, $25 million of volunteer services have been provided to 24,000 needy people by almost 7,000 volunteer dentists.

This program focuses on dentists providing services in their own offices with help from participating dental laboratories. This year, the NFDH expects to help more than 4,000 people with $5 million of dental care.

These are but a few of the "giving" programs staffed by dentists volunteering their services. One JADA Question-ofthe- Month respondent asked whether there was a way to publicize the large amount of donated dental care. Could this be achieved, he asked, without being viewed as self-serving?

To be sure, it's hard to beat your own drum and expect to get credit. Perhaps industry could assist by highlighting dentists' public service contributions in their institutional advertising. A cause-related marketing effort might also do the trick. How about recognition plaques for dental offices? Might the ADA serve as a clearinghouse for such a program?

With no easy answers, it behooves those who make dental policy to be aware of the facts and share them with their influential constituents. The ADA report on charitable services provided by dentists deserves wide distribution. Read it. Share its message. Keep it from becoming just another document on the shelf. ∎

# Outrageous

*Originally published in JADA 1999 130: 308-309*

How long does it take for a community to speak out? To become incensed? To become outraged enough to demand action?

Just a few hours, in the case of the 10-year-old honor student whose mother inadvertently left a kitchen paring knife in her lunch box. The girl was expelled from school, even though she turned in the knife to her teacher. A supportive community quickly rose to her defense, rallying against a school board that held her to a zero-tolerance standard for bringing a weapon to school.

Consider a similar community outpouring of support for a 13- year-old honor student who volunteered to her teacher that her book bag accidentally touched off the fire alarm. She was expelled for her truthfulness. Faced with growing community antagonism, the school board reluctantly reversed its decision.

Well, it's time for the communities throughout America to rear their heads and speak out—this time, against the great American sell-a-thon—our schools and their precious charges being sold to commercial interests. I refer to the intrusion of a $54 billion commercial soda-pop interest into the public school setting.

Few doubt the importance of a public K-12 education. All the statistics point to better jobs, less crime, fewer people on the public dole—more opportunity in general for those who are educated. Yet, public education is costly, accounting for major chunks of local and state budgets. Personal, out-of-pocket taxes are the main source of support for education. To many, especially those who have no children in the school system, education takes too much of their spendable income.

Thus, it's no wonder that when a large corporation offers big bucks for an exclusive marketing deal with a school system, it often finds ready takers. For the schools, the "biggies" are Pepsi and Coca-Cola. The bidding between these two giants often resembles the professional sports free-agency wars, as evidenced by these excerpts from the local Denver newspaper. Doesn't this sound familiar?

The suburban school superintendent "would not discuss the specific figures but did confirm that the soda companies were willing to pay more than $3 million for the exclusive rights to the district's 80,000 students." Such deals have been lucrative for other districts. Earlier this year, Denver signed a deal that guarantees the district at least $5.7 million over five years—perhaps a better agreement than the $3.9 million, sevenyear deal signed by an adjoining suburban school district.

Other types of deals are also available. As I mentioned in November 1997, one of Colorado's largest school districts entered into a partnership with Pepsi and U.S. West to build a $5 million football stadium. Pepsi gets exclusive rights to sell its products in the district's 140 schools, and U.S. West will get naming rights for the stadium and become the district's preferred phone carrier, selling its credit card imprinted with the district's emblem.

> **Some of these corporate/school partnerships are so commercial that the propriety of the public-supported institutions that enter into them becomes questionable.**

These are not hands-off arrangements. Indeed, some of these partnerships are so commercial that the propriety of the public-supported institutions that enter into them becomes questionable. Just a few months ago, a top official in one of these school districts with a soft-drink contract sent a letter to all the school principals warning that if their schools didn't "dramatically" increase sales, the district's schools could lose significant revenue from their soft-drink partner.

While stating that he didn't want to pressure teachers, the administrator suggested that the principals "allow students virtually unlimited access to soft drink machines, move them where they would be accessible to the students all day, permit students to purchase and consume vended products throughout the day," and even "consider allowing students to drink their soft drink products in class."

The school district's contract calls for the sale of 70,000 cases of the soft drink by the third year. What will these schools get if they sell their quota? Just $32.59 per student to "supplement" educational materials. If schools don't meet their quota, they will get "only a fraction" of the payment outlined in their contract with the industrial giant.

The top administrator's edict—let the students have unlimited access—generated little debate. According to one school principal who moved a vending machine from the cafeteria to the hallway where it would be more accessible, "There were some eyebrows raised, but not much discussion."

The president of the local education association, which hears complaints, noted that no teachers contacted the organization about the administrator's letter. This appears to be the norm for all of these school district agreements. Taxpayers seem pleased—there's been only a smattering of letters in the newspapers challenging these commercial relationships.

Why be concerned about what appears to be a mutually beneficial relationship between public education and industry? Simply stated, the continual ingestion of soda pop may be detrimental to the health of children. These are the facts: The average 12- to 19-year-old male who consumes soda pop will drink more than two cans each day—868 cans a year—ingesting 15 or more teaspoons of sugar

daily as the byproduct of his soda habit. Females, averaging one-plus cans and 10 teaspoons of sugar, aren't far behind. Soft drinks, it appears, may be replacing low-fat milk, fruit juice and other healthful foods.

Indeed, teen-age boys are drinking twice as much soda as milk—a reversal of the trend 20 years ago. There is genuine concern that osteoporosis in females may be getting a jumpstart with the substitution of soda pop for calcium-containing drinks.

Is this also a dental problem? You bet! With the well-documented increases in dental caries and erosion of teeth that result from highly fermentable carbohydrates and the low pH of carbonated drinks, we have a major dental health problem—a problem that is not only going unattended, but is being actively promoted by the schools and industry. Interestingly, in all the negotiations between the school districts and industry, not one of the school districts has sought input from local dentists.

I don't think it's a stretch to classify the active promotion of soda pop in schools as child neglect. If this isn't blatant neglect, then how can you rationalize the increased incidence of caries and erosion of teeth that can be traced directly to excessive ingestion of soft-drink products—products that are actively promoted in and by the school? Shouldn't dentists be actively campaigning against these soft-drink contracts? Isn't it time for the dental community to show outrage at these education/industry alliances and demand changes?

America's children deserve better. ∎

# A debt service

*Originally published in JADA 1999 130: 460-461*

With more than $250,000 needed to educate just one dental student, who pays the bill is becoming more than an academic question. Skyrocketing educational debt reported by recent dental graduates indicates that they are assuming greater responsibility for the cost of their educational program— and many just can't afford it.

It's no secret that more than a few graduates are leaving dental school with debts in excess of $150,000. Indeed, 29.3 percent of private school graduates report debt at that level, and that doesn't include their noneducational debt for cars, home mortgages and so on.

Public dental school graduates are not immune. Even with significant subsidies from the state, 13 percent of public dental school graduates reported educational debts of more than $100,000. And these figures are growing. In 1996, average educational debt climbed 11.8 percent. Average debt rose another 7.8 percent in 1997.

That's not inflation.

For many, a dental education has become too costly. Yet, unless you are one of the thousands of recent dental school graduates laboring to repay massive educational debts, the cost of educating future dentists probably is of little concern. It should be.

Consider the following.

Findings from a recent ADA survey of dentists in practice five years or less indicate that this educational debt is having a major impact on practice options and practice selection. The survey was conducted by the ADA Survey Center, the Committee on the New Dentist and the Council on Dental Practice.

Comments from the survey illustrate how pervasive the debt situation has become. Ninety-five percent of respondents stated, "I could not afford to start my own practice." Ninety-one percent said, "I could not afford to purchase a practice," and 78 percent said they had to accept a position as an associate.

There has always been some professional conjecture that high student debt forced new graduates to select dental delivery systems outside of the traditional fee-for-service modality. Perhaps that is correct. Thirty-eight percent of private school graduates and 23 percent of public school graduates indicated they derived more than 25 percent of their billings from contracts with PPOs, capitation plans and straight risk pools.

These graduates don't see their debt disappearing in the near term. More than 75 percent say their student debt will have "somewhat" or "substantial effect" on them financially for the next 10 years.

The ADA is cognizant of this negative impact on its young membership. In 1997, its House of Delegates voted to address the issue of student debt and educational financing. A response from the new dentists' group advanced six directives focused primarily on handling debt.

While recent graduates agree with this initiative, they also give equal ranking to a statement calling on the ADA to "encourage dental schools to keep the cost of a dental education low." Reductions in dental school education costs, they believe, could be passed on to students, resulting in less debt.

As dental schools are presently structured, cost cutting is not an easy task. Dental education's primary expenditure comes from its labor- as well as technology-intensive patient clinics. Medical education is less costly because medical schools don't have to run their own outpatient hospital. Medicine sends its students into the community hospital.

On a number of occasions, I have presented proposals that examine how efficiencies can be achieved that will result in substantial cost reduction, not just holding the line. Basically, my suggestions call for a restructuring of how preclinical and clinical dental education is delivered.

> **Educational debt is having a major impact on practice options and practice selection**

Initial cost savings in the preclinical area will come from the use of virtual reality and other computer-driven simulations. The goal of educating a student to the level of a second-semester junior without involving live patients is not unrealistic.

Addressing the major clinical cost still remains. How can an institution extricate itself from running its own high-cost clinics? The answer, while not simple in execution, is to mimic the medical model and send students out into the community for a major portion of their training.

The concept of using extramural clinics for training students is not new. For more than three decades, most dental schools have sent their students into the community to gain experience in treating patients not normally seen in dental school clinics. What is presently missing is a formal program that delivers substantial portions of the clinical program outside the walls of the dental school.

The logistics of instituting such a program are challenging. Dental faculties will be uneasy with any program that doesn't give them direct physical control over the assessment of student competencies. Yet, there is a working model for this type of program that has demonstrated its worth.

The University of Colorado's School of Dentistry was created, not only to train dentists for Colorado, but also to enhance service to underserved populations. To comply with the state mandate, dental educators, organized dentistry and the state legislators brought forth a program that places students in an external clinical program for one academic year.

Students participate in about 50 community health clinics, hospital-based and private dental practices in underserved areas throughout the state.

Since its inception in 1986, 220 dentists—about 10 percent of all the state's dentists—have participated in the program. With this type of involvement, town/gown conflicts are virtually nonexistent.

All clinics and practices involved in the program are operated independently of the university. While each mentor/ participant holds a faculty appointment, he or she is not compensated by the university. Retreats and other in-service training mechanisms ensure that participating volunteer faculty members are knowledgeable about dental school clinic policies.

While calculations of the costs saved through such a program need to be refined, a rough estimate would be that a combination of advanced simulation, plus six months of an extramural program, could reduce the cost of a dental school education by 20 percent.

I'm sure that today's graduates would gladly accept debt relief of $15,000 to $25,000. Savings of that magnitude would reduce their monthly debt service while increasing their ability to make practice decisions independent of oppressive debt.

This is not just an educator's issue. Practitioners also have a vested interest. Without the understanding and input of the practicing profession, the issue of dental school financing will languish. Collective solutions need to be advanced and supported. Action starts with knowledge. ∎

# Foxes in the henhouse

*Originally published in JADA 1999 130: 612-613*

The right to search for truth implies also a duty. One must not conceal any part of what one has recognized to be true.

**—Albert Einstein**

A recent eye-catching media report noted that an unexpectedly high percentage of American men and women was experiencing sexual dysfunction.

The source of this information was a study published in the scientifically respected Journal of the American Medical Association. Soon after its publication, an Associated Press report out of Chicago said the AMA admitted that its journal "failed to disclose that the authors of the sex study had been paid by Pfizer Inc. to review clinical trial data on Viagra before the impotency drug was submitted for government approval."

Does this mean the results of this "sex" study were invalid, misleading or even false? No, but without any information on the authors' potential conflict of interest, JAMA readers were denied critical knowledge that might have tempered their interpretation of the published results.

A more overt example of scientific conflict of interest comes from records made public during Minnesota's lawsuit against cigarette manufacturers. Thirteen scientists were paid upwards of $156,000 for letters and manuscripts aimed at casting doubt on a 1993 report that linked secondhand smoke to lung cancer. It appears that none of the journal editors who published this material knew that the authors were paid to write it.

These examples are not isolated incidents. A recently presented study at a meeting of the American Association for the Advancement of Science addressed the issue of conflict of interest in publications.

The researchers noted that of 62,000 scientific articles published in 1997, less than 1 percent included information on authors' research links with their for-profit supporters. This percentage is not even close to an expected 35 percent noted in a previous study by the same research group.

Perhaps the reason many authors don't offer up conflict of interest declarations is that doing so goes against their academic research code. To them, allowing bias to creep into their interpretation of research results would be unethical and unthinkable. So be it, except that many, including this editor, believe that judgment should be left to the reader—not to the researcher.

What exactly is conflict of interest? In the scientific arena, it has been defined as a situation in which professional judgment regard- ing the outcome(s) of research might be compromised or unduly influenced by a secondary interest. Such interests are often linked to the potential for financial gain—stock holdings, consultantships, payment for scientific presentations and so forth. But conflicts of interest could take a variety of other forms, including personal relationships that also might influence judgment.

> **The potential for conflict of interest appears to be on the rise because of an increasing volume of university-based research being supported by for-profit companies.**

The ADA has addressed the concept of conflict of interest in two sections of its Principles of Ethics and Code of Professional Conduct. The first calls on dentists who present educational and/or scientific information "to disclose to readers or participants any monetary or special interest the dentists may have with a company whose products are promoted or endorsed in the presentation. Disclosure shall be made in the promotional material and in the presentation itself."

The Principles of Ethics also covers the sale of products in the dental office. Dentists who, "in the regular conduct of their practices, engage in the marketing or sale of products to their patients, must take care not to exploit the trust inherent in the dentist-patient relationship for their own financial gain."

The potential for conflict of interest appears to be on the rise because of an increasing volume of university-based research being supported by for-profit companies. Dentistry, a materials-dependent profession characterized by rapid turnover in technology and new generations of dental products, appears to be a likely source for increased researcher/industry contracts.

JADA has noted a growing number of research manuscripts that have some relationship with for-profit companies. The most common situation involves a company providing funds to a research scientist at a university. Less frequently, the research actually is carried out in the for-profit company's laboratories.

Because of the potential for greater conflicts of interest in either of these situations, we have tried to minimize the number of manuscripts that are selected for review in these categories. This policy has proved unsatisfactory. Journal subscribers have said they want more peer-reviewed product information, and they want to read it monthly in JADA.

To address these needs, we have introduced a new section in The Journal titled Advances in Dental Products. It contains short, peer-reviewed reports published in a timely fashion. This section should assist practitioners in their quest to assess, objectively, new generations of dental materials and technologies.

Most submissions to this category will have had some commercial sponsorship. JADA readers should carefully examine the noted research support and industry affiliations of the clinicians and researchers.

JADA also will increase its vigilance to ensure author compliance with the conflict of interest standards. These author/industry affiliations will be displayed in a prominent and newly accented position in the article. Our peer reviewers will be informed if a manuscript contains conflict of interest disclosure( s), even though doing so may compromise the anonymity of contributors.

Success in this area requires full disclosure by authors. Peer review itself offers no defense against undisclosed conflicts of interest. The review process also is vulnerable to the accuracy of the submitted data. Omissions or distortions, either by accident or purposeful, are almost impossible to detect. Ultimately, it will be the patients who suffer if practitioners do not have all the facts necessary to make a best judgment of a product's true effectiveness.

Mark Twain said those who don't read are no better off than those who can't read. Perhaps this statement should be amended to state that those who read but don't have all the information could be worse off than those who don't read at all. ∎

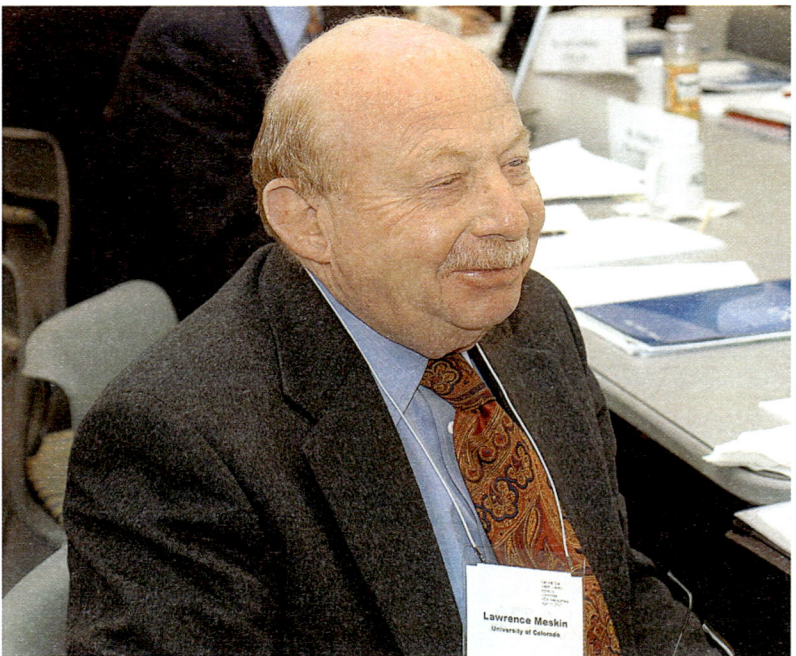

Dr. Meskin enjoys a light moment during a dental meeting.

# Capricious nonsense

*Originally published in JADA 1999 130: 770-771*

The very core of dentistry's preventive oral health message is under attack. Unbelievably, a suit has been filed in a Cook County, Ill., circuit court alleging that toothbrush manufacturers are making unsafe devices and that the ADA is complicit because it gives certain brushes its Seal of Acceptance.

In our litigious society, almost anything can become the subject of a legal suit. But toothbrushes?

The plaintiff and his lawyers claim that toothbrushes cause tooth abrasion and should carry a warning on their packages. They further claim that the ADA, because it gives a Seal to this type of product, is misleading the public into believing that the toothbrush is a safe device.

This claim implies that dentists and hygienists have endangered the oral health of the hundreds of millions of people to whom they have taught proper toothbrushing techniques to control or prevent dental caries and periodontal disease.

Now, if toothbrushes are as dangerous as the participants in this legal suit contend, national and state legislators should be considering the introduction of laws to protect the public.

For example, should a device as dangerous as a toothbrush be allowed out of homes and into the workplace? Speaking about homes, shouldn't toothbrushes be equipped with safety devices to keep them away from vulnerable children? What about concealed toothbrushes in the workplace, on school grounds—even in the school classroom?

Indeed, if the plaintiff's allegations are correct, shouldn't toothbrushes be banned in the dental office? And shouldn't anyone who promotes such a dangerous device demonstrate special training and certification? Would a D.D.S. or R.D.H. be sufficient?

Dangerous! That's what they say. I say ludicrous, capricious and frivolous. This suit amounts to legal hogwash.

Toothbrushes are not a recent invention. The concept of brushing goes back thousands of years, when primitive societies devised ways of cleaning teeth. Many employed the softened ends of twigs, thus ensuring that their toothbrushes were only a bush away. But if blame is to be placed, it rests with the Chinese who, in 1490, designed what became today's toothbrush, with the bristles perpendicular to the handle. We now have about 500 years of experience with these instruments. So how come we are just finding out how potentially dangerous they are to oral health?

Unlike the classic studies by Dr. Harald Löe, who produced and reversed gingivitis by taking away and replacing toothbrushes, ethical considerations preclude conducting similar studies to test the production of toothbrush abrasion. While it is conceivable that an overzealous brusher might abrade away portions of tooth structure over time, the available research literature cannot conclusively indict the toothbrush as the culprit.

In fact, perhaps the majority of lesions once considered toothbrush abrasion may be the result of tensile force created by excessive occlusal force.

These forces are said to bend the tooth with disruption of chemical apatite bonds on the opposite side of the flexure, causing lesions that we may have identified erroneously as toothbrush abrasion. This process would help explain why "toothbrush abrasion lesions" often skip teeth that should have shown wear from the continuous longitudinal stroking of a toothbrush.

Let's also not forget that tooth abrasion might also be the result of a highly abrasive toothpaste—but that's another issue and, sensing the intent of our legal system, perhaps another lawsuit!

At best, the pathogenesis of these cervical (noncarious) lesions needs further investigation before anyone incriminates the toothbrush, the toothbrusher or the dental professional who instructed

> **In our litigious society, almost anything can become the subject of a legal suit. But toothbrushes?**

the person in brushing techniques.

Unfortunately, even a frivolous suit of this nature can have serious negative repercussions. By creating unwarranted fear that toothbrushing can be harmful, an unknown but potentially large number of regular brushers may reduce the frequency and time spent cleaning their teeth. Parents, now concerned that their children might "brush away" their teeth, may become less diligent in supporting good toothbrushing habits in their children.

With the growing amount of evidence that periodontal disease may be linked to systemic illnesses such as cardiovascular disease, stroke and low birthweight, a reduction in brushing frequency conceivably could be life-threatening.

The media continue to view this suit as humorous material for tongue-in-cheek satires. One of their editorials raises the question: Will advocating brushing for children now be considered child abuse? This whole issue is talk-show material, nothing more.

For those seeking a quick way to make a buck, look elsewhere. Perhaps the citrus industry. We do know that sucking on lemons can cause tooth erosion, so why not a warning on each lemon? And how about those popcorn manufacturers and their farmer suppliers? Shouldn't there be a warning about popcorn hulls that can cut into the gingiva?

Outrageous nonsense. Let's hope the judicial system agrees. ∎

# One more time

*Originally published in JADA 1999 130: 910-911*

Physicians are doing it. So are nurses. But how many dentists are doing it? If it's diagnosing oral cancer—not enough.

It appears that the warning of a previous editorial—"do it or lose it"— already may have become reality. A recent report from Maryland's cancer registry indicated that, at least in that state, 83 percent of oral cancers are diagnosed by nondental personnel.

For a disease that is dentistry's to prevent and treat, this new information is just one more example of the continuing evidence that our profession appears to be botching its role. Our abysmal record speaks for itself.

Dentistry has demonstrated a singular lack of progress in controlling the morbidity and mortality associated with oral and pharyngeal cancer. Each year 30,000 U.S. citizens are diagnosed with oral cancer and 8,000 die—numbers that have shown no meaningful decrease in the last three decades.

This lack of progress has not gone unnoticed. Those responsible for determining the nation's health goals for the year 2010 are determined to bring national attention to this problem. You will soon see the results of their collaborative efforts.

Titled "Healthy People 2010," the report lists more than 200 health objectives designed to add years of healthy life and to eliminate health disparities among all Americans. Two of its objectives are aimed exclusively at oral cancer.

To achieve the first oral cancer objective by 2010, 35 percent of adults aged 40 years and older must report having had an exam to detect oral and pharyngeal cancer within the last 12 months. The present baseline is a paltry 7 percent. That's right—just 7 percent of this age group reported having had an oral cancer exam.

> **Dentistry has demonstrated a singular lack of progress in controlling the morbidity and mortality of oral and pharyngeal cancer. Each year 30,000 U.S. citizens are diagnosed with oral cancer and 8,000 die—numbers that have shown no meaningful decrease in the last three decades.**

The second objective is linked to the success of the first objective: early detection, greater survival. Policy-makers are shooting for a goal of having 50 percent of oral and pharyngeal cancers detected at the earliest stage. Presently, the percentage is about 35 percent. Clinical evidence says this makes sense. Survival rates with cancers detected in early stages reach 80 percent. Only 19 percent of patients survive for five years if the cancer has reached an advanced stage.

How realistic are these objectives?

At first glance, both appear to be easily achievable, since every oral examination should include a thorough search for tissue abnormalities. However, the very low percentage of Americans who presently report having had such an exam indicates that either dentists aren't doing it or patients don't know that they've had an oral examination.

As one who has been responsible for instructing thousands of dental students in the pathologies of the oral cavity, I can neither understand nor accept the continuing reports that dentists aren't routinely performing oral cancer examinations.

I would rather believe that the following comments of a JADA reader are a truer reflection of what takes place in the dental office. This dentist wrote, "After examining 50 patients [for oral cancer] I asked patients if they realized they had just had an oral cancer exam ... 43 out of 50 told me they were not aware I had just done an oral cancer examination." The writer concluded, "So perhaps we are doing our job, but we forgot to tell the patient."

Why would dentists "forget" to tell the patient? Are they concerned that such a disclosure will generate fear in their patients and that they will not return in the future? That shouldn't be an issue, especially if the dentist explains that early detection can almost ensure a positive long-term outcome.

Aside from informing patients that they have been screened for oral cancer, the dental profession's challenge is to reach those who do not make annual dental visits and who may be at higher risk of developing oral cancer.

Unfortunately, the message on the importance of early detection of oral cancer has not been effective enough to cause public concern. A search of information from the mass media from 1987 to 1998 supports that contention.

During that entire period, just 50 items were noted and they often contained incomplete or misleading information. For example, only 50 percent mentioned any warning signs of oral cancer, and less than 15 percent noted the need for periodic clinical oral cancer exams by health professionals.

Only a well-financed, ongoing national campaign to "have a yearly oral cancer exam" will move this issue from the shadows into the forefront of health education. While this issue may not have the emotional "pull" to attract funds from conventional sources, new sources for funding may be available.

For example, tobacco use is cited as a pathologic agent in at least 75 percent of cases of oral cancer. Therefore, requesting a portion of the tobacco settlement payouts to discourage tobacco use appears to be a bona fide use of those dollars. While the bulk of any request should be dedicated to prevention programs directed specifically at America's youth, funding programs that stress the importance of annual cancer exams also should get high priority.

In addition to education, perhaps the fiscal requests might also include support of continuing education for health professionals to assist them in keeping current in the diagnosis of oral cancer. The infrequent occurrence of many of these lesions justifies yearly refresher courses for the dental professional.

Accordingly, financial support also needs to include provisions for oral cancer exams available to all, regardless of ability to pay. Why then not consider lobbying for expanded Medicare benefits to include routine oral cancer exams for the older adult?

Once again, I have used this column to wage war on oral cancer. I will not stop. I hope that as practicing dental professionals, you are as offended and troubled by the oral cancer statistics as I am.

Our profession has the knowledge, ability and skill to reduce oral cancer morbidity and mortality. Now is the time to dedicate yourself to the initiation and support of public education campaigns for the prevention and detection of oral cancer. ∎

# Dentistry's best and brightest

*Originally published in JADA 1999 130: 1154-1155*

*The following is adapted from a graduation address delivered May 29 by JADA Editor Lawrence H. Meskin to the class of 1999, University of Colorado School of Dentistry, Denver.*

Today is truly a day for celebration. For our graduates, it marks the achievement of a major career goal. For those who contributed to their academic success over the past two or four years, the exhilaration generated by this ceremony easily compensates for past sacrifices.

And on a personal level, all of our graduates should enjoy the inner satisfaction generated by the knowledge that they have joined the select ranks of a major health profession.

But with this newfound status comes new responsibility. No longer can you turn to an instructor and ask, "What should I do?" The dental school has determined that you have the basic information and technical skills necessary to become practitioners of dentistry.

An awesome responsibility. But even more so when you consider you have also inherited dentistry's covenant with society. That agreement says that, in return for giving the dental profession a virtual monopoly to provide the public with dental services, you as practitioners have the responsibility of placing society's dental needs ahead of your own personal concerns—a potentially challenging and difficult responsibility.

In that regard, let me share a true story with you. A few years ago, one of America's foremost structural engineers designed the support structure for a 59-story New York City skyscraper. Built to house the headquarters of one of America's largest multinational companies, the skyscraper became the work home of thousands.

One day a young student challenged this noted engineering guru, questioning the safety of his girder design for the skyscraper. Nonsense, scoffed the engineer. The design has been tested in wind tunnels, and it has a special safety device to ensure its structural viability.

Determined to show his young critic where he was wrong, the engineer privately re-examined the structure. To his great dismay, he discovered that the building was not safe—that high winds coming from a specific angle could topple it. He learned, too, that the odds were that such winds would occur once every 16 years. And odds being what they are, such winds could arrive tomorrow or never in the building's lifetime.

> **In return for giving the dental profession a virtual monopoly to provide the public with dental services, you as practitioners have the responsibility of placing society's dental needs ahead of your own personal concerns.**

The engineer was faced with a terrible decision. He could blow the whistle on himself and face bankruptcy and professional disgrace. Or he could keep quite and bet people's lives against the odds. He was distraught and actually considered suicide.

What would you do?

The engineer decided not to hide the problem. He devised a method—although costly—that could shore up each of the building's 200 supports. Working at a feverish pace, workers were able to reinforce the structure before the hurricane season could test the odds. The building was saved.

In the ensuing years, the engineer often shared his experiences with prospective structural engineering graduates. He spoke of his initial despair, the question of what to do, the totality of the personal consequences.

But he also addressed the issue of professional responsibility. He reminded the students that they have a societal obligation, that "in return for getting a license and being regarded with respect, you must be self-sacrificing and look beyond the interests of yourself and your client. You must look to society as a whole."

It's really a matter of professionalism. For him and now you.

What will the future hold for you as emerging members of the dental profession? With the millennium rolling toward us, dental futurists will soon be filling the professional media and lecture halls with their predictions.

Taking advantage of my academic pulpit, I'll start the process by predicting that we will see a healthier, wealthier and wiser profession that will offer great professional satisfaction to hygienist and dentist alike.

First, let's consider "healthier."

Despite continued exposure to a variety of hazards, dental professionals appear to be thriving. In a recent survey that asked dentists about their health and well-being, all but a few checked "good" or "excellent."

At a time when poll after poll indicates widespread dissatisfaction with work environments, a recent survey of practitioners indicated that 88 percent of dentists were satisfied with their choice of profession. Fully one-fourth of them, when asked when they planned to retire, answered, "Never." They said they enjoy the practice of dentistry too much.

Next, a look at "wealthier."

After years of flat or even declining take-home income, substantial increases in dentists' income have been noted recently. In fact, the average real income of general practice dentists has surpassed that of physician family practitioners.

It's always good news to hear that the economic status of your profession is on an upward curve—even better if you are sharing in that prosperity. But will the good times continue?

Dental care is a price-sensitive health service. With little anticipated growth in dental insurance, any downturn in the economy could have a negative impact. However, increases in esthetic dental procedures, coupled with treating a newly dentate, older population, should help offset any economic slowdowns.

And what about the emerging relationship between periodontal disease and systemic health? Hygienists, take note: this should give enhanced visibility to the need for preventive dental care.

Finally, the question of "wiser."

On this, there is no doubt. Look to your left, then to your right. Dentistry is attracting the best and brightest, and you represent the top of that ladder. Entrance to the dental program at the University of Colorado is unbelievably competitive. The future of your profession is in your hands, and

I'm sure you will provide the necessary leadership for its success in the new millennium.

To you, emerging dental health professionals, trained to be perfectionists in an imperfect world, consider the following advice:
- maintain your skills so that they never become outdated;
- don't, regardless of the situation, attempt too much at the expense of yourself or your patients;
- if your work ever ceases to be enjoyable, reexamine your criteria for success.

In the main lobby of the San Antonio Hilton Hotel, there is a wall plaque entitled "My Philosophy," written by the hotel's architect, H.B. Zachary. It's about work, and it's about life. Its contents are both poignant and inspiring, and I often reread my copy. While coping with the complexities of today's world of work, perhaps you, too, will find its contents worthy of your thoughts.

This is what Mr. Zachary wrote:

"I do not choose to be a common man. It is my right to be uncommon if I can. I seek opportunity, not security. I will refuse to be a kept citizen, to be humbled and dulled by having my state and nation look after me. I want to dream and to build, to fail and to succeed, never to be numbered among those weak and timid souls who have known neither victory nor defeat.

"I know that happiness can come only from the inside through hard constructive work and sincere positive thinking. I know that the so-called pleasures of the moment should not be confused with a state of happiness. I know that I can get a measure of inner satisfaction from any job if I intelligently plan and courageously execute it.

"I know that, if I put forth every iota of strength that I possess—physical, mental, spiritual—toward the accomplishment of a worthwhile task, ere I fall exhausted by the wayside, the Unseen Hand will reach out and pull me through. Yes, I want to live dangerously, to plan my procedures on the basis of calculated risks, to resolve the problems of everyday living into a measure of inner peace. I know if I know how to do all this, I will know how to live and, if I know how to live, I will know how to die."

Let me give my final salute to this year's dental and dental hygiene graduates. Your university and your school are proud of you for your outstanding accomplishments. Go forth. Enjoy today, tomorrow and forever. ■

# HIV update: misinformation persists

*Originally published in JADA 1999 130: 1260-1261*

A few months ago, a retired 71-year-old dentist took his life. With a higher-than-average rate of suicide supposedly characteristic of the dental profession, such an event would hardly rate a mention on the national wire services. But this one did. It seems that just before ending his life, this dentist had been involved in a highly controversial dental screening of elementary school children.

News reports indicated that the dentist allegedly failed to change gloves and instruments between patients as he examined rural fourth graders. A parent, noticing this, alerted other parents who later hired lawyers and threatened to sue the dentist, the school system, the county health department and the state board of health.

These parents were concerned that such diseases as acquired immunodeficiency syndrome could be transmitted via saliva from one child to another, placing their children at risk of infection. These troubled parents called for the dentist to be tested for the human immunodeficiency virus. They also had their children tested.

The likelihood that any of these children were HIV-positive before the dental examination would be infinitely small. If they were infected, the chance that the virus would spread by exchange of saliva would have been even more remote. In fact, the federal Centers for Disease Control and Prevention has just stated, "In the absence of visible blood in the saliva, exposure to saliva from a person infected with HIV is not considered a risk for HIV transmission." Indeed, certain salivary proteins have been shown to have antiviral properties.

Nevertheless, the fear that their children could be infected with HIV drove these parents to excessive action. Did the public outcry and legal intimidation contribute to the dentist taking his life? If so, this is a tragedy that should not have happened.

HIV infection, once considered a death sentence,

> **Fear of an HIV infection is still pervasive in many sectors. That fear must be checked!**

has been rendered less threatening thanks to the successes of infection control and drug research. For example, since the onset of HIV almost two decades ago, there have been only two documented transmissions from infected health care workers, or HCWs, to patients. These include the infamous Acer group of six patients and a French surgeon who apparently infected one patient.

Minimal evidence of transmission from infected patients to HCWs is equally promising. According to data collected by the CDC through December 1998, only 54 HIV-positive HCWs in the United States could trace exposure to an HIV-infected source. What's more, none of these seroconversions was a dental HCW.

The risk of seroconversion in HCWs exposed to HIV-infected blood through the percutaneous route remains at 0.3 percent or less. The incidence of percutaneous injuries, as measured through the ADA Health Screening Program, dropped from an average of 11.4 incidents per year in 1987 to 2.2 in 1993.

The news is equally good for those who are infected. The development of a number of antiretroviral drugs has dramatically reduced morbidity and mortality. These drugs have been shown to stop HIV replication completely.

By controlling the replication of the virus through chemotherapy, HIV doesn't have the opportunity for "mutational escape" from the antiretroviral therapy. Thus, it is possible to control the virus for years, rather than six months, as was once the case. Data from the University of Colorado HIV investigation show a decline in mortality rates from 12 percent to 2 percent in the last three years.

Of major importance to dental practitioners and their office personnel, nosocomial transmissions can be reduced by 80 percent with a single drug. Multidrug regimens can achieve even greater reductions. But timing is critical. Dentists must have a plan in place if a nosocomial injury occurs. A needlestick late on a Friday with no plan of action could be disastrous.

Despite these positive statistics and developments, some still question the safety of treating an HIV-infected patient. A Maine dentist who was cited for failing to treat an HIV-positive woman has continued to insist that treating her in his private dental office would have posed a "direct threat" to his health and safety. That contention, which has been heard in a number of courts (including the U.S. Supreme Court), has been consistently rejected.

Still, it appears that this dentist is not alone in his concerns. In the April issue of the American Journal of Public Health,[1] researchers report findings from a survey of 6,000 Canadian dentists. One in six of the dentists responding said they would "refuse to treat any patient with HIV," claiming that doing so would place them at personal risk. (Both the Canadian and American Dental Associations hold that dentists should not deny care to any patient solely because of his or her HIV status.)

Concerns about treating HIV-infected patients appear to be driven by a lack of information or, more accurately, by misinformation. When asked, "What is the risk of contracting HIV infection from an HIV-contaminated needlestick injury?", only 12 percent of the Canadian dentists queried knew the correct answer was less than 1 percent. And more than 25 per-

cent believed the risk was greater than 50 percent.

In sharp contrast is the survey of U.S. dental personnel examined during the 1997 ADA Health Screening Program. Ninety-five percent of the dentists, 98 percent of hygienists and 98 percent of chairside assistants examined in the program said they believed current infection control practices are effective. These responses—not those reported in the Canadian study—are what would be expected from a well-informed group of professionals.

Regrettably, this type of positive information has been slow to reach the public and some dental practitioners. In gathering the background information for this editorial, it became apparent that fear of an HIV infection is still pervasive in many sectors. That fear must be checked!

Eradicating prevalent misconceptions about HIV will require the combined efforts of all the health professions, not dentistry alone. The challenge will be to develop and present convincing scientific data offered in a comprehensible fashion to health professionals and the public. Only with the widespread dissemination of this information will prevailing attitudes change.

Let this editorial be a start in that direction. ∎

1. McCarthy GM, Koval JJ, MacDonald JK. Factors associated with refusal to treat HIV-infected patients: the results of a national survey of dentists in Canada. Am J Public Health 1999; 89:541-5.

# Take aspirin and call 911

*Originally published in JADA 1999 130: 1411-1412*

**W**ere you the dental student who asked your basic-technique laboratory professor for evidence supporting the validity of G.V. Black's extension for prevention? Or perhaps the student who questioned the same purveyor of knowledge as to why an occlusal isthmus for a Class II amalgam must be one-third the faciolingual width of the occlusal surface?

Probably not—you graduated.

Besides ... scientific evidence—who needed it? A respected authority figure's words were all that was necessary to perpetuate a standardized outline form. For some, this doctrine has persisted long after evidence-based science indicated that the preservation of sound tooth structure is critical in maintaining the lifelong integrity of the tooth.

Other professorial "in-my-hands" philosophies of care have been challenged and set aside when scientific evidence indicated that they were no longer correct. Still, many treatment decisions continue to be based solely on the practitioner's clinical experience.

Is that the way it should be?

Yes, if the practitioner's judgment represents the "best evidence" for that treatment at a point in time. No, if the scientific evidence indicates there is a more desirable "best" treatment for that patient.

Consider this example from medicine.

Store-brand aspirin is probably prevention's biggest bargain. The American Heart Association says that aspirin, taken when signs of heart attack are present, has been shown conclusively to reduce mortality in a myocardial infarction, or MI, event by 25 percent vs. 7 percent for thrombolytic drugs—at 1/10,000th the cost.

Yet, even with this information, emergency-department physicians are not using aspirin to treat all patients who have experienced MI. According to a recent study,[1] only 45 percent of these patients received aspirin in the ED setting. Worse yet, those who were given aspirin often did not receive it within the recommended time for most effective action: within 30 minutes of the MI.

In the unlikely event that you experienced an MI, wouldn't you want your ED physician to be knowledgeable about the literature's evidence on aspirin?

Examples such as this give substance to the arguments of those who are advocating greater involvement of evidence-based medicine, or EBM, in physicians' treatment decisions.

In fact, EBM is the hottest buzzword in medical circles. While it is hardly a new concept, it is receiving a great deal of professional attention from the National Institutes of Health, the Agency for Health Care Policy and Research, medical schools and—you guessed it—third-party payers.

In essence, the process of EBM calls on the health care practitioner to continually confirm the validity of his or her service offerings with new scientific information.

To achieve medicine's goal of providing the best health care to the patient, EBM requires that new information be available to the practitioner in a timely, accurate and understandable form. Practitioner willingness to change to a "better" way of practice, if appropriate, completes the successful cycle.

Dentistry has not been immune to suggestions that it, too, use evidence-based dentistry, or EBD, as a basis for treatment decisions. The Reader's Digest exposé[2] pointed out dentistry's vulnerability: so many different treatment plans for the same case. Asked for specifics, proponents of EBD point to such treatment issues as the prophylactic removal of third molars and occlusal adjustment to treat bruxism as prime examples of present clinical treatments that would benefit from an evidence-based approach.

> **The chronic nature of dental disease often means that decades might pass before a prospective study can offer information on the merits of different treatments.**

However, the solution is simply not a matter of analyzing existing data. Additional research needs to be done on outcomes of clinical dental treatment. Compounding the problem, the chronic nature of dental disease often means that decades might pass before a prospective study can offer information on the merits of different treatments.

Furthermore, new dental products emerge daily and when they do they are hyped as "better" or the "best." How can the EBD concept be applied to reveal the truth?

Unfortunately, much of the information on dental products comes from those who have a financial interest in the promotion and sale of these products. Also, clinical research testing often is done by highly specialized clinicians, not grassroots dentists. EBD must strive to include more practice data collected by the dental practitioner.

EBD has its critics. A major and justifiable concern with the EBD concept is that its misuse could compromise practitioners' ability to deliver the best treatment for the patient. Treatment decisions based on EBD will not necessarily be the best option for every patient. The ability of practitioners to exercise their own judgment after considering the patient's needs and preferences must be an integral part of any EBD practice effort.

Another legitimate concern is that those with interests in containing costs could misuse treatment protocols that evolve from EBD. Denial of "necessary" treatment by benefit managers continues to be the major criticism of health plans by patients and health care practitioners. Under these circumstances, it isn't difficult to visualize payers selecting only EBD that supports the cheapest treatments.

Even apart from potential third-party interference, the everyday use of EBD in dental practices faces an uphill battle. While seeking new knowledge is part of the dentist's ethical responsibility, practitioners' reluctance to change the way they have always done things could be problematic.

If EBD is to become an integral part of dental practice, practitioners will need to interpret the scientific literature. Since many dentists lack the statistical skills and/or the available time to filter through the literature, they need assistance.

To facilitate this educational process, let me suggest that the dental profession focus on developing a centralized site capable of storing, translating and transferring scientific clinical information. I envision the creation of dentistry's own electronic search engine housed at the ADA. The ADA's divisions of Science, Dental Practice and Dental Informatics and the ADA library would be an ideal team to develop this initiative.

Using this mechanism, practitioners could quickly call up EBD information on any clinical subject—even while they are treating patients. An unobtrusive computer screen located in the operatory would be the only additional cost to the dentist implementing an EBD practice.

To create and maintain this high-quality EBD system will necessitate a major buy-in from the practicing dental community. Development and maintenance of a user-friendly EBD system will not be cheap. A back-room operation underwritten by a few passionate dental supporters will not do. The EBD concept needs your vocal support!

Information—timely, accurate, transferable and useful—will be the underpinning for success in the 21st century. Where will you be? ∎

1. Saketkhou BB, Conte FJ, Noris M, et al. Emergency department use of aspirin in patients with possible acute myocardial infarction. Ann Intern Med 1997;127(2):126-9.
2. Ecenbarger W. How honest are dentists? Readers Digest, February 1997: 50-6.

# 'I think I can ... I thought I could ... I did'

*Originally published in JADA 1999 130: 1549-1550*

**Editor's note:** On Oct. 7, 1999, the U.S. House of Representatives passed an ADA-supported comprehensive managed care reform bill sponsored by Reps. Charlie Norwood (R-Ga.), a dentist, and John Dingell (D-Mich.). The bill contains all of the same provisions as last year's bill; there was no compromise. This represents a major victory for the profession and the public.

To acknowledge your Association's efforts in successfully promoting what promises to be a landmark decision in the delivery of health care, we are reprinting here an editorial published in April 1998.

"No battle was ever fought where one person won it, and this one wasn't either," Rep. Norwood told the ADA House of Delegates. "It would not have happened without you, and I am very grateful to you."

The battle is not over. As of press time, the House and Senate still had to reconcile different bills, and if that process is continuing as you read this, your assistance is needed.

**R**emember that classic childhood story of the Little Blue Engine that, against immeasurable odds, successfully chugged up and over a mountain to bring toys to deserving children? Of course. Who could ever forget "The Little Engine That Could"?

"I think I can," and then "I thought I could," the Little Blue Engine cried out, imparting an inspirational message for all ages: what initially appears to be impossible may, with superlative effort, be achieved.

Dentistry and the American public are witnessing a replay of the Little Blue Engine's ride to success. Following that story line, it appears that a few years ago a group of distraught townspeople gathered together to discuss how to stop the continued erosion of their relationships with their health care providers.

They were especially concerned that administrators of their health plans were denying or delaying needed care, often refusing to allow referrals and then claiming they were not accountable when deleterious outcomes resulted.

The concerned citizens debated what to do. "Our rights as patients are being violated, and we have no one to protect us," they said. "We need a spokesperson. We need action. We need legislation. But who will represent our interests? Who is willing to speak for us? Who can move us out of this quagmire?"

Turning to the biggest engine—the insurance companies—they asked, "Will you help us?"

"Why should I?" the insurance companies replied. "Helping you will adversely affect our bottom line." And the insurance companies chugged off.

The townspeople then turned to the next biggest engine—the largest association of American physicians—and asked for help.

"No!" it replied. "That agenda is way too complex to support, especially the antidiscrimination clause. Besides, I'm a very important engine indeed. I won't pull the likes of you." The physicians' group huffed and puffed, and it chugged off.

"Who can we turn to now?" cried the people. "We need help!"

Then they saw the American Dental Association engine coming down the track. "Could it help us?" they wondered. "No, it's not big enough to carry our message because it represents just over 4 percent of the $1 trillion U.S. health care expenditure."

But they asked anyway. And to their surprise, the ADA engine said, "I think I can." And so, led by one of their own, Rep. Charlie Norwood of Georgia, the ADA three years ago became one of the primary supporters of the Patient Access to Responsible Care Act (PARCA, HR1415).

Carefully constructed to address the concerns of a growing number of patients, PARCA proposes to

> **PARCA supporters want those making medical decisions to be held responsible for their actions— even if they are not physicians.**

re-establish the patients' right to choose health providers within a plan. It also offers the option of joining a point-of-service plan outside the network. Additionally, patients would be assured of prompt care, access to care within reasonable distances from their home and emergency care without prior authorization from their health plan.

PARCA would ensure that patients would not be denied specialty care and would eliminate the use of gag rules prohibiting health care workers from providing patients with information on appropriate treatment options not covered by the plan.

Quality of care also would be emphasized under the proposed legislation. Through periodic assessments of the health plan's review and administrative operations, PARCA is designed to protect patients from health plans that place bottom-line profit ahead of quality and access to care.

The accountability components of PARCA call for sweeping changes over present-day practices that restrict many patients from pursuing legal action for negligence against health plans. This option currently is denied to 125 million workers enrolled in employer self-insured health plans.

This inability to hold employer self-insured plans liable for negligence springs from the Employer Retirement Income Security Act, or ERISA. Initially designed to protect employee pensions, it unfortunately contains language allowing self-insured health plans to bypass state accountability laws.

PARCA has attracted the support of 221 bipartisan members of the U.S. House of Representatives and scores of national health organizations. Adding to PARCA's momentum has been the highly visible letter-writing campaign and personal visits with legislators by ADA grassroots members.

This support has not gone unnoticed by the bill's opponents. Powerful politicians in the House of Representatives have begun a vocal bombardment against the bill. Insurers and employers also are lining up to defeat the bill, claiming that its provisions could drive up the cost of insurance by 23 percent to 39 percent.

The naysayers argue that if this bill became law, it would cause "thousands" of employers to stop offering insurance. They also maintain that the higher cost of premiums will force millions of lower-income workers to drop their insurance.

PARCA supporters say these cost estimates are exaggerated. They point to a recent study by a national actuarial firm estimating premium increases only in the 0.7-to-2.6 percent range. They also cite the recent experience with PARCA-like legislation in Texas where premiums climbed just 1 percent—nowhere near the 28 percent increase forecasted by those against patient protection.

What may derail PARCA is not the threat of increased premiums but its liability provisions. The insurance companies are obviously concerned because PARCA will hold them liable. Employers also are fearful, even though Rep. Norwood has added a provision that would protect them from malpractice suits.

The battle lines have been drawn. PARCA supporters want those making medical decisions to be held responsible for their actions—even if they are not physicians. Opposing them are the heavily financed insurance and business lobbies, who are stepping up their efforts to defeat PARCA.

It's conceivable that PARCA might not survive in its present form—only time will tell. But even if it doesn't, it has placed the issue of patients' rights on the nation's front burner. Eventually some form of legislation will pass—that's a given. Additional legislative actions will follow and will continue until patient rights are fully acknowledged and protected.

The American Dental Association—its Washington office and its grassroots supporters—should take pride in bringing this issue to national prominence. Others, far better positioned, were unwilling to do so. The ADA's efforts truly represent the wisdom professed in "The Little Engine That Could."

"I think I can ... I thought I could." ■

# Great expectations

*Originally published in JADA 1999 130: 1690-1691*

With the year 2000—the dreaded Y2K—only days away, those anticipating cataclysmic outcomes have already purchased generators, stocked food and planned to have plenty of cash on hand. They're ready! The rest of us are still wondering what, if any, inconveniences will accompany the transition to Y2K.

Lost in all this hoopla are the prognostications that futurists normally offer at such a historical juncture. Similarly ignored have been references to the accomplishments of the last century.

This is truly unfortunate for the dental profession. Looking back at dentistry's last century, I can't help but be impressed at the exciting developments that have taken place, and I look forward to even greater achievements in the future.

What might they be?

It's often stated that you can't predict the future without exploring the past. I agree. For the moment, let's push aside any Y2K concerns and examine our profession—where it's been and where it might go in the new millennium.

The year is 1900. Dr. G.V. Black is elected president of the National Dental Association (forerunner of the American Dental Association). At this time, professional concerns focus on the poor quality of dental students, what constitutes an appropriate dental curriculum, and the entrepreneurial nature of dental education.

Addressing the quality-of-student issue, the National Association of Dental Faculties has just increased the entrance requirements for prospective dental students to three years of high-school education.

For-profit dental schools in 1900 are proving to be a major barrier to improving the quality of dental education. Because of what are viewed as commercial opportunities, 57 dental schools are in operation, up from 43 in 1880. (It isn't until 1929 that the last for-profit dental school ceases operation.)

Expectations for an outstanding future for the dental profession are high in 1900. This excerpt from an editorial of that year, titled "Another Century" and written by A.W. Diack, D.D.S.,[1] reflects that optimism.

*"In scientific progress the coming century certainly appears at its birth to be fraught with great possibilities. When we cast a backward glance over the last half century and realize what has been done in the scientific development of dentistry; when one sees the substitution of rational ideas for the baldest empiricism; when it is seen that we are nearly on the threshold of practical application of newly discovered natural laws, it is no wonder that the future seems so bright with promises of untold advancement."*

I'm sure that Dr. Diack, even in his most enthusiastic projections, could not have perceived that in the ensuing century, U.S. dentistry would evolve into the world's premier exemplar of the dental health profession.

Think about just a few of these advances:

- the introduction of procaine hydrochloride in 1905, making painless dentistry possible for all;
- the development of the turbine in dental handpieces, a discovery that revolutionizes dentistry for both patient and dentist;
- the development of antibiotics in the mid-1940s, which gives the dentist the ability to control and prevent infection;
- the discovery and promotion of fluoridation, one of the major contributions to health worldwide;
- the development of resins as a dental restorative material;
- a 700 percent increase in the number of dentists along with major changes in the profession's ethnic and sex composition;

> **Dental futurists examining the past can only be in awe of the unprecedented number of discoveries that characterized the 20th century. What would they say about dentistry's future?**

■ revolutionary changes in the dental school curriculum brought about by the Gies report of 1926,[2] calling for a closer integration of the basic sciences into clinical practice;

■ the development of the computer and its related products, with an impact on dental practice that no one could have imagined.

Dental futurists examining the past can only be in awe of the unprecedented number of discoveries that characterized the 20th century. What would they say about dentistry's future?

Aside from the unpredictable, said to account for 90 percent of future progress in dentistry, three areas stand out. The first is self-evident: computers and their byproducts will continue to change how dentistry is practiced.

Second are biological innovations. With genetic engineering of enamel and dentin an accomplished fact, their use in dental tissue rehabilitation will completely transform the practice of restorative dentistry.

Third, information and how to use it effectively will greatly affect professional success throughout the 21st century. Unfortunately, with new knowledge pouring out daily from a variety of sources, dentists have neither the time nor the training to evaluate its utility. The solution? Dental "filters" will be needed to collect, analyze and report, in a user-friendly mode, the most current knowledge on specific products and treatments.

A few high-quality filters already exist. JADA's peer-review system ensures vigorous oversight of its published materials. The ADA's Seal of Acceptance program, which has been evaluating products for decades, serves both practitioners and the public. Additionally, a number of dental organizations publish quality journals and newsletters that assist practitioners in making treatment decisions.

Aside from the product and treatment filters, there is a growing need for a filter that will assist practitioners in evaluating technological advances. With the explosion of technology, the average dentist has difficulty making costly purchase decisions without the opportunity for hands-on evaluation.

In a past editorial, I suggested the development of regional dental technology demonstration centers where dentists could receive— prior to purchase—an indepth experience with new technologies. Fortunately, a prototype to address this need will be developed at the University of Minnesota School of Dentistry. Generous financial support for this technology center will come from an educational grant donated by a dental industry leader. Others need to follow!

With a new millennium approaching, dentistry is positioned between what was and what will be. We can anticipate a future that will be even better than the past. I am confident that, with a past so superb, the profession of dentistry and the public it serves will witness a 21st century of even greater progress.

Happy New Year. ■

1. Diack AW. Another century (editorial). Dent Reg 1900;417-29.
2. Gies W. Dental education in the United States and Canada (bulletin 19). New York: Carnegie Foundation for the Advancement of Teaching; 1926.

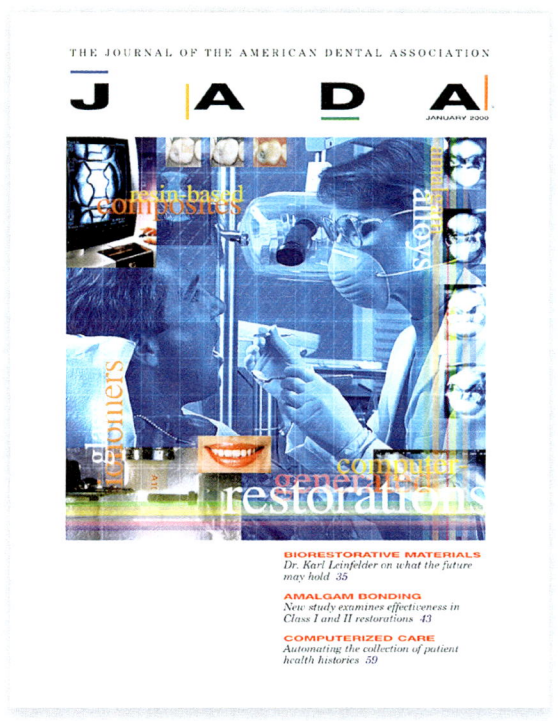

# 2000

"If strength can be measured by numbers,
then today the ADA is strong. Will it remain so?
Not without creative thinking and risk taking."

# Thinking outside the box

*Originally published in JADA 2000 131: 12-14.*

With membership at just over 71 percent of eligible dentists, the ADA has earned distinction as the gold standard for national professional organizations. Neither the American Medical Association nor the American Bar Association, with membership numbers hovering around 40 percent, can compete.

This strength in numbers has served the Association well. However, a slow but continuous erosion in the percentage of those qualified to join the organization but not doing so may signal trouble ahead. Between 1993 and 1998, the ADA's market share decreased from 74.3 percent to 71.4 percent, with a 1.2 percent loss noted in 1998.

A continuation of this downward trend over the next decade could tarnish the ADA's image as the representative of the dental profession's interests. One hopes this will not occur, but an examination of present and future membership components should sound an alarm.

Consider: In 1993, ADA market share of those who classified themselves as nonminority was 75.5 percent. By 1998, that percentage had dropped to 73.4 percent. The ADA's minority market share declined even further, dropping from 61.7 percent of those eligible in 1993 to 57.6 percent last year.

The 1998 market shares for those reporting themselves as minorities were 41.8 percent for African-Americans, 57.3 percent for Hispanics and 65.4 percent for Asians and Pacific Islanders. Sex differences were also noted. Less than 65 percent of women eligible for membership belonged to the ADA.

These market-share percentages take on added significance when the following facts are noted:
- Of the 20,000 minority dentists presently in active practice, approximately 50 percent graduated from dental school less than 10 years ago.
- Of this year's dental freshmen, 24 percent are Asian or Pacific Islander.
- Future sex ratios will be profoundly altered as the cohort of recent dental graduates, of whom 40 percent are women, moves through the membership ranks.

Minorities and women are critical to the future of the profession, but many have not responded to current membership incentives. Not that the ADA hasn't tried. Our membership division puts forth extraordinary efforts to capture both the emerging and the older non-member. Its creativity appears to have no limits, yet market share still falls.

Perhaps what ADA membership offers is insufficient to affect commitment. Today's dentists want to know what the organization does for them; otherwise, the feeling runs, why join?

Credit cards, insurance, home mortgages and loan consolidations can be attractive membership inducements.

It is right and appropriate for the Association to offer such services, but they alone will not attract and hold new members.

The ADA should emphasize highly relevant, practice-directed benefits with broad appeal to all dental practitioners regardless of age, sex or racial background.

A review of the ADA's programming indicates there are at least two activities that presently fit these descriptions: continuing education and political advocacy. Both need only to be enhanced to increase their present effectiveness. To this grouping, I would add a creative program of information transfer plus the creation of a new structure within the ADA that will allow for enhanced recognition of special interest groups.

Continuing education is an ADA benefit that could affect ADA members at all stages of their careers. It could become the hook that attracts and

> With membership at just over 71 percent of eligible dentists, the ADA has earned distinction as the gold standard for national professional organizations.

maintains members for life.

It's not that the ADA isn't already active in this field. Outstanding clinicians pack them in at the national meeting. With assistance from Sullivan-Schein Dental and 3M Dental Products, more than 50 half- and full-day seminars are available to individual dentists and dental organizations. The JADA continuing education program counted more than 18,000 dentist enrollments last year.

Today's dentists want to know what the organization does for them; otherwise, the feeling runs, why join?

The suggestion here is to think beyond the traditional. Expand! Expand! Expand! Make an ADA membership synonymous with continuing education. Say the words "continuing education"—think ADA. Lectures, hands-on instruction, fellowships, masterships, distance learning—even, perhaps, a virtual university that grants continuing education degrees—are potential components of an ADA education program.

An initiative of this magnitude challenges the resources of the ADA. But I believe that by partnering with education, industry and the ADA's component and constituent societies, the Association could accomplish such a venture.

The ADA's Washington advocacy program tops the list as a membership benefit that addresses the interests of all ADA members. Consider: What member would deny that practice life is so much better now that dentists do not have to fear an unannounced visit by an Occupational Safety and Health Administration inspector? What young practitioner isn't enjoying the enhanced student loan interest deduction?

The ADA's advocacy continues. Through its efforts, there are no ergonomic restrictions for dental offices; patients' rights, including the patient's right to choose his or her dentist, are being championed; and dentists can play music in the office without being taxed. Can this benefit be enhanced?

Not by increasing the activity; it already operates at a high level. Perhaps the ADA's accomplishments in advocacy could be more broadly communicated, perhaps through newsworthy inclusions in the nonmember issues of ADA News. These are accomplishments worth mentioning more than once.

In a previous editorial, I suggested that the ADA serve as the search engine for members seeking up-to-date information on products and clinical treatment. This concept has unbelievable potential as a membership benefit. Imagine tens of thousands of ADA members hooked up electronically and communicating daily with the ADA's Division of Science and with each other. Now, that's a membership benefit!

Finally, addressing the oft-stated concerns that the ADA is not appropriately addressing the needs of its minority and female members requires a new initiative tailored to recognize ethnic, sex-related and cultural issues.

Dentists who fall into these categories need to have the opportunity to develop special interest groups within the ADA structure. This does not mean abandoning their present external organizations. On the contrary, they could bring the thoughts of these external organizations directly to the ADA through the special interest mechanism—thus ensuring that their voices would be heard at the highest organizational levels. This is not a radical proposal. Such organizations as the American Association for Dental Research and the American Association of Dental Schools have successfully acknowledged the special interests of their constituents, giving them both position and voice.

If strength can be measured by numbers, then today the ADA is strong. Will it remain so? Not without creative thinking and risk taking. The current catch phrase, "thinking outside the box," takes on real meaning when applied to the critical issue of how to build the ADA's future membership base. ∎

# Strictly personal

*Originally published in JADA 2000 131: 140-141.*

I'm on record as an unwavering advocate for more efficient dental delivery, for technological change, for hardware solutions to many of dentistry's challenges. I've also championed the computer revolution in dentistry and the multiple benefits the profession stands to reap in its technological future.

But a growing feeling of uneasiness brought about by the seemingly unending number of electronic discoveries competes with my support of this technological future. I'm wary that as many of our daily tasks are replaced by electronic substitutes, the personal will become the impersonal, nonverbal communication will become extinct, and human touch will become low-level electronic buzz.

Take telephones, for example. I'd guess 60 percent of my phone calls are now answered by machines. I can buy a car, lock in a mortgage, order a prescription or transfer my bank balance from one account to another without ever speaking to another person. I now spend inordinate amounts of time punching the telephone buttons in response to a recorded menu. Make an entering mistake and you start all over again.

Consider computers. You can log on to one or more Internet e-commerce sites and buy an international airline ticket, seats at a New York City theater or the latest best-selling book without ever hearing a human voice. That unseen face somehow monitors my every entry, apparently building a constant record of my buying habits, personal banking and reading interests.

On a daily basis, computers, through their analyst programmers, control my options, channel my behavior, dictate my choices—nudging me further and further away from the people with whom I used to interact personally.

Sometimes you reach the point where you just want to type in "E-NOUGH."

This depersonalization is at dentistry's doorstep. October's ADA Technology Day speakers inspired their listeners to conjure up a dental office of the future. Envisioned was a beautifully appointed office with no receptionist. Instead, a computer unit registers patients via "card swipe."

Electronically stored voices inform patients of their projected waiting time. Patients are entertained with customized dental health education programming tailored to their individual health profile. Behind the terminal is an incredibly fast, efficient system managing all medical, dental and financial information—including treatment planning.

Dentists draped in gowns, hidden behind masks, glasses and gloves, dictate clinical observations into a voice-recognition system and document their observations with minute video cameras. Those same cameras verify patient consent and document clinical procedures to ensure against potential malpractice suits. One more swipe of a credit or debit card and patients can be on their way.

Efficient? You bet. Personal? Hardly.

The dental profession can hardly tolerate further depersonalization of the office visit. For almost a decade, dentists have been required to cover themselves with gowns, gloves, masks and eyeshields in response to stringent federal infection control regulations.

While this attire may assure patients that their visit will be a safe one, it essentially destroys the dentist's ability to communicate in a nonverbal manner. Patients no longer are able to perceive the dentist's facial mannerisms. Hidden behind the mask and eyewear are smiles that once exuded warmth, caring, interest and even safety.

Modern dental practice always has relied on a

> **As many of our daily tasks are replaced by electronic substitutes, the personal will become the impersonal, nonverbal communication will become extinct, and human touch will become low-level electronic buzz.**

strong personal relationship between practitioner and patient. Disrupting that relationship can result in less satisfying experiences for dentists and patients. Avoiding further technological changes that might adversely affect the personal relationship between dentist and patient should rank high on each dentist's list of priorities. Rather, dental offices need to accentuate strategies that enhance the human touch.

For a start, just consider having a live voice answer the office phone during all of the office hours. There is nothing more disconcerting than trying to share a dental problem with an answering machine that plays, "We are busy right now, but if you leave your name and number we will get back to you as soon as we can," or "Our office hours are from 8 to 12 and 1:30 to 5. Please leave a voice message, and we will get back to you."

Those messages may be OK for a library or an auto-repair shop but not for a medical or dental office. Can you imagine calling a hospital emergency room phone that says "We are busy at the present time; please leave a voice message at the beep."

For all practical purposes, dental practices are miniambulatory outpatient dental hospitals. Voice recordings just aren't acceptable during office hours.

A relatively inexpensive way to put the personal touch back into the office is to get rid of your voice-messaging system during lunch and breaks. Purchase a cellular phone for staff use. Assign a different staff member to phone duty each day. During the times the office was previously closed for lunch or whatever, a staff member would be available to answer the phone and respond to patient needs. She or he need not be in the office to carry out this task. Simple and inexpensive! Plus, no more of the "press 1" stuff if you wish to leave a message.

The personal touch. It's critical. Keep it! Restore it! Find new ways to offer it! ∎

# Ready or not

*Originally published in JADA 2000 131: 284-285.*

"My worst day in the office is better than my best day on the golf course."

—One dentist's twist on a familiar golfing expression, offered as his response to a JADA Question of the Month

**M**ore than 30,000 dentists are inventoried as "professionally inactive," the bureaucratic term for retired. That amounts to 16 percent of all registered dentists—a percentage expected to dramatically increase over the next 15 years as baby-boomer dentists leave their dental practices.

In 1995, 23.4 percent of professionally active dentists were 55 years of age or older. That percentage is projected to reach 33 percent by 2005 and 40 percent by 2010. Except for the occasional stalwart who vows to "work till I drop," dentists generally assign a high priority to the financial and psychological issues surrounding their eventual retirement from dental practice. For many, as the statistics indicate, that departure date isn't far away.

Having a comfortable retirement is a high priority for the majority of Americans, and dentists are no exception. How well these dentists have planned for retirement will determine their future options. As small business entrepreneurs, they must initiate most of their retirement programs themselves.

How are they doing?

Last April, JADA's Question of the Month asked, "In your view, are you adequately prepared for retirement?" Forty-six percent of responding dentists checked "No." Another 10 percent answered "I don't know" to the same question. While surveys of this type hardly can be construed as representative of all dentists, the preponderance of "No" and "I don't know" responses can't be ignored.

> For many dentists who have made dentistry the total focus of their lives, the prospect of closing the office door for the last time fills them with trepidation, even if they're financially secure.

Comments from respondents with 20 to 30 years in practice give some indication of their frustrations. "Not even close," wrote one dentist. Another who said he was not ready asked, "But who is?" A number of young dentists practicing less than 10 years echoed one another by pointing to high student debt as a barrier to initiating a retirement savings plan.

How much is enough? The inability to accurately define what would leave a dentist comfortable in retirement makes them fearful that quiting practice prematurely may result in outliving their financial resources.

Financial advisers agree that 70 percent to 80 percent of present adjusted gross income should be sufficient to maintain an "excellent" retirement life style. Assuming that percentage is correct, the average dentist may have difficulty meeting that mark. According to a 1995 ADA Survey Center report, exclusive of any proceeds anticipated from the sale of a practice or from Social Security, the average total amount of savings in all retirement plans for those aged 55 to 65 years of age was $563,433.

Depending on whether these savings are invested in high- or low-risk investments and what amount, if any, the dentists wish to preserve over a specific period will greatly affect their yearly retirement payoff.

For example, dentists who wish to preserve their entire capital over a 20-year period by investing it in a 10-percent yielding portfolio would receive an annual return of $56,000. Add to these dollars about $13,000 from Social Security and the total falls far short of the $110,000 estimate needed to reach the suggested 80 percent of total present income.

While most dentists have additional assets, such as their homes, these become liquid only when sold.

What about the sale of the dentist's practice? For years, many dentists considered those proceeds an integral part of their retirement assets. Apparently that's not so any more. Just 9 percent of dentists indicated they were depending "heavily" or "exclusively" on the sale of their practices to finance their retirements. Thirty percent said they were "moderately" reliant on practice sale, while 41 percent said, "just a little."

A "little" may be all many dentists will receive for their practices.

An experienced broker of dental practices estimates that applying an average sale factor of 60 percent to a practice with $500,000 in annual collections would yield $300,000 from a successful sale. Subtracting the necessary income taxes and the 10 percent sale commission, the practitioner receives about $190,000.

That $190,000 is only available if you can sell your practice. Demographic projections for 1999 through 2020 show that retirees will outnumber graduates by the year 2008. The gap will widen steadily after that. These projections are based on maintaining the present number of graduating dentists at 4,200 per year.

That number may be too high. Even with the present economic boom, the number of dental schools has declined by 4 percent and 7 percent, respectively, for the past two years. Based on the number of people who have taken the Dental Aptitude Test, educators expect the drop in applicants to continue for the year 2000.

This translates into negative pressure to increase dental class size. The result? Fewer candidates available to purchase dental practices. Under these circumstances, the value of dental practices will decline.

If, in the future, you are unable to sell your practice at the right price—or sell at all—you might consider donating it to your dental school. If the tax ramifications of a recent proposal on this issue prove favorable, they may provide at least a few dentists practicing in underserved areas with an unusual opportunity.

For many dentists who have made dentistry the total focus of their lives, the prospect of closing the office door for the last time fills them with trepidation, even if they're financially secure. Imagine the retirement anxiety of those dentists whose finances are insufficient. Some dentists may even be pushed to practice long after their physical abilities have been compromised.

The nation is presently enjoying an unprecedented economic boom. Most dentists have shared in the good times. However, instead of following the national pattern of increased consumer spending and reduced savings, this is the time for dentists to funnel more of their assets into retirement investments—building an infrastructure that will ensure a secure and desirable retirement. ■

# Those who can, do

*Originally published in JADA 2000 131: 428-42.*

The derogatory "Those who can, do; those who can't, teach" sends the blood pressure of committed educators soaring, and dental faculty are no exception. In dentistry, this disparaging comment is aimed at the supposed lack of clinical deftness of those selecting a dental educator's role. The inference: educators couldn't "make it" in private dental practice.

For dentists who hold this view and have concerns that the future of dental education lies in the hands of the clinically inept, worry no longer. Now it appears that everybody "can." Few dentists, it seems, are opting for an academic career. In fact, the number of dentists selecting academic pathways has fallen to crisis levels, with projections for even greater disparities if something isn't done.

While this appears to be a problem solely for dental education, closer examination indicates a broader issue with major ramifications for present and future dental practitioners.

Dentists seeking quality dental education programs for their children, attempting to hire qualified dental associates, or wishing to sell their practices will find it difficult to meet their needs. Left unsolved, a reduction in the quality of dental education with a corresponding negative impact on dental practice and its public can be expected.

Let's examine the evidence of this faculty "crisis."

Between 1992 and 1997, full-time academic vacancies in the clinical dental sciences increased 75 percent, from 139 to 244. This latter number expands to 300 full-time opportunities when the basic science and allied health programs are counted.

Intensifying the present shortage will be the rising number of retirements of an aging dental faculty. Today, 47 percent of all dental faculty members are 50 years of age or older, with 20 percent more than 61 years old.1 With this "graying"

> **The number of dentists selecting academic pathways has fallen to crisis levels, with projections for even greater disparities if something isn't done.**

of the dental faculty, a worst-case scenario would be that more than half of present faculty members will retire within the next decade. With no plan to replace this huge contingent, "faculty crisis" is an appropriate term.

With all these faculty vacancies, it might be expected that young dentists would welcome the opportunities available to them as future academics.

Not so!

While survey responses do not necessarily reflect eventual behavior, in 1995 only 1.1 percent of dental school graduates said they would pursue an academic career. Three years later, just 0.5 percent indicated a similar interest.2 With 4,000 graduates a year, that means only 20 will enter the education pipeline—not the 200 needed each year for faculty replacement.

The opportunities and benefits of an academic career should have greater appeal. Far more than 20 recent grads should be interested in sharing knowledge, influencing students, savoring the joys of satisfying their intellectual curiosity through research, having the opportunity to travel, and meeting and collaborating with colleagues throughout the world.

How many private dental practitioners can receive a six-month sabbatical to seek new knowledge every seven years—at full salary?

Yet, as a recent dental graduate comments, "Perhaps the stark contrast of the high-financial rewards, independence and power to control one's practice makes the private practice too fundamentally appealing to the majority of dental students, when compared to their perception of life at the university."

There is little question that the economic issue is central to the young dentists' decision making. Recent dental graduates leave school with upwards of $100,000 in debt. While debt often can be deferred until the completion of advanced training—a necessity for most academic careers—entry-level academic salaries don't appear sufficient to justify the further time commitment.

For example, consider a young dentist who has completed a one-year general practice residency and a three-year specialty program. He or she would be hired at the assistant professor rank with an average salary, after two or three years in that rank, of $65,000 in a public school and $59,000 in a private school. Compare that with the $187,000 average net income for a specialist who graduated from dental school less than 10 years ago. Disparities in earning power of this magnitude do not go unnoticed.

The American Association of Dental Schools, or AADS, recently released a report of the President's Task Force on Future Dental School Faculty.[1] A number of its recommendations are worthy of comment. Recommendation Two, for example, to "promote debt forgiveness and other means of funding those who pursue education and research careers," is a must if there is any chance of minimizing the negative impact of student debt on choosing an academic career.

Recommendation Five, to "establish methods for developing, nurturing and retaining faculty," addresses the concept of recruiting private practitioners into academia. Here lies one of dental education's biggest opportunities to address the faculty crisis. I personally know a number of dentists who, after satisfying private-practice careers, have made successful transitions to academia.

The AADS report also calls for the ongoing collection of data to "clarify the magnitude and reasons for faculty shortages." While doing so, it would be worthwhile for them to examine how increasing the amount of community-based education can bring in new faculty, while decreasing the dependence on full-time faculty.

How about the impact of simulation as an educational tool? Will it decrease the need for preclinical faculty? Also, in this era of electronics, must every dental school "own" and "pay" for a full complement of, for example, oral pathologists? Could they not share?

While not replacing managed care, OSHA, waterlines and other hot topics, the dental faculty crisis is starting to make its way to the forefront of crucial issues facing the dental profession. In addition to becoming knowledgeable and conversant on this subject, some of you also could become part of the solution.

Dental education needs seasoned practitioners to move into its full-time ranks. If you have the desire, energy and perhaps the financial wherewithal, now is a good time to investigate an academic career.

Yes, let those who can, "do." But let "do" include teaching, as well as private practice. ∎

1. American Association of Dental Schools. Future of dental school faculty: Report of the President's Task Force, Aug. 13, 1999. Washington: American Association of Dental Schools; 1999.
2. American Association of Dental Schools. 1988 survey of dental school seniors. Washington: American Association of Dental Schools; 1988.

# The noble lie

*Originally published in JADA 2000 131: 556-557.*

**D**o you always tell the truth? What about the ghastly paperweight given to you by your office staff as a means of honoring you on Boss's Day? Overwhelmed by their thoughtfulness (you didn't even know there was such a thing as Boss's Day), how could you say anything but, "Thank you, what a beautiful gift."?

Fortunately, dentistry has not reached the point where its practitioners are pressured into gaming the system.

These little "white lies"—daily occurrences in everyday life—function not to deceive but rather to spare the feelings of a person loved or respected. They are distinguished from so-called "black lies"— untruths specifically designed to mislead, often for personal gain.

What about the situation in which a falsehood is told on behalf of another person without any personal benefit to the fabricator?

Can there be such a thing as a "noble lie"?

Yes, if you ask a significant number of physicians. Motivated by an altruism that derives its interpretive support from their medical ethic that places patient needs ahead of their own, many health professionals are filing less than truthful diagnostic claims to qualify their patients for the treatment they feel is best.

As evidence, consider the results of three recent studies of physician behaviors. In the first investigation, 169 board-certified internists were asked, through a series of hypothetical vignettes, whether they would sanction a colleague's deception of a third-party payer.[2]

Fifty-seven percent of physicians condoned subterfuge in the vignette that would result in a patient being approved for bypass surgery. Forced to change companies, the patient's new health con-

> "Doctors have to get over their old-fashioned idea that they are advocates for individual patients. Now [a physician's] job is to manage a population of patients, and that means finding what works for most of them, most of the time, at a price everyone can accept."

tractor would not pay for her preexisting condition even though the angiogram indicated severe three-vessel coronary occlusion. Only if the physician would lie and say her chest pains had increased in frequency would the surgery be granted.

What would you advise?

Percentages in favor of deception for the other vignettes ranged from 48 percent in a case authorizing a diagnosis sufficient to get intravenous pain medication for a terminal cancer patient to just 3 percent in a case involving cosmetic rhinoplasty.

Against that hypothetical framework are the results of a Kaiser-Family Foundation survey in which almost 90 percent of physicians reported having experienced some form of denial of coverage for their patients' health services.[3] For example, 79 percent claimed that during the last two years, a plan had disapproved coverage for a prescription drug they believed a patient needed.

These physicians believe that between one-third and two-thirds of these denials resulted in serious decline in a patient's health status. It's no wonder, then, that 26 percent of these physicians reported exaggerating a patient's condition, either often or sometimes, to get needed care. Another 22 percent admitted doing this on "rare" occasions.

Similar percentages were noted in a study of 400 physicians conducted by the American Medical Association's Institute for Ethics. In that survey, 39 percent of physicians said they sometimes, often or very often used deception to help patients obtain coverage for needed services.[4] Twenty-six percent reported exaggerating the severity of a patient's condition to avoid premature hospital discharge, 23 percent changed a billing diagnosis, and 9 percent reported symptoms patients did not have to secure additional coverage.

So much for good deeds! Physicians who act with their hearts instead of their minds—tampering with health policies they view as unreasonable—could be undermining future benefits for other patients as well as setting themselves up for potential medical board and litigation problems.

"Gaming," the name given to this practice of acting against a distribution system that the physician believes is unfair to his or her patients, has its own share of critics. They suggest that gaming could interfere with the future trust patients have for physicians. They ask: Would the physician who lies for the patient also be capable of lying to the patient?

Distributive justice—getting resources to those who have a right to them—is undermined by gaming, some health ethicists contend. By going against the health plan to get more service for their patient, the physician is either directly or indirectly taking future resources from other health plan patients.

Furthermore, this new health system requires the physician to recognize the contractual obligation the patient has with his or her plan. Because physicians no longer own the resources, as distributors they must follow the rules.

Not all physicians readily accept this "materialistic" philosophy. One wrote, in response to a Denver Post article, "Is the decision I make for this patient made independently of any financial impact that decision may have on me or any entity other than my patient? That question must be answered in the affirmative for truly ethical care."

The ADA's "Principles of Ethics and Code of Professional Conduct" could be interpreted as lending support to that position. It states: "The same ethical considerations apply whether the dentist engages in fee-for-service, managed care or some other practice arrangement. Dentists may choose to enter into contracts governing the provision of care to a group of patients; however, contract obligations do not excuse dentists from their ethical duty to put the patience's welfare first."

Depending how "welfare first" is interpreted, dentists could find themselves in the difficult position of acting against a distribution system that they believe is unfair. Fortunately, dentistry has not reached the point where its practitioners are pressured into gaming the system.

Credit the lack of penetration by health maintenance organizations into the dental marketplace for this enviable position. Dentistry's solo and small group practices continue to compete successfully with alternative dental delivery systems.

Surveys of dentists and patients demonstrate the high satisfaction levels with fee-for-service programs when compared with alternatives. Indeed, in the next few months, studies conducted by the ADA and the highly respected Rand Corp. will be published in JADA. You will be heartened by their conclusions.

It appears that for the immediate future any gaming dentists are involved in won't be with insurance claim forms. ∎

1. Hubler E. Ill at ease: physicians finding pain in bid to heal themselves. Denver Post Jan. 16, 2000; Business Section:L-01.
2. Freeman VG, Rathore SS, Weinfurt KP, Schulman KA, Sulmasy DP. Lying for patients: physician deception of third-party payers. Arch Intern Med 1999;159:2263–70.[Abstract/Free Full Text]
3. Kaiser Family Foundation. Survey of physicians and nurses. Available at: "http://www.kff.org/content/1999/1503". Accessed April 14, 2000.
4. Is it OK to lie to your patients? AMA News Sept. 6, 1999:1, 30.

# Blueprint for the future

*Originally published in JADA 2000 131: 714-715.*

"Look at the future, because it's where you'll spend the rest of your lives."
— ADA President Richard F. Mascola's charge to the ADA Future of Dentistry panels

A man was walking through a field when he came upon a fence on which three targets were nailed. All three had been shot with perfect bull's-eyes. He asked a young man standing nearby, "Who is the extraordinary marksman who never misses his mark?"

"I am," said the lad.

"How did you learn to shoot like that?"

"I shoot first," said the young man, "and then I draw the circle."

With the "predictive" hoopla surrounding entry into the new millennium, it was no surprise when ADA Immediate Past President Tim Rose's promotion of a "new" Future of Dentistry, or FOD, planning effort gained collegial support. His vision: look beyond the ordinary; anticipate, plan, then act. The ADA, he maintained, has the expertise and resources to construct dental blueprints that will lead to the coveted bull's-eyes. And no need to draw circles after the fact.

The ADA House of Delegates supported the FOD project by an overwhelming margin—but not before thoroughly airing concerns that the finished document not be allowed to sit on a shelf gathering dust. Their message to the ADA hierarchy: Do it. Do it well, but make sure the end product is relevant, understandable and useful to all of the profession's constituents.

Prophecies alone will not suffice. The final document must contain action plans, steps to achieve potentially favorable outcomes and (if the predicted trends are not considered in dentistry's best interest) action plans to alter the unfavorable direction.

> The major drawback of the 1983 Future of Dentistry report was not its content but that so few dentists actually used it. That won't happen with the forthcoming document.

To develop this plan, experts have been selected from all areas of dentistry. While some have been drawn from dentistry's affirmed leaders, a significant number of the FOD panelists represent the "new guard," chosen to offer fresh perspectives on the future dental environment. Led by Dr. Leslie Seldin, a full-time practicing general dentist, the majority of the oversight committee and panel members are actively involved in the clinical practice of dentistry.

The timetable for the FOD panelists is tight. A draft product of their initial efforts will be circulated to communities of interest late this year. It will be followed by public sessions to ensure communitywide participation. This will be an open process, no secrets, no surprises.

This present initiative is not without precedent. In 1983, the ADA published a Future of Dentistry document that, had the profession adhered to its projections and recommendations, could have been the basis for proactivity.

Consider a couple of the forecasts from the 1983 report:

■ Computer use was predicted to develop at an accelerated pace. It did. In 1984, only 11 percent of dentists had a computer in their primary dental practice. By 1994, 67 percent did. Today, the rate is probably close to 90 percent.

■ Changes in licensure requirements were given little chance for success. Actually, a great deal of movement has been noted since that time. Thirty-four states presently offer provisions for licensure by credentials, compared with just 16 in 1979. Yet, some would still agree with the 1983 panel's vision and say even that pace is far too slow.

■ In the area of dental research, the 1983 panel's prophecies were on target. The report predicted that "unless dentistry can secure more funding for research, the profession will have decreased ability to generate new knowledge." This is exactly what happened.

Many dental research grants with high scientific scores are not funded owing to lack of sufficient funds. This dearth of support dollars, coupled with a growing shortage of early- and midcareer dental researchers, does not bode well for dentistry's continued need for new knowledge.

The 1983 FOD panel also was correct in its prediction that dental education would have problems in its financial support structures. What's more, the panel successfully predicted that dental schools would reduce their class sizes in response to market forces.

The panelists who studied dental work-force trends 17 years ago may have been correct in predicting large-scale reductions in the numbers of dental graduates, but they missed the mark when they predicted that a shortage of auxiliaries was not expected throughout the rest of the century.

Had they heeded the thoughts of their panel on dental practice, which forecast that oral hygiene and prevention activities in the dental office would increase dramatically, perhaps there would have been more encouragement for the training of additional dental hygienists. In 1980, 5,184 dental hygiene graduates entered the marketplace. In 1997, even with population increases, only 5,023 dental hygiene graduates joined the work force, obviously not enough.

The major drawback of the 1983 FOD report was not its content but that so few dentists actually used it. I can assure you, that won't happen with this forthcoming document. Plans are already under way to ensure that the new report will reach each ADA member in a variety of user-friendly formats.

Getting insider information in today's fast-paced world often has proved to be the road to financial success. The FOD document will do just that for you. There are a number of recent documents focused on specific segments of dentistry—The Institute of Medicine's "Dental Education at the Crossroads" and the soon-to-be-released "Surgeon General's Report on the Oral Health of America." None addresses the specific future needs of practicing dentists. The FOD will. ∎

# A Cinderella story

*Originally published in JADA 2000 131: 844-845.*

The exceptional value of an ADA membership has been extolled in JADA's Views section many times. Whether it's low-interest, multipurpose credit cards, insurance programs, a strong Washington lobby, new e-commerce initiatives, electronic records, JADA and ADA News, or hundreds of other tangible benefits, today's ADA members have definitive proof that their membership dollars are at work.

To its credit, the ADA does not rest. It continues to pursue additional programs to satisfy the expanding needs of its constituents.

Why doesn't the ADA consider offering a program that would monitor the personal health status of dental professionals? In today's complex world of dental practice, a system providing continuous data on health risks associated with clinical dental care is essential. Results from this health monitoring could be used to develop policies and recommendations that would make dental offices safer for providers and patients.

No need!

The program already exists—and has existed for more than 36 years. Under the rubric of the ADA Health Foundation's Health Screening Program, or HSP, dentists and auxiliary personnel have been participating in a screening program at the ADA annual session since 1964. Data from that program have provided the dental profession with priceless information.

Unfortunately, this program has remained virtually unnoticed except by a small number of registrants who partake of its services during the yearly convention. Considering that the HSP is the vehicle that continues to provide the largest body of data on the health of the dental profession, this is a program that should be flying high on the ADA membership benefits flagpole.

Today's dental participants are offered expanded serum clinical chemistry with differential choles-terol analysis; hepatitis B and C screenings; anonymous HIV screening; urinary mercury analysis; head and neck examinations; electrocardiograms; skin-prick testing for immediate hypersensitivity to latex proteins; patch testing for delayed hypersensitivity to examination glove processing chemicals and other chemicals commonly found in the dental office; and, recently added, screening for carpal tunnel syndrome.

All at no charge to the participant.

Data from the HSP do not sit on a shelf. Besides the direct health status feedback offered to dental participants, the aggregation of their laboratory findings has provided excellent material for the development of a number of ADA policies.

> The ADA Health Foundation's Health Screening Program should be flying high on the ADA membership benefits flagpole.

One example is the area of mercury toxicity. A major reduction from 15 micrograms per liter in the HSP data of the 1980s to the present 4 µg/L vividly demonstrates the efficacy of ADA recommendations in reducing mercury vapor in the dental practice environment.

Needlestick injuries, with their potential for subsequent infections such as human immunodeficiency virus, were a cause for concern in the late 1980s. HSP data indicated that the average dentist reported 11.4 such injuries in 1987. Careful monitoring through the HSP indicates that ADA recommendations for reducing percutaneous injuries have been a success. By 1991, HSP participants were reporting just 3.4 such injuries per year.

Information yielded by the testing and recording of the seroprevalence of hepatitis B, hepatitis C and HIV in HSP participants assuaged the fears of dentists and patients regarding routine dental visits. Only one of the 19,000 dentists tested had a positive test for HIV.

Similarly, tracing antibody titers to HBV indicates that 85 percent of health screening participants have received the HBV vaccine—the highest rate of compliance among all the health professions. More good news from the HSP screening: HCV rates for general dentists were found to be comparable with those of the general population.

Allergies to latex are becoming a major concern for health professionals, and dentistry is no exception. HSP data gathered from tests of more than 2,000 dentists, dental hygienists and assistants indicate type I hypersensitivity rates in the 6 to 9 percent range—far less than earlier reports of up to 50 percent. These results are being used to devise recommendations for the use of latex products during dental treatment.

Remember a few years back, when the lay press was reporting that dental sealants and resin-based composites were able to mimic the effects of estrogen? What parent would agree to have sealants placed if that information proved true? HSP to the rescue. On testing, no HSP participant with either sealants or composites in his or her mouth showed the presence of bisphenol-A, the supposed guilty party.

On occasion, new products of potential benefit to the health of dentists have been tested at an HSP event. For at least one dentist, that policy may turn out to be a lifesaver. Through the use of a brush biopsy—a computer-based diagnostic system—at the 1999 HSP, at least two innocuous oral lesions that normally would not have been candidates for a surgical biopsy demonstrated aplastic changes. Subsequent surgical biopsy validated the earlier HSP findings.

It is difficult to fathom how the HSP manages to escape the limelight it so justly deserves. It has no competitor. It has no equal. The HSP has repeatedly demonstrated its ability to serve the profession and the public. Yet, it remains an unsung hero. Indeed, there have been times when curtailment of one or more of its programs has been considered because of lack of support.

Funding for the HSP comes mainly through contributions from the dental industry, channeled through the ADA Health Foundation. Association staff and local volunteers account for the remainder of the program's resources. Frankly, the HSP budget is mighty lean. Here lies a major funding opportunity for a constituent or component dental society—or even an individual wishing to make a visible contribution to dentistry.

It's time to give this Cinderella story the accolades it deserves. It has served the profession silently but well. ∎

# Simply not simple

*Originally published in JADA 2000 131: 1106-1107.*

A controversial state educational testing program has supplied the Colorado press with extraordinary editorial opportunities—and, through analogy, provided insight in evaluating the recommendations of the recently released "Oral Health in America: A Report of the Surgeon General."

Colorado legislators have proposed that teachers be rated according to their students' performances on standardized tests. One newspaper writer, arguing that these legislators were "misguided," used an interesting tongue-in-cheek analogy to make her point. She "reported" on a program that would gauge dentists' effectiveness by the caries levels in their young patients.

The number of cavities in each patient at different ages would be recorded, wrote the columnist. On the basis of these numbers, the dentists then would be rated on a scale from "excellent" to "unsatisfactory." Just as has been proposed in the case of Colorado teachers, these ratings would tell parents who the best dentists were. Furthermore, she wrote, it ostensibly would "encourage the less effective dentists to get better, and poor dentists who don't improve could lose their licenses."

The columnist went on to describe the response of a hypothetical dentist who had been subjected to this "let's improve the oral health of everybody" program.

"That's terrible," she "quoted" him as saying. "That's not a fair way to determine who is practicing good dentistry. So much depends on things we can't control.

"For example," the hypothetical dentist continued, "I work in a rural area with a high percentage of patients from deprived homes. Many of the parents I work with don't bring their children to see me until there is a problem. Also, many of the parents let their kids eat too much candy, and many of

my patients have well water, which is untreated and has no fluoride in it.

"My work is as good as anyone's," the dentist said in conclusion, "but my average cavity count is going to be higher than a lot of other dentists' because I choose to work where I am needed most."

The columnist's summation: "A performance evaluation that ignores the vastly different conditions under which people work is unfair and doomed to fail."

We in dentistry know well how true this is.

Difficulties in accessing dental care, especially for underprivileged children, have received nationwide attention with the recent publication of the surgeon general's report. While citing dramatic improvements in oral health during the past 50 years, the report pointed to a "silent epidemic" of oral disease that "burdens" some population groups.

> **Not all Americans, even those who have the resources to achieve optimum oral health, will avail themselves of the opportunity.**

These "profound" health disparities, the report continues, are to be found primarily among "those without the knowledge and resources to achieve good oral care." Specifically mentioned were poor Americans, especially children, the elderly, members of racial and ethnic groups, and those with disabilities and complex health conditions.

Disadvantaged children's oral health has dramatically improved. In the 1970s, children at or below the poverty line had 2.14 untreated carious permanent teeth. By the 1990s, that statistic had dropped dramatically to 0.46, a 78 percent reduction. Similar reductions were noted for primary teeth.

Nevertheless, challenges remain. In a recent issue of Pediatrics, a nationwide study of unmet health needs showed that 7.3 percent (4.7 million children) experienced at least one unmet need for health care annually. Those in need of dental care topped the list with 5.3 percent (3.4 million); the percentage with unmet medical needs was 1.6 percent.

The surgeon general's report calls for a national partnership that would provide "opportunities for individuals, communities and the health professions to work together to maintain and improve the nation's oral health."

It is encouraging that oral health is now receiving the attention warranted by its importance to overall health. But expectations should be tempered with reality. Not all Americans, even those who have the resources to achieve optimum oral health, will avail themselves of the opportunity. For some, it will take years of innovative programming before oral health becomes a major priority.

Still, there are many actions that can be taken to break down existing barriers to obtaining dental care—adequate payment to dentists, for example. In many states, Medicaid is underfunded, in some instances paying the provider less than overhead costs.

Compounding the payment issue are administrative constraints and snafus that frustrate even the most committed dentist. Eligibility verification, inordinate payment delays and complicated preauthorization requirements often find dentists treating without even bothering to submit a claim.

Increasing dentist reimbursement does appear to increase provider participation. One state appears to be aggressively attacking the reimbursement issue by enrolling its residents who are eligible for the Children's Health Insurance Program in private dental insurance programs that pay the dentist's usual-and-customary fee, with no patient copayment.

For those enrolled, utilization rates approximate those of patients with private dental insurance. But even with extensive recruitment initiatives, enrollment has lagged behind expectations.

Thus, even with insurance, some children have unmet oral health needs. This suggests that insurance alone is not sufficient to close the gap between higher-and-lower income children.

Income, education, ethnicity, immigration, acculturation, language, public transportation, location of the health facility, travel costs, child care, parent(s) taking time off work—these are just a few of the factors that affect access.

The same energies dedicated to achieving sufficient provider remuneration also need to be directed at removing barriers to access. Even assuming uniform access and utilization, it is still conceivable that differences in oral health status may continue. As evidence, consider recently published research that points to the relationship between lead ingestion and dental caries. This research offered evidence that significant amounts of dental caries could be attributed to moderate and high lead levels in children.

While one report is not sufficient to establish a cause-and-effect relationship, the strength of the lead-caries association may help explain the higher caries rate noted in certain populations.

The surgeon general's report on America's oral health paints a generally positive picture of our country's oral health status. While it points out the past success of American dentistry, it also encourages public-private partnerships to take oral health to the next level. This lofty goal will not be achieved in minutes, days or months. It will require vision, leadership energy, resources, persistence and commitment.

It's simply not simple—but ultimately worthwhile. ∎

# Dentistry's other secret

*Originally published in JADA 2000 131: 1234-1235.*

**M**ost dental water's so dirty, no wonder they tell you to spit," cried the Newsweek ad for the "20/20" exposé on dental office waterlines, which first aired Feb. 18. Promising to tell all about dentistry's "dirty secret," the actual program fell far short of its prebroadcast hype.

Hindering the TV muckraking was the fact that the ADA had been publicly seeking and promoting solutions to this problem for years. So much for the secret, which proved to be not so "dirty" and hardly "secret."

But dentistry does have an authentic secret of its own. Don't expect to see it on any TV exposé. It doesn't have the necessary emotional pull. But if ignored, it could cause irreparable harm to the dental profession and its members.

Few dentists have knowledge of this internal time bomb. Indeed, my own awareness of it came only after observing this year's commencement activities for the University of Colorado's 34 dental graduates.

The dental school dean had invited immediate relatives of the graduates who were dentists to participate in the hooding process. It was this ceremony that gave me the first inkling that dentistry had its own "family" secret. As each dental student came forward to receive his or her hood, I marveled at the large number of dental relatives. Fifteen fathers, two brothers, three husbands and one grandfather hooded their sons, daughters, grandsons or significant others. That's more than 60 percent of the class.

Remember not that long ago when dentists were saying, "I'd never want a child of mine to go into dentistry"?

What's changed?

For many dentists, it's the economics. After suffering for decades with negative or minimal real increases in their income, dentists are now seeing incomes that exceed those of many of their physician counterparts. Don't think dentists haven't passed that message on to their children or relatives.

The paradox is that, except for those connected to dental families, there has been a drop, rather than the expected increase, in applications for dental school.

According to the widely accepted economic formula of "rate of return"—which factors time, cost of education and lost income against anticipated future earnings—the recent increases in dentists' income should have translated into increased dental school applications. Not so! In fact, the opposite is occurring.

> **Remember not that long ago when dentists were saying, "I'd never want a child of mine to go into dentistry"? What's changed?**

The number of applications for dental school has dropped significantly in each of the last three years. There may be an even more precipitous drop in the next few years, as judged by the unexpected reduction in prospective dental students taking the dental aptitude test, or DAT. Consider these figures: five years ago, 11,314 took the DAT; last year, only 6,645 did so.

What's going on?

■ Demographers would say this is simply a birthrate issue. With fewer 18-year-olds presently available in the cohort of those who might select college and professional careers, dentistry's percentage drops accordingly.

■ Characteristically, dentistry has served as an upwardly mobile profession, offering those who enjoy working with their hands an opportunity to become health professionals. The present tight job market is drawing many of these prospective dental students into immediately high-paying work opportunities in the trades.

■ The economic return of other professions offers shorter time in school for immediate high returns. This is especially true for minority and under-served people whose families may not have had experience with paying long-term debt in hopes of eventual high returns.

■ There are insufficient scholarships and low-interest loans to lessen the cost of a dental education.

■ The health professions have experienced a drop in status. For the first time in decades, dentistry has fallen out of the top five in the annual "Honesty and Ethics in Professions" poll conducted by The Gallup Organization.[1]

■ There is no major recruitment effort promoting the dental profession as a desirable career path.

The good news is that even with these unexpected reductions in dental school and DAT applicants, the grade point averages of those entering dental school continue to increase, as do their DAT scores.

So for the present, we're doing OK with less. But what about the future?

The ADA's Dental Workforce Model: 1996-2020[2] predicts a modest increase—less than one-half percent—in the number of dentists. This is well below the projected growth rate for the U.S. population during the same period. Will the dental education system continue to find sufficient qualified applicants to meet the dental needs offered by the ADA projections? If not, practicing dentists can expect increased difficulties in hiring associates and even greater problems in finding buyers for their practices.

On a national level, those who believe that a dentist shortage already exists will use any weakness in the number and quality of new dental graduates as evidence that the government should provide incentives to increase the availability of dental services. That might include pressure to add duties to segments of the dental auxiliary work force, especially to those looking for nonsupervised practice opportunities.

We've seen the results of that strategy before.

Sharing dentistry's secret can prevent the problem. The biggest and best group of recruiters for dentistry is dentists themselves. It's time for them to get dentistry's "good-news" message out to their patients and friends.

Consider this: if only 10 percent of all ADA members were able to recruit just one person a year to become a candidate for dental school, the number of applicants would be almost triple the present number. That's just one prospective student every 10 years for each ADA member—surely not an insurmountable task.

It's time that dentistry's "other secret" remains a secret no longer. ■

1. The Gallup Organization. Honesty and ethics in professions. Princeton, N.J.: The Gallup Organization; 1999.

2. American Dental Association Survey Center. The American Dental Association dental workforce model: 1996-2020. Chicago: American Dental Association; 1999.

# The perfect patient

*Originally published in JADA 2000 131: 1395-1396.*

Although managed care continues to grab the headlines, licensure issues still account for the largest flow of unsolicited e-mail and letters to the editor. The profession's entry examination has consistently drawn the wrath of young graduates, who perceive the examination as unfair. Licensed dentists cite barriers to mobility as their objection to present dental licensure requirements. Nothing new. This issue doesn't even recycle. It just keeps on rolling.

Admittedly, some progress has been made. All licensing bodies accept Part I of the National Boards, and just maybe, with a big push, they soon may accept Part II. The problem that remains—the big barrier—is the clinical examination. Four independent regional boards and 12 separate licensing bodies all require their own examinations.

High expectations accompanied consolidation of two of the largest regional boards in 1994 when the Northeast Regional Board, or NERB, and the Central Regional Dental Testing Service, or CRDTS, came together in offering a common clinical examination. The two boards represent 23 states.

Unfortunately, the agreement between the two lasted only one year. Reasonableness has not prevailed, and the two agencies are showing little inclination to reconcile their differences.

While licensing is totally within the jurisdiction of the states, dentists continue to look to the ADA for some formal action. Not forthcoming, dentists lay the blame on the Association.

The lack of an acceptable solution to the licensure issue has generated side effects that go beyond inconvenience and cost. According to an article published in last year's Journal of Dental Education,[1] some dental board candidates are displaying behaviors unacceptable to the ethical standards of the profession.

A nationwide survey of general dentists who graduated between 1980 and 1994 pinpointed some unacceptable professional activities in connection with these dentists' clinical board experiences. For example, 24 percent failed to arrange for indicated follow-up care for their board patients. One-third took unneeded radiographs, 20 percent pointed out colleagues who allegedly provided premature treatment before the examination, and 8 percent claimed definite knowledge of colleagues who intentionally created a lesion for the board examination.

These results raise obvious questions about the ethics of using live patients for clinical board examinations. Forget the unneeded X-ray exposure or the lack of follow-up treatment. Ignore the creation of "new" carious lesions. Consider answering this larger question: Is it ethical to use human subjects for the purpose of discovering incompetence?

While examination failure rates don't seem to be exceeding 80 percent, as they did for some schools early in the 1990s, even a 25 percent failure rate on the examinations translates into more than a thousand dental board patients receiving substandard treatment.

A commentary in the March/April issue of Dental Abstracts substantiates the practitioner survey. Titled "Dental Licensing Revisited,"[2] a former dental board examiner confides that while he was "impressed with the dedication of individuals responsible for the design and administration of the exam," there was "significant" variability in the examiners, despite previous calibration exercises.

He also asserts that board examinations provoke a number of behaviors among the graduates being examined that are "less than professional and, at worst, unethical." Ascribing these behaviors to the need to pass at any price—many of these new graduates have already signed on with dentists as associates or have placed down payments on equipment, practices or both—the creation of the perfect board patient becomes an obsession that

> **Is it ethical to use human subjects for the purpose of discovering incompetence?**

promotes unacceptable ethical behavior.

This former dental examiner questions the validity of the licensing examination. He notes that he is unaware of any instance in which an entry-level candidate at his institution failed the regional examination three times. Where, he asks, did their new skills come from? Most, if not all, of these candidates are graduates who have no way to remediate their deficiencies.

His solution: A single uniform clinical test given several months before the student's graduation. This would allow for remediation if necessary. In a good/better/best rating, I'd rank his suggestion as "good." But it still doesn't address the use of live patients during the clinical examination.

There was a time when the lack of uniform educational standards created vast differences in the quality of dental graduates. Many dental schools operated on a for-profit basis. Safeguarding bottom lines was more important than turning out quality students. No wonder that state licensing agencies sought to protect the health and welfare of their citizens by testing the clinical abilities of these dental professionals.

Those days are long gone. For years, the ADA, working with the Commission on Dental Accreditation, has established standards that ensure the highest-quality dental training in the world.

I have previously suggested that we place more trust in the accreditation process. Let our faculties determine the competence of the potential graduates and follow the leadership of the Canadian dental schools, which link the accreditation process with the licensing authority. Both groups formally participate in the dental schools' on-site evalua-

tions. And no further examination is required for licensure.

Why not adopt the Canadian model? Involving the licensing bodies in the accreditation process makes sense. But for entry-level dentists judged clinically competent by their faculties, I would add an examination consisting of interactive simulations (National Dental Board Part III). This patient-free examination would eliminate past ethical problems and could offer solutions to the mobility issues of the already licensed.

To date, the licensure debate has focused on initial entry and mobility. No longer. The explosion in technology and the globalization of the world's economy already are expanding that horizon.

Consider the practice of tele-dentistry. Licensure issues have already surfaced in that area, with 20 states requiring health practitioners to have a full license if they participate in Internet practices. The global issue of dentists freely moving from country to country has surfaced in the discussions of the European Economic Community and the North American Free Trade Association.

It's time to resolve the issues surrounding licensure. While any solution depends on the states' agreeing on a common policy, that requirement should not be a rationale for inaction. The ADA's activity in this area should step up from "encouragement" to aggressive jawboning. There is just too much at stake to accept the present slow "progress" as the pathway to an eventual solution. ∎

1. Feil PF, Meeske J, Fortman J. Knowledge of ethical lapses and other experiences on clinical licensure examinations. J Dent Educ 1999;63:453–8.[Abstract]
2. Stoller NH. Dental licensing revisited. Dent Abstr 2000;45:52–5.

# Leveling the playing field

*Originally published in JADA 2000 131: 1531-1532.*

**D**entists involved in collective bargaining with insurers? Not today! But that could quickly change. Faced with perceived third-party intrusions into patient/dentist relationships, dentists are supporting actions that will help maintain the integrity of this critical practice component.

One such response has been the ADA's support of the Quality Health Care Coalition Act of 2000, also known as the Campbell bill (HR 1304). Embraced by the American Medical Association and representatives of other health professions, this bill sought to improve patient care through federal legislation that would give self-employed practitioners the right to negotiate collectively with insurers and other health plan administrators.

This endorsement did not signal a new policy direction for the ADA. Approval for the concept of collective bargaining rights for dentists can be traced to a 1994 ADA House of Delegates action that advocated for changes in federal antitrust laws.

The Campbell bill, which had strong bipartisan backing, gained overwhelming approval in the U.S. House of Representatives. However, lack of a companion bill in the U.S. Senate erased its opportunity to be adopted into law during the 2000 legislative session.

It is gone—but definitely not forgotten.

Advocates of the Campbell bill want to ensure that the concepts of collective bargaining expressed in past legislation will be resurrected in future law-making activities. They believe that even though practitioners may be self-employed, the insurance industry has such great power over their livelihood and professional decision-making process that they are de facto employees and should have negotiating rights.

The present antitrust laws say no! Indeed, dentists who inadvertently have become involved in collective bargaining attempts have paid a stiff legal and financial price.

Any new legislation will have its opponents. The insurers will continue to oppose any bill that would give practitioners the right to bargain. Two previous detractors of the Campbell bill, the Federal Trade Commission and the U.S. Department of Justice, suggest patient protection legislation as a preferable way to address the patient/provider concerns.

Within the dental profession, new and emerging information may slow or alter policies that favor collective bargaining.

Legally, collective actions that don't precisely follow the letter of the law could place practitioners in serious legal difficulty. Under I Campbell-type legislation, dentists considering participating in collective bargaining activities might, by necessity, incur significant administrative costs. Conceivably, some dentists may not be willing to pay these costs, thereby creating schisms that negatively alter professional relationships.

Dental economists also mention some potentially serious fiscal concerns regarding the impact of dental collective bargaining. For example, unlike medicine, in which catastrophic insurance is considered a must, acceptance or maintenance of dental insurance plans often is discretionary and exceedingly price-sensitive.

There is concern that increases in reimbursement fees achieved through collective bargaining might have adverse consequences on dental plans. Faced with increased costs, the insurer could pass the fee increases directly to the plan's sponsors, who might reduce benefits or even eliminate the

> **Advocates of the Campbell bill believe that even though practitioners may be self-employed, the insurance industry has such great power over their livelihood and professional decision-making process that they are de facto employees and should have negotiating rights.**

program.

The economists also point out that the environment for collective bargaining, with its organizational costs and unknown impact on payment plans, may be less necessary in dentistry than in medicine, which derives 85 percent of its payments from insurers. Dentistry, in which less than 50 percent of payment is derived from insurers, is less susceptible to the adverse impact of fee discounts.

Organized dentistry knows that the passage of collective bargaining legislation would open the door for unions to solicit the self-employed dentist. Their other benefits notwithstanding, dentists paying union dues might not continue their ADA membership. New dental graduates might not join. And any serious reduction in the number of ADA members could severely weaken the ADA's legislative, educational and scientific agendas.

Finally, there is a question as to how the public would regard unionized dentists who were depicted as "greedy" tradespeople by their third-party adversaries. Would just a few dentists' becoming unionized paint the entire profession with that brush? Would dentistry be viewed as a trade rather than a profession?

Last year, the AMA voted to endorse a medical union that could represent more than 100,000 employed physicians in their negotiations with health plans, hospitals and universities. Monitoring the professional impact of that action, the JADA Question of the Month asked readers to comment on whether they thought the AMA unionization action would detract from physicians' professionalism.[1]

We received an unprecedented large number of replies, equally divided between "yes" vs. "no" answers. Supporters of the AMA actions directed their comments to combating the power and money of the insurers. Phrases such as "it's time to fight back" were constantly noted. The underlying theme was that medicine's professionalism already had been compromised by insurance companies, so physicians had nothing to lose by unionizing.

Those who felt that unionization would compromise professionalism thought the AMA action was "stupid"—that unionized "rich doctors" would appear as a bunch of self-serving, money-hungry professionals.

If a bill similar to the Campbell bill is introduced in the next Congress, the AMA surely will support it. Collective bargaining is a critical companion piece to the AMA's previous union action.

Organized dentistry's future position is not as clear. With the need for collective bargaining not nearly as established as it is in medicine, some are saying, "Let's reevaluate before we go forward." Others contend that strong patient protection legislation could solve some of the pressing dentist/patient concerns, thus negating the need to seek collective bargaining rights.

The "let's-go-for-it-all" group wants both patients' rights legislation and collective bargaining. They point out that even though the Campbell bill did not emerge from this Congress, it has served notice to the insurance companies that members of the health professions value their patient/provider relationships and will use appropriate legislation to preserve and defend them.

Legislation to provide self-employed health professionals with the right to participate in collective bargaining presently sits on the congressional back burner—but not for long. Ultimately, dentistry will have to decide how it will proceed.

Only a knowledgeable and vocal ADA membership can ensure that its leaders make the correct decision. ■

1. Lund A. E. Question of the month: do you think that physicians' being unionized detracts from their professionalism? JADA 1999; 130:1573.

# Spreading the word, or the three R's

*Originally published in JADA 2000 131: 1666-1667.*

When is good news not necessarily good news? When it doesn't get published. Until last month, Denver's two independent newspapers were locked in a pitched battle for circulation supremacy. During that period, The University of Colorado's Health Science Center, attempting to improve its community image, approached the competing newspapers asking what they could do to receive some favorable press.

"Little" was the response. Good news doesn't sell newspapers. Now, a misappropriation of Medicare funds or a botched medical procedure—that's acceptable reading material, but don't try to get space for anything less.

Too much "good" news—could this be the problem that haunts professional acceptance of the "Oral Health in America: A Report of the Surgeon General"?

Released to its various publics in May 2000, "Oral Health in America" was the first surgeon general's report to be specifically focused on oral health.

JADA's special report on "Oral Health in America" (page 1721) is an executive summary tailored to the interests of the practicing dentist. The full document, representing a three-year effort by hundreds of consulting experts, was released with great fanfare by the surgeon general's office seven months ago.

Its good news: the United States has seen great gains in oral health by almost all of its citizens. Its bad news: disparities in disease and treatment opportunities still exist, especially among indigent children and older adults.

Major communications campaigns to reach all communities of interest with these messages followed the report's release. A California dentist assisted in securing reports in 24 daily newspapers, 30 television stations and 18 radio stations. Other major venues such as the annual scientific sessions of the American Association of Dental Research and the American Public Health Association exposed public health workers and dental researchers to components of the surgeon general's report.

The desired outcome of this publicity would be support of programs that make oral health an integral component of general health. This goal would be realized through the creation of public/private partnerships dedicated to actions that address this purpose. The involvement of the dental profession in these activities is essential.

But if my informal and unscientific poll of dentists is correct, Dr. Average Dentist knows very little about this report. When speaking before a group of 51 dentists attending a continuing education course last month in Colorado, I asked how many had heard of the surgeon general's report and what their thoughts were regarding its contents. Only three could recollect hearing or reading about the report—and none was conversant with its recommendations.

This is not good news. While Colorado is not necessarily representative of the universe of U.S. dentists, those assembled for this continuing education course would be expected to be more knowledgeable on matters of dental importance than their nonparticipating counterparts.

The contents of this document are too important to be relegated to a shelf. Yet it appears that the traditional means of exposure aren't working. Is it because the report's good news doesn't sell newspapers and its bad news isn't bad enough to print?

Perhaps the surgeon general's report will not join past documents that sit on shelves or in boxes. I hope it won't. But I have doubts. If it fails to garner the attention it deserves, it sends a negative message to those engaged in similar efforts.

As a member of the oversight committee for the

> If my informal and unscientific poll of dentists is correct, Dr. Average Dentist knows very little about 'Oral Health in America: A Report of the Surgeon General.'

ADA's Future of Dentistry, or FOD, Initiative, I am concerned that the output of its 60-plus consultants, who are working to develop a document to guide the profession for the next 15 years, could suffer the same fate.

Insight into dentistry's future—along with action plans that direct the profession to a desired outcome—is critical to the profession's future success. Plans to ensure that the FOD's recommendations get into the hands and head of each ADA member should be an integral component of the initiative. Unfortunately, the present FOD's scope of work ends with the submission of the report to the 2001 House of Delegates.

To stimulate discussion of this critical issue, I am proposing a unique dissemination plan based on employing the three R's: relevancy, repetition and reputation.

Creating relevancy for the FOD material should be the product of the various expert panels and the oversight committee. These FOD recommendations and subsequent action plans must be presented in a clearly understandable format to the practicing dental professional.

Repetition of the FOD message should follow. One or two media "mentions" appear to be insufficient. The dental professional must be offered information from the FOD report in a variety of different venues. Furthermore, the sender of the message must have the reputation as an opinion leader who can command the practitioner's attention and respect.

I would suggest these people be chosen from three groups. The first of these would be former ADA trustees. During my tenure as editor, I have had the opportunity to work with many talented volunteers. When their terms are over, succession rules dictate that they be "gone." This policy is understandable, as it allows new leaders to emerge, but what a waste of knowledge and experience! I propose we solicit ex-trustees to serve as FOD advocates and to participate in the process of explaining the merits of FOD recommendations to ADA constituents.

To add to this group of opinion leaders, I would solicit the assistance of gurus on the lecture circuit. These people come in contact with thousands of dentists. Imagine the impact if each speaker would include some aspect of the FOD report in his or her presentations.

I also would advocate for a similar organization for retired dentists. With their numbers constantly increasing—estimates now exceed 30,000—even a 1 percent participation rate could produce a powerful advocate group for the FOD report.

Will these initiatives work? Will they ensure that the FOD's recommendations reach all who have an interest? Only time will tell. But failing to make a special effort to share the future directions of our profession abdicates our responsibility to our constituents and their patients. ∎

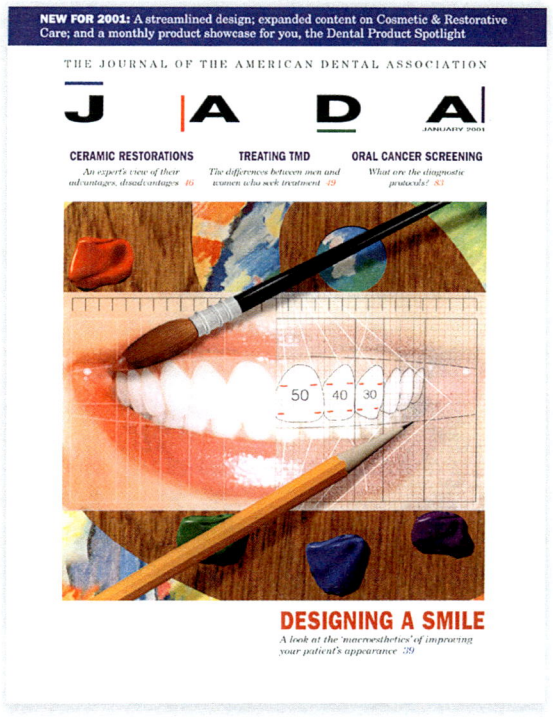

# 2001

"Writing 131 editorials was a real joy.
Each was centered on the principles that actions
starts with knowledge and that the success of an
editorial resides in its ability to be insightful
and predictive; to be a step ahead of what is
considered correct; to explore issues that may not
be mainstream; to go where others fear to go."

# Outrageous II

*Originally published in JADA 2001 132: 10-11.*

If one is good, two must be better. This axiom, offering a rationale for indulgence, may cause more harm than good. Visualize the adverse effects of pharmacological overdosing or the impact of binge eating on those predisposed to obesity. Similarly, apply the concept to business ventures; how many sequels to movies have been as good as or better than the original? "Godfather II" and ... ?

In March 1999, I wrote an editorial titled "Outrageous." The theme focused on the need for dentists to speak out against the cancerlike growth of commercial interests that appear to pervade every niche of the K-12 curricula. The editorial was well-received—prompting the usual number of letters to the editor. So, considering the history of sequels, why revisit the subject?

Simply, the topic is critical to the oral and systemic health of America's schoolchildren. And while a growing number of dentists appear willing to take on leadership roles in addressing this issue, many more dental supporters are needed. Now!

Pouring rights—a term used to describe exclusive contracts between school districts and soft-drink manufacturers—is where dentistry becomes involved. The commercialism of schools by industry is the umbrella issue that allows and promotes such contracts.

School systems, seemingly underfunded to carry out all the activities demanded of them, seek non-public financial support for their programs. Industry, sensing an opportunity to establish brand loyalty, becomes a willing partner and a ready source of funds. Pizzas, hamburgers, athletic shoes, candy and soda pop—all have become excellent candidates for "exclusive" marketing deals with schools.

If these commercial deals cause no harm, so be it. However, if one of these "pouring" contracts can

> **With more schools entering into 'pouring rights' contracts with soft-drink manufacturers, the highspeed handpiece and anesthetic syringe could again become symbols of a dental visit by America's youth.**

be shown to adversely affect the health of schoolchildren, dental health professionals have an ethical responsibility to intervene. The excessive promotion of soft drinks falls in that category.

Consider the following excerpt from that earlier editorial. A high-ranking official of a school district with a lucrative soft drink contract sent a letter to his school principals warning that if their schools didn't "dramatically" increase sales, the district's schools would lose significant revenue.

While indicating that this was not to pressure the teachers, he did suggest "allowing students virtually unlimited access to soft-drink machines." To facilitate this access, he suggested moving the soft-drink dispensers closer to the classrooms. The letter also urged teachers to "consider" encouraging students to consume their soft drinks in class.

Amazingly, the edict generated little concern among the teachers. No teachers contacted the local education association, and the local dental society appeared to be out of the loop.

Not any more. In Michigan, Wisconsin, Ohio, Pennsylvania and New York, local and state dental societies are saying "we care" and are taking action. Both Michigan and Wisconsin submitted to the 2000 ADA House of Delegates resolutions directed to contractual arrangements that "inappropriately influence consumption patterns of soft drinks by schoolchildren."

Their combined efforts, plus testimony from a group of impassioned dentists during Reference Committee hearings, led to a resolution that attracted almost unanimous support from the 2000 ADA House of Delegates.

The resolution (73RC) calls on the ADA to "gather scientific facts and supportive data concerning consumption of soft drinks in schools, develop educational material for the public and school districts on this subject, encourage cooperation with various medical and school constituencies to increase awareness of the nutritive issues, and specifically endorse a policy directed to the opposition of 'pouring rights' contracts."

Some positive actions already have occurred.

Pennsylvania's Fifth District dental leaders reported in a letter to JADA that "dentists are contacting school nurses, boards of education and administration. Already soda machines are being eliminated, restricted to non-school hours or limited to natural fruit juices. ..."

In Michigan, a special education teacher acknowledging organized dentistry's involvement on the soft-drink issue wrote in the local paper, "Thanks ... for taking a stand and speaking out in our schools. I have long anguished over the availability and consumption [of soft drinks] at the school in which I teach special education and am happy to see a community member taking action."

The Jackson, (Mich.) Citizen Patriot's May 28 editorial on this issue, called "Liquid Candy," stated, "Bless the men and women of the Michigan Dental Association who have drawn a line in the sand on the surrender of one school district after another to easy money from soft drinks. ... Dentists might have a reason to applaud the increased consumption of soft drinks, for it generates more tooth decay and thus more business. But, of course, that isn't the way dentists look at it. Their professional goal is to educate, inform, and attack the factors promoting tooth decay."

Well stated.

The Lansing (Mich.) State Journal also praised the Michigan Dental Association's efforts to promote good nutrition in schoolchildren. Pointing to the "pouring" contracts, they lamented, "Is this the price our children must pay so adults can make their budgets work?"

Outrageous? You bet!

Dentists are noting an increase in the caries rate in their teenage and young adult populations. While evidence remains anecdotal, ongoing research looks to increases in refined sugar consumption as the culprit. Fluoride-protected teeth can resist only so much acid before succumbing to decay. With more schools entering into pouring rights contracts (150 at last count), the highspeed hand-piece and anesthetic syringe could again become symbols of a dental visit by America's youth.

Isn't this sufficient reason for all dentists to become involved? ■

# A fluid issue

*Originally published in JADA 2001 132: 138-139.*

Americans are abandoning tap water as their primary source of drinking water, and safety isn't the issue. Thanks to tough Environmental Protection Agency, or EPA, regulations, water from the tap rarely poses a disease threat. The same cannot be said for its taste, color and odor, all of which can make the drinking experience less than enjoyable. It's no wonder that so many now seek filtered or non-public sources of water for their daily requirements.

Consider that in 1992, just over 2 billion gallons of bottled-water products were sold—about nine gallons per capita. Beverage industry statistics for 1999 show that U.S. per capita consumption skyrocketed to almost 16 gallons.

With sales doubling over the previous year, the bottled-water industry now claims 8.1 percent of all beverages sold. These percentages don't include individuals and families who have chosen to filter their home tap water. According to a marketing report, the top seller of home water filters sold more than 4 million in the first six months of 1999.

For regular purchasers of bottled water, a recently published report indicates that they may not be getting the extra benefits they desire.[1] In laboratory tests, 57 samples of five categories of bottled water were analyzed for coliform organisms. Bacterial counts in the bottled water samples ranged from less than 0.01 to 4,900 colony-forming units per milliliter. In contrast, tap water demonstrated counts ranging from just 0.2 to 2.7 CFU/mL.

However, it's not coliform levels that make bottled water an issue for dentistry. Rather, it's determining the fluoride content of these alternative water supplies. Suboptimal levels might be detrimental—especially for high-risk children and

> If the Environmental Protection Agency requires community water suppliers to provide their customers with yearly drinking water quality reports, why shouldn't the U.S. Food and Drug Administration require similar information for bottled water?

adults whose oral health depends on receiving adequate amounts of fluoride.

Seems that determination would be a no-brainer—just read the fluoride level on the label of the bottled water container. Wrong! Only a few manufacturers' labels contain this information. Indeed, one study noted that of 78 different bottled waters examined, not one had fluoride concentrations on the label.[2]

Where is the EPA? Nowhere. Since water is classified as a food, it's the U.S. Food and Drug Administration, or FDA, that has oversight responsibility for bottled water. If fluoride is added during processing, the FDA requires the fluoride content of bottled water to be listed on the label. But that regulation doesn't apply to bottled water that already contains fluoride. In this circumstance, both consumer and dentist must rely on optional labeling or must contact the bottling company for fluoride information.

The ADA doesn't like that situation and has been lobbying the FDA to require fluoride-concentration information on all bottled-water labels. Its argument is cogent. If the EPA requires community water suppliers to provide their customers with yearly drinking-water quality reports, why shouldn't the FDA require similar information for bottled water?

Producers of bottled water cite cost and monitoring difficulties as the two major reasons for not labeling their products. They claim that fluoride levels of the same product can vary according to the source of the water, seasonal variations, different fluoride testing methods and inconsistencies in fluoride concentration tests even within the same batch.

The industrial concerns appear to have been

heeded by the FDA, which, under the direction of Congress, recently completed its final study on the "appropriate" and "feasible" methods of informing consumers about the contents of bottled water.

Two suggestions were made. The first called on bottled-water manufacturers to offer a phone number or address on the label directing consumers to where they can receive information from the company. The second offered a combination approach in which some information is placed on the label "provided that [it] does not result in excessive information," with the remainder of the information available through contact with the company by phone or mail.

Will these "suggestions" ensure that consumers will get ready access to information regarding whether their bottled drinking water contains fluoride and, if so, how much?

I think not. Searching for a phone number (which, according to the FDA, need not be toll-free) is hardly user-friendly. Most consumers wouldn't bother.

While Congress could ask for more explicit labeling or the FDA could consider making further rules, it appears that a more definitive labeling of the fluoride content in bottled water will not be coming in the near future.

The ADA can be expected to continue its lobbying efforts but will face an uphill battle unless it can show that the use of bottled water with reduced fluoride content is associated with increased caries in children or adults.

With only anecdotal reports linking increased caries to the ingestion of bottled water, this type of research would require costly investigations of large population groups. However, dentists know

that fluoride, especially in a topical role, is critical to the remineralization process that can retard or stop caries. Good sense says that removing a well-documented preventive agent like fluoride cannot be beneficial.

Dentists interested in ensuring that their patients are not harmed by drinking bottled water or filtered home drinking water should include questions in their patients' health history questionnaire pertaining to their water-drinking habits. Daily amount ingested, origin of water for cooking and other sources of liquid consumed during the day also require documentation.

For people at high risk of developing caries who are unable or do not wish to discontinue use of waters containing a suboptimal amount of fluoride, supplementary fluoride office procedures or use of home fluoride products should be considered.

In addition to continuing its lobbying activities with the FDA, the ADA also should consider alerting bottled-water manufacturers that labeling the fluoride content of their products actually may give them a sales advantage. Many parents purchasing bottled water still want their children to have caries protection.

Eventually, I envision packagers of bottled water asking to be included in the ADA Seal of Acceptance program. Why not an ADA Seal for bottled waters that contain the optimal amount of fluoride? Safe and effective? History says yes! ∎

1. Lalumandier JA, Ayers LA. Fluoride and bacterial content of bottled water vs. tap water. Arch Fam Med 2000;9:246–50.[Abstract/Free Full Text]

2. Van Winkle S, Levy SM, Kiritsy MC, Heilman JR, Wefel JS. Water and formula fluoride concentrations: significance for infants fed formula. Pediatr Dent 1995;17(4):305–10.[Medline]

# Declaration of independence

*Originally published in JADA 2001 132: 266-268.*

Two years ago, the American Medical Association fired the celebrated editor of its flagship journal, The Journal of the American Medical Association. AMA leaders said George Lundberg, M.D., JAMA's editor of 17 years, "went a step too far" when he published findings from a survey on what physical acts college students said qualified as having "had sex."

While the subject may or may not have major medical implications, the AMA brass thought it more than coincidental that the article appeared during the Clinton impeachment hearings. They intimated that the JAMA editor had, in this instance, used the journal to make a political statement.

Dr. Lundberg, they said, "through his recent actions, has threatened the historic tradition and integrity of The Journal of the American Medical Association by inappropriately and inexcusably interjecting [JAMA] into a major political debate that has nothing to do with science or medicine."

Dr. Lundberg's dismissal provoked many of his fellow editors to pen strong letters of protest, alleging that the AMA had violated JAMA's editorial independence. Dr. Lundberg himself claimed AMA leaders had "inappropriately intruded into the historically inviolable ground of editorial independence in scientific journalism."

If you've been keeping up with the news lately, you may know that I will step down at the end of this year after 10 years as JADA editor. I've always enjoyed strong support from the ADA leadership. Mine is an amicable departure. I am the one who decided it is time to go, no one else.

The search for my successor has been in progress now for several months. Indeed, the deadline for candidates to submit their credentials is March 31.

It seems appropriate then, during this transitional period, to explore the issues and challenges that all editors face—to take stock of what we really think and really believe about such matters as editorial independence, scientific integrity and an editor's responsibility to the organization. And vice versa.

Candidates seeking the JADA editorship and those charged to make that selection should consider the issues raised in the Lundberg debacle. And so, JADA reader, should you. You have a stake in this as well. It is, after all, your professional journal we're talking about.

As I see it, the first order of business is to define what actually constitutes "editorial independence." This raises a number of questions. For instance, is it inconsistent with editorial independence if a journal solely represents the views of its constituency—the organization and its members? Is editorial independence violated or altogether lost if a manuscript is rejected because it is considered politically unfit? And if this ever happens, will readers be able to accept with confidence that what is published represents the best knowledge available, served up without institutional bias?

Obviously, as a scientific journal, JADA's publication goals should not be confused with those of the public press. JADA is dedicated and funded to serve the needs of the members of the American Dental Association. The Association's dual mission—to serve the interests of both the public and the profession—challenges its editor to determine the proper balance between editorial integrity and professional responsibility.

When you are not the editor, it may be easy, even comforting, to imagine that you would always make the right call and fight the good fight. But that assumes that you could invariably discern clear-cut distinctions between right and wrong, good and evil, black and white. In publishing, I

> **Is editorial independence violated or altogether lost if a manuscript is rejected because it is considered politically unfit?**

submit, the predominant color is gray, and it comes in an ever-widening variety of shades.

Let us now play a game. Call it "What's My Choice?" Described below are a number of situations that require an editor's judgment. These are fictitious, of course, though they represent the kinds of decisions the editor of a major scientific journal is called on to make everyday. You are that editor. You make the call.

1. You have published a peer-reviewed article on the instrument sterilization practices of the dentists in a particular state. Findings from this study, which involved more than 400 dental offices, show that 80 percent of the offices in the state were doing a poor job of sterilizing their instruments. However, the study also showed that once staff were instructed in how to "pack" instruments properly, the sterilization failure rate was reduced to 2 percent.

Shortly after the study is published, you get a call from the president of the state's dental association, who says he's swamped with complaints from his membership. He says his member dentists are concerned that the article could invite unwanted attention from investigative journalists from programs like "20/20" and "60 Minutes" who might use the article to characterize the dental office as an unsafe place.

How do you respond to these concerns?

2. You have received a well-crafted report on the dental profession's participation in Medicaid from a dentist who is universally disliked by his peers. This dentist often is insulting and dismissive of his colleagues, and is well-known for criticizing dentists who are reluctant to treat Medicaid patients. Still, the paper is well researched and presents a number of solid suggestions on how to increase dental participation in Medicaid. You know you won't win any popularity contests by publishing his material. In fact, it's conceivable you might lose your editorship if the dental community challenges your judgment.

Do you publish the article?

3. A research manuscript on the safety of an infection control product has passed through the peer-review process with flying colors. Without exception, the reviewers recommend that the paper be published. The study explores the efficacy of a well-known product used in dental offices across the country. The study concludes that this product is not particularly effective; it even identifies other products that clearly work much better. But the maker of this apparently ineffective product is your major advertiser. Most likely, if the article is published, the manufacturer will cancel his ads. Your journal is expected to turn a profit, and you depend on that revenue.

Do you follow your reviewer's suggestions and publish the research?

4. Your dental association's executive committee has decided it will seek approval of a dues increase at its next annual meeting. You have been an outspoken critic of such an increase, arguing that it would harm membership among younger dentists—encouraging them to quit or not to join in the first place. The association's officers predict that the loss of membership resulting from the dues increase would be minimal, and they think you're something of an alarmist. But your own research shows that, in fact, the membership loss would be substantial, and you're thinking about writing an editorial to that effect. This, of course, would pit you directly against the association's hierarchy.

Do you write the editorial?

As an ADA member and JADA reader, you are a stakeholder in a for-profit enterprise that is driven, as its mission states, to deliver high-quality, accurate and relevant information on matters related to dental care and dental practice. That information should reach you in a timely fashion, and it should be presented without external and internal influence. The ability of the editor to function in a censorship-free environment is critical to fulfilling The Journal's mission.

All of us accept it as a basic tenet of our profession that dentists should have the right to treat their patients as their knowledge and experience dictates, within the limits of accepted dental practice. Is the profession willing to apply that same principle to the work of the editor of its flagship journal? Will the ADA bestow on the editor the right to make difficult, sometimes unpopular choices?

I urge those seeking the JADA editorship to pose such questions to their interviewers. ∎

# Back to the future

*Originally published in JADA 2001 132: 421-422.*

**M**ost JADA readers were still in high school when President Lyndon Johnson launched his "War on Poverty." Designed to cure the country's social ills, the program included a goal of improving access to health care. Dentistry, believed to have a serious shortage of personnel, was spotlighted as a profession needing extensive financial assistance to achieve the nation's health goals.

What followed was a massive influx of federal funds for dental education. New dental schools were built. Existing schools were renovated. Curricula were shortened to allow for early graduation. The results: too many dental personnel for a delivery system that would be adversely affected by two economic recessions, miscalculated predictions of U.S. population increases and a failure to account for the impact of fluoride on dental needs.

It took years for the dental marketplace to recover from these ill-conceived presidential initiatives. For dentists who suffered through those less-than-professionally-satisfying times, the recent decade of prosperity has just started to remove the bad memories of the "oversupply" days.

Now, almost a half-century later, voices are being raised to say that we may again have a shortage of dental personnel. Gear up the institutions and increase dental class size, some insist. Lack of access to dental care is a national problem, and national solutions are necessary, say others.

Whether valid or not, such phrases recall a past filled with well-intentioned but misdirected initiatives.

Let's examine the present situation. The U.S. surgeon general's report "Oral Health in America," while acknowledging dramatic improvements in

> **For dentists who suffered through the less-than-professionally-satisfying times of the 1970s and 1980s, the recent decade of prosperity has just started to remove the bad memories of the 'oversupply' days.**

oral health over the last 50 years, notes "profound" health disparities mainly among those "without the knowledge and resources to achieve good oral care." Specifically mentioned in the report were poor Americans—especially children—the elderly, members of various racial and ethnic groups, and those with disabilities and complex health conditions.

Would enlarging the pool of dental practitioners necessarily improve the health status for these populations? Probably not.

For example, the lack of access to dental care for Medicaid patients most often is a remuneration issue, which will not be solved by simply increasing the number of dentists. Regardless of how many dentists are serving a community, a system that asks them to deliver care at rates that are lower than their costs cannot be sustained. When the cost barrier is obviated, access improves, often dramatically.

In Michigan, for example, the state's Children's Health Insurance Program converted its Medicaid program to a private administration that paid the dentists' usual and customary fees. The result: a 50 percent increase in the number of children receiving care.

Even adequate compensation, however, often will not be enough to eliminate disparities in oral health status. Last month's JADA cover story demonstrated that even with a universal, publicly financed dental insurance care program for children, oral health disparities among specific children's groups still remain.

Improving access to dental services entails more than educating more dentists or even offering a just payment system. Access involves complex interactions, often requiring the attention of the social scientist as well as of the health care professional.

Still, some opinion leaders insist there should be

an immediate increase in the number of dentists. In addition to anecdotal reports of shortages, they point to work-force models that purportedly show more dentists leaving than entering the profession over the next two decades. They predict more early retirements and an increase in the number of part-time dental workers set against an overall rise in U.S. population. Within these observations, they see the potential for a major dentist/population imbalance.

Is this the time for preemptive action? Should dental schools be encouraged to increase their class sizes? I think not.

Remember the overproduction of dentists that occurred in the 1970s and 1980s. We learned from that period that the complex variables affecting the demand for dental care and dental personnel are exceedingly difficult to understand. While the prediction process has been refined over the years, few would assert that today's estimates will prove correct. Unfortunately, false prophecies that cause us to produce more dentists can become a 35-year mistake spread across the entire profession.

In 1977, I published an opinion piece titled, "Too Many Dentists? If So, What Then?" At that time,

dental care system "improvements" driven by LBJ's "War on Poverty" were starting to show some obvious cracks.

Acknowledging the difficulty of predicting dental personnel needs, I proposed a system that expands or contracts by altering the number and duties of auxiliaries, not by increasing the numbers of dentists. Auxiliaries would be provided with continuing education programs that offer upward mobility, skill enhancement and retraining as cost-effective components of the delivery system.

For more than two decades, I have persisted in promoting this concept, firmly believing that it displays an inherent flexibility capable of responding quickly to changes in consumer demand. While minimizing the chance of a dentist oversupply, the model is responsive to the professional needs of the dental team member, offering a meaningful opportunity for professional advancement.

I've heard it said that a profession that ignores its past has no future. That's a bit strong. Rather, focusing on the issue of the dental work force, I would say that a profession that ignores its past fails to secure its future. ∎

# Hidden treasure

*Originally published in JADA 2001 132: 572-574.*

Until two or three decades ago, displays featuring antiquated dental equipment intermixed with local historic memorabilia could be found in almost every U.S. dental school. They often were housed in spaces far away from student, faculty or patient traffic patterns, and a visitor to these minimuseums was a rare event.

Usually it was either a dental dean emeritus or some aging faculty member who was designated curator—a title that, in most cases, came without responsibility. Eventually, as space in the dental schools became premium, a faculty vote to rid the school of this dusty and ill-used space resulted in its contents being packaged and sent to some off-campus storage space.

Few dentists mourned the exit of these vestiges of their profession's historical past. Dentistry, it appeared, was moving up the professional ladder so rapidly that it was willing to ignore that not so long ago, its members had been barbers or blacksmiths.

This attitude was not unexpected. Millions of immigrants who came to America during the same period in which dentistry was becoming one of the health sciences' foremost professions wanted no part of their heritage. Assimilation into the American mainstream was the desired goal.

That perspective has changed. More and more Americans are looking back to their roots, examining their heritage and building personal histories into their daily lives. Could the creation in 1996 of a national dental museum in Baltimore signal that the dental profession is following suit?

Whether the answer is yes or no, the existence of this new museum, with its outstanding professional and public programs, should be promoted.

Building on the University of Maryland's already well-stocked collection of historic dental items and bolstered by a million-dollar grant from Dr. Samuel Harris, the Samuel D. Harris National Museum of Dentistry, or NMD, opened its doors in 1996. The museum is appropriately housed in a building that served as the University of Maryland Dental Department from 1904 to 1929. The fact that the Baltimore College of Dentistry was the site of the nation's first dental school adds to the importance of the museum's location.

The concept of a national museum of dentistry to showcase the profession's historic and scientific achievements is one that has intrigued me for many years.

In fact, a number of years ago, thinking I had the ear of the ADA president at the time, I suggested starting a national museum of dentistry in Colorado Springs, Colo.

My argument—that the site where fluoride's dental effects were first identified would be an appropriate place for such a museum—was not received with enthusiasm. There were too many more pertinent needs, I was told. So be it. But my interest remained, and I was delighted when the NMD opened its doors.

The museum's eclectic collection includes our first president's dentures, an Andy Warhol silkscreen of St. Apollonia (dentistry's patron saint), Queen Victoria's tooth-cleaning paraphernalia and examples of antiquated dental equipment—including some bone-chilling extraction instruments that explained why so many in the past saw dentists as purveyors of pain.

On the lighter side is something designed especially for children: a video jukebox. This popular attraction, shaped like a giant mouth, projects vintage toothpaste commercials on a large screen when the visitor pushes one of the teeth. The backdrop for this display includes a number of out-

> **The Samuel D. Harris National Museum of Dentistry is a jewel, but it lacks national recognition and the financial resources it needs to realize its potential.**

standing examples of classic dental poster art.

Hands-on opportunities are in abundance, especially for children. A small theater, interactive computer displays of oral anatomy and a setting in which children have the opportunity to play dentist with scaled-down dental chairs are only a few examples of adventures and activities that the museum offers throughout its two exhibit floors.

New exhibits are introduced continually; this year, the museum featured women in dentistry and a major exhibit entitled "Watch Your Mouth! Sports and Dentistry," which featured mouth and face guards used by sports celebrities.

The visitor is struck by the multiple offerings for adults and children. On my visit, I found a number of older people, like me, trying out the children's interactive displays.

A classy newsletter and an attractive Web site round out the museum's offerings, thus allowing the nonvisitor or the infrequent visitor the opportunity to share in dentistry's history.

The museum has become such a popular attraction that the Sun, in an assessment of the city's 40-plus museums, gave it four and a half stars of a possible five. "They did the impossible," observed the Sun in August 1998. "They made a dental museum bright, colorful and fun. [It] houses an entertaining mix of gear, gadgets and lore associated with dentistry and teeth."

The museum is a jewel, but it lacks national recognition and the financial resources it needs to realize its potential. I hope this editorial will alert the profession to this treasure, but more publicity is needed.

The museum is seeking federal designation as a national museum. This recognition is a political one that would increase public awareness, under-standing and appreciation of dentistry. Such special recognition is warranted; in fact, the museum already is a national resource, having loaned a number of exhibits to the Smithsonian Institution in Washington.

To help in its quest for "national museum" designation, the NMD's board of visitors is seeking assistance from such notables as Rep. Charles Norwood (R-Ga.), a dentist. I hope the ADA's Government Affairs office also will lend its support.

While the ADA, as early as 1988, endorsed the concept of a national museum and reaffirmed its endorsement of the NMD as the official museum of the dental profession, it left the door open for recognition of other museums as well. No problem. Other national museums have not precluded the development of new museums.

Finally, let me make a pitch for your financial support. The NMD has a board of visitors and a national advisory committee whose members make up a who's who of dentistry. With the support of these people, plus the contributions from the University of Maryland, national fund-raising activities have been able to support the basic operations of the museum. Elevating the museum to the next level, however, will require additional funding. Procuring an official "national" designation will help, but the museum still needs many more friends.

The NMD is offering contributors the right to have their names engraved on a brick to be permanently displayed in the courtyard at the museum's entrance. For a $100 contribution, you can help pave the way to dental history. Greater or lesser dollar amounts would be welcome. Take pride in your profession—become a partner in this exciting endeavor. My check is on its way. ∎

# Forever vigilant

*Originally published in JADA 2001 132: 716-717.*

Considering a surgical operation? You might want to check who's going to deliver the anesthetic—and assess your own comfort level with that person if he or she is not a physician. If a new Health Care Financing Administration ruling is allowed to stand, a long-standing policy requiring physicians to supervise nurse anesthetists will be history. Physicians aren't pleased.

Commenting on the new ruling, the president of the American Medical Association remarked that the action "ignores the substantial differences in training between physicians and nurse anesthetists." To emphasize his point, he contrasts the physician's minimum of seven years of training, including hands-on hospital residence experience, with the lack of even bachelor's-degree education for one-third of the nurse anesthetists.

Physician anesthesiologists have been even more vocal, commenting that "the underlying motivation for the rule was political, totally ignoring safety and science." The anesthesiologists plan to take their fight to the states where state medical practice acts still can impose legal constraints against the unsupervised practices of nurse anesthetists.

The movement toward unsupervised practice is hardly confined to nurse anesthetists or nurse practitioners. In Illinois, pharmacists want to "initiate, monitor and modify prescribed drugs." Physicians say "no" to these pharmacists, who want to practice medicine by having "patients" come in and describe their symptoms, followed by the pharmacist prescribing a drug or changing a dosage. Illinois also has added physician assistants to the list; they're seeking legislation to conduct and sign off on school physical examinations.

The growing issue of nonphysician clinicians' becoming independent practitioners is particularly disturbing to me. For years, I have advocated that, at least in the first stages of a perceived work-force shortage, additional allied dental personnel, not dentists, should be trained to help address inequities in work-force numbers and distribution. Unfortunately, there is a potential danger in pursuing this course of action.

History demonstrates that having obtained the expanded clinical training, one or more members of the newly trained group will argue that they can provide the same service as the original provider to more people and at lower cost. Vocal and well-organized, they often have been able to convince lawmaking bodies to change state practice acts in their favor.

Take denturists, for example. Because of their small number, their clinical activities rarely attract nationwide attention. In fact, a recent ADA survey indicated that the dental profession is "not at all concerned" about these independent practitioners. Perhaps it should be.

Ask the Montana State Board of Dentistry, which recently advised several denturists not to use the acronym D.D.M. or the title Doctorate of Medical Denturity. Close to dentistry's D.M.D., isn't it? Undaunted, Montana denturists sought a ruling that would allow them to evaluate temporomandibular joint disorders. Again, the board of dental examiners ruled that denturists cannot diagnose or treat these disorders. Similarly, the board of education responded negatively to a denturist request to be the accrediting agent for denturism education programs.

These issues aside, my personal concern rests in the potential fragmentation of care, especially in the detection of oral lesions by unsupervised denturists. Maine recognizes the issue and requires that a dentist examine the patient within 30 days before a denturist can begin fabricating the pa-

> **Professional vigilance must never be relaxed. Intrusions by lesser-trained people into the dentist/patient relationship should not be tolerated.**

tient's denture.

In Oregon, the denturist must obtain an oral health certificate from a dentist or physician before initiating treatment, but that requirement can be waived if the denturist has had additional training in oral pathology. That exemption troubles me. What level of training for these unsupervised denturists will bring them to the competence level of a dentist?

I have the same issue with the unsupervised practice of dental hygiene. New Mexico, one of the six states that allow the hygienist either limited or total unsupervised practice, provides that "qualified hygienists may own and manage a hygiene practice and may advise a patient of suspected pathology and periodontal status, though they may not diagnose dental disease."

What differentiates advising a patient of suspected pathology from actually making a diagnosis? Ultimately, the issue is this: do unsupervised hygienists have the same level of training in oral medicine and oral pathology as dentists? If not, then it's the patient who suffers.

Contrary to statements often made by hygienists seeking unsupervised practices, dental hygiene students or graduates do not receive the same level of basic science and clinical training as dental students. While technical proficiency in certain procedures can be achieved equally by dentists and allied dental personnel, diagnosis, treatment planning and outcome evaluation cannot.

Then there is the issue of continuity of care—dentistry's one big claim of supremacy over medicine. Because we are a profession dominated by general practitioners, the bulk of care provided to any one patient is delivered by one professional. Start taking off a little chunk here and another piece there and it doesn't take too long until no one is in charge of the patient's health needs—and again, the patient suffers.

If branching off from the parent and creating independent domains is inherent in systems that allow delegation of duties to lesser-trained people, how can the dental profession minimize the number of expanded-duty allied dental personnel who seek unsupervised practice?

Foremost, dental practitioners need to provide a stimulating work environment, with sufficient reward systems to acknowledge the performance excellence of dental team members. Continuing education opportunities supported by the dental office should be built on the concept of upward mobility. The ideal endpoint of professional advancement should be admission to dental school with advanced standing. Becoming a dentist, not an independent nondentist clinician, should be the desired outcome.

Professional efforts need to focus on legislative actions that ensure that expanded duties for allied dental personnel do not infringe on the dentist's unique abilities to diagnose conditions and plan treatment. While this has been the prevailing philosophy of the dental profession, continued oversight is needed to guard against capricious political actions that would lead to lower standards of care.

If the dental work force is to be augmented mainly with expanded-duty allied dental personnel, implementation of these two suggestions should alleviate many of the previously noted problems. Regardless of any successful programmatic outcomes, professional vigilance must never be relaxed. Intrusions by lesser-trained people into the dentist/patient relationship should not be tolerated. ∎

# Pluses

*Originally published in JADA 2001 132: 848-849.*

I have been asked repeatedly, "What will you miss most when your JADA editorship comes to a close?" Without hesitation, I answer, "I will miss no longer producing the monthly JADA editorial."

Imagine having an ongoing opportunity to share your thoughts with a potential audience of 150,000. After 11 years and 131 editorials, there will be a void.

Each of the JADA editorials is built on the philosophy that action starts with knowledge. A commitment to that principle requires continuous searches for issues that are professionally relevant and have a broad appeal to the JADA audience. The results of thorough searches and collation of pertinent background material precedes the creation of the editorial's narrative. Most editorials end with a problem-solving proposal.

If that format attracts reader interest—whether they agree with it or not—I consider the editorial a success. In the instances in which communities of interest take actions suggested in the editorial, that's a real plus. As my editorship draws to a close, I have examined past editorials for potential "pluses." Let me share my selections with you and see if you agree with my assessment.

Two editorials, "Outrageous" (March 1999)[1] and "Outrageous II" (January 2001),[2] focused on the growing number of "pouring rights" contracts between schools and the heavyweights of the soft-drink industry. Both editorials described the exclusive contracts and the potential proceeds for the schools that reach millions of dollars, depending in many cases on the children's drinking the "required amount of cans" specified in the contract.

The statement of a high-ranking school official imploring teachers to get their students to drink more soda by "allowing students virtually unlimited access to soft drink machines"—moving the machines to where they would be accessible to the students all day, permitting students to purchase and consume vended products throughout the day and even "allowing students to drink their soft drinks in class"—compelled me to characterize these actions as examples of "blatant" child abuse. Others consider it outright exploitation of children.

The initial editorial chastised dentists for not becoming involved in opposing the school promotion of products that lead directly to increased oral disease. The follow-up piece praised dentists, as evidence of their involvement in fighting school/industry contracts grew substantially across the nation.

> **Imagine having an ongoing opportunity to share your thoughts with a potential audience of 150,000. After 11 years and 131 editorials, there will be a void.**

No doubt those dentists crusading against pouring rights were heartened to read about Coke's apparently new policy to "aggressively discourage bottlers from making controversial exclusive arrangements with schools to promote the sale of soda." While dentistry's contribution to this policy reversal is difficult to measure, it can be said that we were there!

Opponents of these contracts aren't satisfied with the Coke announcement. Considering the new policy as only a publicity stunt, they believe nothing will change. They may be right. More evidence is needed before pouring rights contracts can be placed in the "plus" category.

The editorials "Do It or Lose It" (August 1997)[3] and "One More Time" (July 1999),[4] which addressed the issue of oral cancer, appear to be bona fide competitors for a "plus" rating. With the message that "for a disease that is dentistry's to prevent and treat, we have demonstrated a singular lack of progress in controlling the occurrence of oral and pharyngeal cancer," the thrust of these editorials was to light a fire under the profession to take an active role in early diagnosis and prevention programs. To detect oral cancer, you have to look for it.

Good news. Grassroots dental activity in establishing programs to recognize oral cancer appear to be on the upswing. Notable is the recent public promotion of free cancer screenings by a coalition of health institutions in the New York/New Jersey region. Their visible success encouraged similar institutions in the Boston area to duplicate their programming. Other states and regions are considering similar programs.

A "plus" score should be considered.

Sometimes a "plus" takes a long time to develop. It was back in August 1992 when an editorial called "The Next Revolution: It's Here"[5] proposed that "because of the sophisticated technology and high cost of these innovations, organized dentistry, in concert with industry, should consider providing its members with a number of regional advanced dental technology centers."

In that regard, the University of Minnesota recently announced the opening of its new clinical center, where "students, faculty and practicing clinicians will have access to the latest technologies in dentistry." Supported by a major corporation that has committed to providing new equipment on an ongoing basis, the clinic promises to offer dental students and dental practitioners training in cutting-edge technologies. What a great model for others to emulate!

Surely deserving a plus, if the legislation ever passes both legislative chambers, is the issue of patient protection. As depicted in the editorial " 'I Think I Can ... I Thought I Could' " (April 1998),[6] organized dentistry helped bring this issue to national prominence when others, far better positioned, were unwilling to do so. As each new rendition of legislation has been offered, the ADA's "Little Engine That Could" has stood firm, unwilling to accept any legislation that does not completely secure patients' rights.

For those disturbed by use of human subjects in licensure examinations, the editorial "The Perfect Patient" (October 2000)[7] would garner a number of votes for a "plus." The ADA's House of Delegates resolution 64H-2000 (calling for elimination of the use of human subjects in the clinical licensure examination by 2005) caused a great deal of excitement among those who have sought licensure reform for years, especially students. Associations in a number of states, Texas being the most recent, have passed similar resolutions.

These are my choices for "pluses." While I'm sure that others would merit equal recognition, I'm equally convinced there are some that would qualify as "minuses"—editorials that missed the mark.

After all, editorial writing is far from an exact science.

Although I participate in an occasional course in editorial writing for dental editors, I have no illusions that editorial achievement can be attained by following a set of rules. Rather, success depends more on the editor's ability to be insightful and predictive, to be a step ahead of what is considered correct and to be willing to share thoughts that may not be mainstream—to go where others fear to go.

Stimulating the reader's mind, that's really what it's all about. "Pluses" are just frosting. ∎

1. Meskin LH. Outrageous. JADA 1999;130(3):308–12.[Free Full Text]
2. Meskin LH. Outrageous II. JADA 2001;132(1):10–2.[Free Full Text]
3. Meskin LH. Do it or lose it. JADA 1997;128(8):1058–60.[Free Full Text]
4. Meskin LH. One more time. JADA 1999;130(7):910–6.[Free Full Text]
5. Meskin LH. The next revolution: it's here. JADA 1992;123(8):8–10.[Medline]
6. Meskin LH. 'I think I can ... I thought I could' (editorial). JADA 1998;129(4):402–4.[Free Full Text]
7. Meskin LH. The perfect patient. JADA 2000;131(10):1394–6.[Medline]

# 'Freshly washed little cherubs'

*Originally published in JADA 2001 132: 1078-1080.*

Unbridled enthusiasm among its American Student Dental Association, or ASDA, sponsors was evident when the 2000 ADA House of Delegates passed Resolution 64H, which called for the elimination of the use of human subjects in the clinical licensure examination. ASDA viewed the action as a "great" move by the ADA to rid itself of a process "that has been embarrassing, unethical and does not serve the purpose [for which] it was intended." Not so pleased were the resolution's detractors, who now are being "encouraged" to work within their jurisdiction to rescind 64H.

Following passage of the live-patient resolution, a JADA Question of the Month asked if 64H was a positive move for dentistry. It elicited an unprecedented number of responses from students and dental practitioners.

Students universally acclaimed its passage, which indicated that many of the problems associated with clinical licensure examinations—such as cost of providing dental assistants, insurance, transportation and lodging—would be eliminated. The clinical board examination without patients would be more fair and predictable, and no one would flunk if a patient was a no-show. The ethical aspects of using live patients for detecting incompetence also would cease to be an issue.

The hundreds of letters received from students can be summed up best by this statement from a student from California: "This is a position which will move to establish greater equity in the clinical licensure exam. Dental schools provide the training and evaluation to ensure students develop appropriate skills in working with the variables associated with live patient interaction. In the ideal world, shouldn't we be like our medical counterparts—placing the responsibility and accountability on the dental school to ensure clinical

> **The clinical board examination without patients would be more fair and predictable, and no one would flunk if a patient was a no-show.**

competency? We need to provide means for all dentists to have full freedom of movement unencumbered by the current restrictions by many states in not accepting all clinical board exams. This is one step in that direction."

The concept that dental schools should confirm and be held accountable for the clinical skills of their students in lieu of clinical licensure examinations was noted by many of the students and dentists who had responded in the affirmative to the JADA question. Many practitioners indicated this action was long overdue; one of these wrote that using "live patients is barbaric, unnerving, and unethical treatment of people—patients and students alike."

Not every respondent agreed that eliminating live patients would be good for dentistry. Comments such as "If students can't handle the pressure of board exams with human subjects, how will they handle the real world of dentistry?" or "Real dentists should prove they can work on real people" and "Treating the live patient in an exam setting gives a more complete look at the applicant's clinical and management skills" are just a few of the antiresolution comments. Concerns that dental schools also might become de facto licensing institutions also were voiced.

An editorial in the spring issue of Bulletin of the American Association of Dental Examiners[1] captured the essence of the dentists' negative comments in an editorial entitled "Ignorance." Implying that 64H was a stupid effort, it questions whether "this was an egalitarian effort on the part of the House of Delegates to spare the dental school consumer from the carnage produced by these future 'competent by graduation' candidates."

The idea that clinical board examinations and dental school accreditation should be considered "redundancies" if dental schools are "teaching what is required of them" is pooh-poohed by the writer, who expresses his contempt by stating, "Duh! My, my, my, it would certainly ease the transition of the freshly washed little cherubs into the ADA fold if we were to have no standards for licensure whatsoever."

The editorial implies that the 64H action was just the ADA's pandering to the students to get them to join the ADA—that it had no relationship to human subjects or measuring competency. Furthermore, it states that the 64H vote was taken late in the day, when delegates apparently were "demonstrating more of a late cocktail desire than an interest in serious debate of issue."

Let's examine the editorial's comments. Was this just a ploy of the ADA to gain eventual members? No. The live patient issue is a troublesome one that continues to plague the students. Just look at what happened at the Central Regional Dental Testing Service's August examination in Kansas City, Mo.: a broken water main leading to clinical facilities resulted in cancellation of the examination. Any clinical procedures not finished at that time had to be completed at a future examination. The examination in Chicago, three weeks later, would be the earliest opportunity. While candidates needn't pay additional testing charges, costs for transporting and housing the candidate, a patient and perhaps even a dental assistant would have to be added to the already existing test expenditures.

This obviously was a very difficult situation for newly graduated students already burdened with a debt of more than $100,000 and no ready supply of cash to pay for the additional expenditure.

And it would be a nonissue if live patients were not involved.

But, yes, it also is a membership issue. Young dentists certainly warrant the ADA's attention. Please consider that by 2010, 40,000 new dentists will have joined the dental work force. For organized dentistry to continue to speak with one voice, it is crucial that these potential members see value in an ADA membership. If they have a valid issue, why shouldn't it be addressed?

The ideal solution to the entry licensure issue would be to have examiners and educators work together to ensure that graduates were competent to practice dentistry. Presently, I get the feeling that "live-patient" licensure advocates do not believe that dental schools are graduating dentists who are clinically capable.

They point to the failure rate on the present licensure examinations as evidence that simply licensing graduates from an accredited dental school does not protect the public from incompetence. I would question whether clinical examinations weed out the incompetent and ask this: where did the dentists who initially failed and then passed the licensure examination gain their newfound skills, since they had no opportunity for remediation?

Personally, I like the Canadian licensure model, which links the accreditation process with the licensing authority. With both entities participating in the schools' onsite evaluations, no clinical examination is required for licensure. We can do that. In fact, we are doing it.

Initiated a few years ago, a member of the dental examining community (selected by the American Association of Dental Examiners) is included as a full participant in all U.S. dental school accreditations. If these examiners detect clinical problems, they are in an excellent position to bring them to the attention of the accreditation team and the dental school.

This could be the solution. But until both education and licensure communities gain sufficient trust in the system and each other, I suggest that if we must give a clinical examination, let's do it in the presence of both faculty and dental board members while the dental student still is enrolled in school. This handles the ethical and remediation issues.

Meanwhile, the world of U.S. dentistry is not waiting for the dental education and licensure community to find some accommodation. The Texas Dental Association has become the latest to support the elimination of use of human subjects in the clinical licensure examination.

Recent action by the board of governors of the New York State Dental Association authorized its organization to seek legislation to eliminate live testing on clinical tests for dental licensure. They are also investigating requiring a fifth year in an accredited general practice residency program as the future criterion for licensure in New York.

Obviously, more than a few dentists think our "freshly washed little cherubs" are real dentists with real concerns. ∎

1. Pattalochi RE. Ignorance. Bull Amer Assoc Dent Exam 2001;Spring:5.

# Do no harm

*Originally published in JADA 2001 132: 1200-1201.*

Amalgam, dentistry's mainstay restorative material, is under fire—again, for the umpteenth time. Controversies fueled by those who question the safety and efficacy of amalgam date to amalgam's introduction in 1833 as the Royal Mineral Succedaneum.

You remember that story. A silver/mercury paste was promoted cleverly by two French dentists who more often than not placed the filling material over carious areas without removing the decay. It didn't take long for patients to develop painful conditions. In light of these unacceptable outcomes, many dentists sought to ban amalgam outright.

The furor between amalgam supporters and detractors, known as the "Amalgam Wars," threatened the existence of the entire profession. Fortunately, for those hundreds of millions worldwide who have enjoyed the benefits of this superb restorative material, "silver" amalgam still remains the dominant restorative material in dentistry.

It's the mercury in amalgam that has its detractors dancing around like the Mad Hatter from "Alice in Wonderland." Attributing almost every conceivable health woe to a person's dental fillings, amalgam opponents state that these restorations release sufficient mercury to cause multiple sclerosis, or MS; Parkinson's disease; Alzheimer's disease; and a host of other conditions.

Regardless of repeated scientific evidence of amalgam's safety—plus the endorsement of all the major national and international public health organizations—amalgam's critics remain vocal and active, often using misinterpretation of facts to promote their cause.

The insidiousness of the antiamalgamist approach was evident in what I call the "throw-away-

> **Dentists have been thrust into the role of having to defend amalgam when their silence on the issue could have had them replacing billions—yes, billions—of amalgam restorations with the more expensive resin-based composites.**

the-crutches" speech delivered in a 1990 "60 Minutes" broadcast on CBS-TV. The presentation featured a woman with MS who declared that she was able to go dancing immediately after her amalgam restorations were removed, giving new, false hope to many MS sufferers.

No TV host tried to explain why her relief was so instantaneous, especially considering that the vapors from amalgam are at their highest during removal. No one described MS as a disease that often is characterized by spontaneous remission. Nor, a few months later, did "60 Minutes" air the fact that the woman in the earlier broadcast was back to using crutches.

How many others suffered a similar fate of false hope, brought by those who choose to ignore the absence of any science linking MS and mercury in dental fillings?

Instances such as this led the ADA to include in its "Principles of Ethics and Code of Professional Conduct" the statement: "... removal of amalgam restorations from the non-allergic patient for the alleged purpose of removing toxic substances from the body, when such treatment is performed solely at the recommendation of the dentist, is improper and unethical."[1]

Apparently failing to develop sufficient "science" of their own to refute safety claims by the U.S. Public Health Service and the ADA, the antiamalgamists are turning to the legal community to assist them in their quest.

A suit filed in May by five dentists and seven patients in a Maryland federal court alleges that dental regulators use "control of dental licenses to punish or threaten punishment of dentists who criticize 'mercury' amalgam."[2] The desire of the antiamalgam activists apparently is to demonstrate

First Amendment interference with the ability of dentists to share with their patients the "hazards" of dental amalgam.

A related legal initiative was filed recently against the ADA and the California Dental Association, claiming that the organizations weren't telling all about what's in amalgam. Adding to the turmoil is a ruckus between California state officials and the California Dental Board over a fact sheet the board is supposed to produce regarding various restorative materials, including the mercury in amalgam.

With all of this brouhaha, one would think that dentists are reaping huge financial rewards from amalgam use. In actuality, the opposite is true. Dentists have been thrust into the role of having to defend amalgam when their silence on the issue could have had them replacing billions—yes, billions—of amalgam restorations with the more expensive resin-based composites.

It's the fluoride story all over again. Dentists continually have been called on to defend the science behind one of public health's most crowning achievements. Had dentistry simply acquiesced to the antifluoridationists' claims, the result would have been a drill-and-fill bonanza of immeasurable proportions.

There still is no sound scientific evidence supporting links between amalgam fillings and systemic diseases or chronic illness.

But the profession has stood fast in both situations, believing that the science behind the restorative material and the preventive value of fluoride support their continued use. The winner, so far, has been the American public, which—as pointed out in the U.S. surgeon general's report on oral health earlier this year—enjoys unprecedented oral health. The report also indicated the importance of oral health to general health, emphasizing that there still was room for improvement in the health needs of certain pockets of Americans who have difficulty gaining access to dental care.

Removing amalgam as a restorative material will make that goal far more difficult to achieve. Considering that many public dental programs suffer from underfunding, using a more costly dental restorative material to replace the durable and low-cost amalgam could result in less care for fewer people.

For example, substituting composite resins for amalgam at 1999 fee index levels would increase the cost of a two-surface restoration by 35 percent. With the present difficulty in boosting present funding levels of public programs to even approximate private-practice levels, imagine the impact of a 35 percent increase just to supply the same amount of service.

Worldwide, removing amalgam as a restorative material would be devastating. Many fledgling dental public health programs presently offering amalgam restorations as an alternative to extraction would collapse under the burden of higher material costs and lack of clinical expertise in placing resin-based composites.

Antiamalgamists, take note. Regardless of what you may think, there still is no sound scientific evidence supporting links between amalgam fillings and systemic diseases or chronic illness. However, if ongoing scientific inquiry ever were to indicate that amalgam is detrimental to the health and welfare of the public, I can assure you that dentistry would need no outside organization, group or individual to remind it of its obligation to do no harm. ■

1. American Dental Association. ADA principles of ethics and code of professional conduct. Available at: "www.ada.org/prof/prac/law/code/index.html". Accessed Aug. 13, 2001.
2. Kranhold K. Dentists battle 'gag' on warning about mercury. Wall Street Journal May 16, 2001:B1.

# Look who's practicing dentistry

*Originally published in JADA 2001 132: 1352-1353.*

**W**ouldn't you think acquiring the knowledge and skills necessary to manage the diagnosis, prevention and treatment of early childhood dental caries would require more than a three-hour continuing education training session?

Not so—at least not in North Carolina.

In sections of that state, pediatricians and family practitioners, aided by their physician assistants, are actively involved in the delivery of preventive dental services. Targeting a Medicaid population of 0- to 3-year-olds, these nondental health care providers are offering screening for oral disorders, fluoride varnish applications and counseling of the children's caregivers.

Encouragement for these medically supplied dental services arose from public concerns regarding inadequate access to dental services for certain segments of North Carolina's Medicaid-eligible children. In 1998, only 12 percent of the state's Medicaid-enrolled children aged 1 year to 5 years visited a dentist.[1] The Health Care Financing Administration (now the Center for Medicare and Medicaid Services) responded by initiating a demonstration program called "Smart Smiles" for 1,000 preschool children in North Carolina. Plans to extend the program to include more than 100,000 children are under way.

The irony: medical auxiliary personnel, with minimal training, are performing preventive dental procedures. Meanwhile, state-employed dental hygienists cannot participate, since their dental practice act requires them to be under the direct supervision of dentists.

This is not the only state in which medical personnel are offering dental services. Missouri recently enacted a law that permits physicians to provide preventive dental services when children receive their immunizations.

Previously, the Washington State Medical Quality Assurance Commission decided that application of fluoride varnish to teeth by physicians and physician assistants was within those disciplines' scope of practice.

Why this medical intrusion into an area where dentistry has been the undeniable leader—the promotion of preventive dentistry for children? It's the need to ensure access to dental services, or the lack of that access, that is the stimulus.

Difficulties in accessing dental care, especially for underprivileged children and older adults, have received nationwide attention with the publication of "Oral Health in America: A Report of the Surgeon General."[1] While citing dramatic improvements in oral health during the past 50 years, the report pointed to a "silent epidemic" of oral disease that "burdens" some population groups.

Specifically, while disadvantaged children's oral health has dramatically improved, a study of unmet health needs of children found those requiring dental care topped the list with 5.3 percent (3.4 million); the percentage with unmet medical needs was only 1.6 percent.[2]

One solution to this problem, cited in both the surgeon general's report, as well as other associated documents, calls for dentistry to partner with other professions and agencies to increase access to dental services.

The North Carolina Smart Smiles program is an example of such a partnership—or is it?

On the surface, it appears to be a "do-good" situation. After all, isn't some prevention better than none at all? Actually, no—not when there isn't evi-

> In North Carolina, medical auxiliary personnel, with minimal training, are performing preventive dental procedures. Meanwhile, state-employed dental hygienists cannot participate, since their dental practice act requires them to be under the direct supervision of dentists.

dence of a "true" dental/medical partnering agreement that ensures continuity of care for the child. Sure, having the pediatric assistant paint fluoride varnish on the child's teeth can be a positive interaction by socializing parents to the importance of obtaining dental treatment for their children. But as an isolated, singular event, it easily could lull the caregiver into a false sense of security, believing his or her child is receiving all necessary dental care. If the perceived lack of access to dental care for underprivileged children continues, can it be expected that additional dental services will be offered by medical personnel?

In previous years, the answer would have been that physicians had more than enough to do without adding dental procedures to the service mix. But now, with mean incomes of dentists greater than those of their pediatric and family physician counterparts—significant differences when hours worked are divided into net income—I could foresee a willingness to expand their dental services offerings.

Interestingly, in many states, these physicians could deliver dental services without taking any additional training. Indeed, they might even consider augmenting their dental offering by hiring a dental hygienist. But can they legally hire a dental hygienist? Considering how careful dental practice acts are in specifying what services and what supervision is required of dental auxiliaries, medical practice acts allow physicians a wide latitude as to what services they and their auxiliary personnel can perform. In contrast, the majority of dental practice acts exempt physicians who deliver dental services.

Will physician-delivered dental services increase? With up to 29 percent of dental service output characterized as "preventive dental procedures,"[3] the entrepreneurial physician might be tempted to venture forth. I wouldn't be surprised to see continuing education offerings for physicians and their staffs featuring instruction in preventive dentistry.

Who knows, we may eventually see medical residencies offering clerkships in dentistry—and perhaps even the development of a full-fledged residency in dentistry consisting of a one-year general medicine internship plus two years dedicated to learning dentistry. This would produce an interesting medical practitioner able to have a step up in the practice of geriatric or pediatric dentistry.

Public solutions to the dental care access issue continue to spring up. Note the present legislative initiative in California, which would allow physicians and dentists from Mexico to "cross the border" without meeting California licensure requirements to expand services to "poor, largely Spanish-speaking patients."[4]

Breaking down cultural and language barriers also are cited as reasons to employ these health professionals, who will be paid at rates commensurate with the clinic's regularly licensed doctors. The California Dental Society opposes the legislation on potential "quality issues," indicating that it allows foreign-trained dentists to practice without any means of evaluating their training. If their training is not comparable to that of U.S. dentists, this initiative could foster a two-tiered health care system, with substandard care being offered to some.

If this proposed legislation passes, will the California legislature be receiving similar legislative requests to allow licensed dentists from other countries to come to the United States to treat underserved people with whom they share similar ethnic backgrounds?

All in the name of access! ■

1. U.S. Public Health Service, Office of the Surgeon General. Oral health in America: a report of the surgeon general. Available at: "www.nidcr.nih.gov/sgr/sgrohweb/welcome.htm". Accessed Aug. 14, 2001.
2. Newacheck PW, Hughes DC, Hun Y-Y, Wong S, Stoddard JJ. Health needs and consumer views: the unmet health needs of America's children. Pediatrics 2000; 105(4):989–96.[Abstract/Free Full Text]
3. American Dental Association. 1999 Survey of dental practice. Chicago: American Dental Association, Survey Center; 2000.
4. Gronke A. Bill would open door to doctors from Mexico. Los Angeles Times June 17, 2001; California Section.

# Strength in numbers

*Originally published in JADA 2001 132: 1494-1496*

Licensure, dental office wastewater, third-party interference with dentist/patient relationships—these are "real" issues guaranteed to grab the interest of the rank-and-file dentist. It's doubtful that the issue of the declining number of dentists choosing to become ADA members would elicit similar concerns.

But dentistry's leaders believe otherwise. They know that only through high membership percentages can an organization exert its strength and power, especially in its advocacy initiatives.

This was recently illustrated during the ADA's testimony on ergonomics to Occupational Safety and Health Administration officials. At the conclusion of the spokesperson's remarks, OSHA was informed of the high percentage of dentists the ADA represents. OSHA's response acknowledged that "by working with [the ADA, they] could reach the vast majority of dentists."

It's understandable why the U.S. Department of Labor officials were impressed. With membership currently at just over 70 percent of eligible dentists, the ADA has earned the distinction as the gold standard for national professional organizations. Neither the American Medical Association nor the American Bar Association, with membership percentages in the 40 percent range or less, can compete.

Whether we are able to maintain this strength in numbers is questionable. The last seven years have seen a continuing decline in the ADA's membership market share. Additionally, there have been major increases in the absolute numbers of dentists located in categories that have demonstrated less-than-average membership histories.

For example, the ADA's minority dentist market share for membership purposes fell from 61.7 percent of those eligible in 1993 to 55.6 percent last year. Specifically, the year 2000 market share for those groups contained in the minorities category was 38.8 percent for African-Americans, 51.7 percent for Hispanics and 62.6 percent and 61.6 percent for Asian or Pacific Islanders and American Indians, respectively. As for women, a major component of the minority category, less than 63 percent have joined the ADA.

The impact of lowered female market share could signal even more difficulty in the future as the older age groups of dentists, which are predominantly male, retire.

The ADA's membership staff is well aware of the importance of courting the emerging and older nonmember dentists. They have directed similar efforts to those dentists who, for a variety of reasons, chose not to renew their membership. Unlimited energies and creative solutions abound; still the market share falls.

Apparently what is being offered is insufficient to affect commitment. Dentists of my era, to whom I have proudly referred as the "pledge-allegiance" generation, dutifully and without question opened each school day with a pledge to the American flag. There was never a discussion as to why we recited this pledge or why America needed or deserved our loyalty.

This willingness to make unqualified commitments to the country translated years later to professional membership in the American Dental Association. Here, too, there was no question as to the benefits of membership. Joining was value in itself. Close to 90 percent of this age group choose to belong to the ADA.

Obviously, this philosophy does not exist today. Dentists now want to know what the organization does for them; otherwise, why join?

So the ADA offers insurance, credit cards, home mortgages and a host of other financial services. Good, but not good enough. I've always believed

> **With membership currently at just over 70 percent of eligible dentists, the ADA has earned the distinction as the gold standard for national professional organizations.**

that loyalty for financial services was only as deep as a one-half percent reduction in interest rates.

No, our dentists want more, and by emphasizing highly relevant, practice-directed benefits, we can deliver it.

Advocacy, for example, is probably the ADA's strongest suit. The aforementioned activity in the ergonomics field has prevented unbelievable punitive actions against the dentist by OSHA. Its new legal initiative, filing a class-action lawsuit (for reduction of benefits to providers) against one of the nation's major dental insurance companies, represents a milestone in the ADA's continuing attempt to preserve the dentist/patient relationship.

Unfortunately, for the same reasons unions demanded closed shops, the value from the ADA advocacy efforts works for members and nonmembers alike. "Why join?" the nonmember might think. "I can get all the benefits without spending a penny."

Sad, but true. Localizing the ownership of advocacy ranges from difficult to impossible. More tangible programs are needed to attract potential members. Since dentists like hands-on action, let's give them hands-on reasons to be members of the ADA. To do that will require moving two of the ADA's already successful initiatives to the next level.

Continuing education, for example. Today, outstanding clinicians are made available to members at the ADA's national meeting. With the assistance of industry, more than 50 seminars have been made available to individual dentists and dental organizations. Online educational instruction has been added recently, and the JADA continuing education program counted more than 18,000 dental enrollments last year.

Adding value to this educational focus is the ADA's Continuing Education Recognition Program, or CERP, which provides guidance to the profession by scrutinizing educational programs for their content.

Once again, I would like to ask the ADA to step up and take a leadership role in formulating the direction of continuing education in dentistry. The suggestion here is to move from the present approval of courses through CERP to a new educational role of advising and mentoring dentists in their educational progress. These activities should be coupled with the development and administration of a suitable reward system that is capable of publicly acknowledging professional growth.

Lectures, hands-on instruction, fellowships,

even perhaps a virtual university that grants continuing education degrees—all could become integral components of this new ADA initiative.

No need to develop new courses. The majority of educational offerings would come from educational presentations already offered by universities, dental societies, study clubs and industry.

The membership payoff would be a visible, ongoing, educational experience only for ADA members. Conceivably, thousands of ADA members would find themselves inextricably linked to the ADA.

I would propose a similar type of program for the science and dental practice areas. Our members say they want more information on dental products—a reasonable request, since new generations of dental materials are coming onto the market constantly.

Why not link thousands of dental offices electronically so that dentists can share product usage information with their fellow dentists? Most dental offices easily could be joined to provide this information, with dentists acting both as clinical researchers and recipients of "hot" information on a daily basis.

Now that would be a membership benefit!

Finally, I would like to address the oft-stated concern that the ADA is not appropriately addressing the needs of its minority and female members, with a proposal for a structural change in the ADA. The initiative would give minority and female members the opportunity to develop special-interest groups within the ADA structure. This would not mean abandoning their present organizations. On the contrary, they could use this format to bring the thoughts of these external organizations directly to the ADA through the special-interest mechanism, thus ensuring that their voices would be heard at the highest levels.

This is not a radical proposal. Organizations such as the American Association for Dental Research and the American Dental Education Association have structured their organizations to acknowledge and give voice to their constituents.

Membership is the foundation of a strong organization. We in the ADA have been fortunate to introduce ourselves as the voice of dentistry. Will it continue? Only if the ADA is ready to programmatically move to new levels that link members on a daily basis with the organization.

Remember: with numbers comes strength! ∎

# End of the line

*Originally published in JADA 2001 132: 1634-1636*

This December editorial represents my last opportunity to share thoughts and ideas with you as JADA's editor. It has been 11 years and 132 issues of The Journal since I assumed the editorship. These have been challenging years for dentistry and for JADA. We've had HIV and infection control, Occupational Safety and Health Administration regulations, managed care, patient protection—one issue after another.

It has been an exciting time in terms of trying to build a professional journal that would be relevant to its readers. It also has been a productive time, if establishing JADA as the world's best-read dental journal is the criterion for success. Independent readership scores now verify that JADA is not only dentistry's best-read peer-reviewed journal, but also is the favorite of dentists who have been in practice 15 years or less.

These favorable statistics, coupled with the hundreds of regular mail and e-mail responses to the monthly editorials, show that JADA is offering its readers up-to-date, relevant material pertinent to dental practitioners.

Writing 131 editorials was a real joy. Each was centered on the principles that action starts with knowledge and that the success of an editorial resides in its ability to be insightful and predictive; to be a step ahead of what is considered correct; to explore issues that may not be mainstream; to go where others fear to go. Foremost, the editorialist must be open to the thoughts of others.

So many issues, so many editorial subjects. A favorite? Perhaps it would be oral cancer. A few weeks ago, while driving through New Mexico, I noticed a billboard that really caught my attention. In front of me was a vivid, full-faced picture of a cowboy with a resected mandible. Superimposed were the words "HALF OFF" and then the word "TOBACCO." Nothing left to the imagination! Use

**Upon my successor I bestow a professional journal that is considered the gold standard for successful health organization publications.**

tobacco; bear the consequences.

It pleased me that the ADA, even in light of the tragic events of Sept. 11, has gone forward with an extensive public service campaign to make America aware of the importance of prevention and early detection of oral cancer.

Reminiscing brings back the importance of conveying the need for JADA readers to go further than blindly accepting the bottom line—to always examine the components of an issue. To illustrate, I used a road sign located in Gold Hill, Colo. It was first pictured in the January 1991 issue, with my first editorial. On the next page, I repeat it for its important message. An editor must be willing to go where others fear to go. That's why I have always been intrigued by the theatrical production of "Man of La Mancha."

"To dream the impossible dream/ To fight the unbeatable foe ... ." Those words from the play's signature song conjure up a picture of an errant knight battling with windmills.

The foundation for this acclaimed musical was the vision of a Spanish philosopher who wrote: "Only he who attempts the absurd is capable of achieving the impossible." What better way to visualize the ADA than as a "David" taking the lead role, clashing with the giants, as it demonstrated early support for patients' rights legislation?

I would be remiss not to mention the inspirational words of H.B. Zachry, an architect responsible for the development of the Hilton Palacio del Rio in San Antonio. His personal philosophy, displayed on a plaque in the hotel, is about work, and it's about life. His observations are both poignant and inspiring. I read them often.

"I do not choose to be a common man. It is my right to be uncommon if I can. I seek opportunity, not security. I will refuse to be a kept citizen, to be humbled and dulled by having my state and nation look after me. I want to dream and to build, to fail and to succeed, never to be numbered among those weak and timid souls who have known neither victory nor defeat.

"I know that happiness can come only from the inside through hard constructive work and sincere positive thinking. I know that the so-called pleasures of the moment should not be confused with a state of happiness. I know that I can get a measure of inner satisfaction from any job if I intelligently plan and courageously execute it.

"I know that, if I put forth every iota of strength that I possess—physical, mental, spiritual—toward the accomplishment of a worthwhile task, ere I fall exhausted by the wayside, the Unseen Hand will reach out and pull me through. Yes, I want to live dangerously, to plan my procedures on the basis of calculated risks, to resolve the problems of everyday living into a measure of inner peace. I know if I know how to do all this, I will know how to live and, if I know how to live, I will know how to die."

Heady words!

All of JADA's successes can be traced to a group that I affectionately refer to as Team JADA. The goal of JADA as the flagship publication of the American Dental Association is to offer its members a print and online scientific journal that represents the best available information on clinical subjects relevant to dentistry. To achieve this requires the efforts of a large and diverse group of dedicated people. Foremost are its contributing authors. Without their willingness to submit written documentation of their clinical and research findings, there would be no Journal.

Next in line are the more than 900 reviewers who donate their time and energies in assessing the relevance and accuracy of the submitted material. Intensely involved in both the review process and the solicitation of cutting-edge clinical research findings are the associate editors who provide everyday input into Journal materials. The editorial board, consisting of members drawn from all facets of dentistry, provides continuing advice on policy issues that affect The Journal.

The ultimate task—the process of turning the submitted words into publishable copy—is the assignment of JADA's editorial, art and production staff. They work directly with authors to produce copy that will be readable and a Journal that is accessible and attractive. Getting The Journal out on time is their responsibility. They have never failed in my 11 years as editor.

The publisher, the associate publishers and their staff round out Team JADA. They provide the infrastructure and protect the editorial integrity of The Journal. My heartfelt thanks for their support.

Oh, yes. No publication would be complete without its readers. To them, I offer the following advice:
■ Maintain your skills so that they never become outdated.
■ Never stop seeking new knowledge.
■ Information—timely, accurate, transferable and useful—will be the underpinnings for success in the 21st century.
■ Don't, regardless of the situation, attempt too much at the expense of yourself or your patients.
■ If your work ever ceases to be enjoyable, reexamine your criteria for success.

Upon my successor—a highly qualified, internationally recognized clinician and researcher—I bestow a professional journal that is considered the gold standard for successful health organization publications; a professional membership whose dedication to patient welfare embellishes its world-class status; and a superb team of JADA staff and volunteers committed to excellence in publishing.

It's the end of the line. Time to get off. But what an awesome run! ■